Working

Cures

Working Cures

Cures

Healing, Health,

and Power on

Southern Slave

Plantations

Sharla M. Fett

The University of North Carolina Press *Chapel Hill & London*

Portions of Chapters 3 and 5 have been published previously in
"'It's a Spirit in Me': Spiritual Power and the Healing Work of African
American Women in Slavery," in *A Mighty Baptism: Race, Gender, and
the Creation of American Protestantism,* edited by Susan Juster and
Lisa MacFarlane (Ithaca, N.Y.: Cornell University Press, 1996), 189–209.

Library of Congress Cataloging-in-Publication Data
Fett, Sharla M.
Working cures: healing, health, and power on southern slave
plantations / Sharla M. Fett.
    p. cm. — (Gender and American culture)
Includes bibliographical references (p.) and index.
ISBN 978-0-8078-2709-3 (cloth: alk. paper)
ISBN 978-0-8078-5378-8 (pbk.: alk. paper)
1. Healing — Southern States — History.   2. Slaves — Health and
hygiene — Southern States — History.   3. Plantation life — Southern
States — History.   4. Slaves — Medical care — Southern States —
History.   5. Health and race — Southern States — History.
6. Slaves — Southern States — Social conditions.   7. Southern
States — Social conditions.   I. Title.   II. Gender & American
culture.
RA448.5.N4 F48   2002
362.1'086'250975 — dc21   2001057016

For my mother, Betty Marie Fett, 1935–1987

Contents

Illustrations

Preface

rising mortality of freedpeople attributed to new can to americ assumed they were too stupid or stubborn to follow public health guidelines)

In the immediate aftermath of slavery, white officials in the South frequently alleged that African Americans rejected white medical institutions and health regulations in the name of their newly won freedom. A judge in Athens, Georgia, accused freedpeople of worsening the 1866 smallpox epidemic by refusing "any attention from the Doctor saying they would manage their own affairs."[1] A leading Charleston physician charged that freedmen and freedwomen disregarded public health restrictions because "any restraint reminded them too much of their former enslaved condition."[2] Far from disinterested observers, these men portrayed African American rejection of white medical supervision as the symptom of a disordered society. Health and healing, it seems, carried political weight for ex-masters as well as ex-slaves.

Richard Arnold, a physician and former slaveholder in Savannah, implied exactly this point in a letter describing how his daughter Ellen had attended Fanny, a cholera-stricken freedwoman who cooked for the Arnolds in 1866. He wrote that Ellen had "boldly nursed her as if she had been her slave, instead of being 'nobody's nigger but her own.'" Regretting that none of the "hypocritical, self-satisfied Pharisees of Massachusetts" were there to witness his solicitude for the sick woman, Arnold found vindication in the incident for the entire social order of southern slave society. By taking possession of Fanny's medical care, and thereby symbolically asserting ownership over her person, Richard Arnold believed he had spared Fanny the fate of many freedpeople whose rising mortality he attributed directly to their new status.[3] At stake was not just the public health of Savannah but the uncertain nature of race and class relations in the postemancipation South.

While freedpeople's alleged rejection of white medical care during Reconstruction requires further research, it is clear that African Americans entered the new terrain of freedom with a critical analysis of medical care under slavery. Across the antebellum South, health and healing stood at the nexus of plantation social relations. Far from being an isolated sphere, slave health intersected intimately with black labor, religion, sexuality, and family. Indeed, conflicts between slaves and slaveholders over matters of health often held stakes much higher than the proving of any particular therapy. It is not surprising, therefore, that newly freed men and women would claim self-determination in health care as one of the fruits of emancipation. In doing so, African American communities acted upon a dual legacy forged in the antebellum period. African Americans emerged from enslavement with, on one hand, a storehouse of healing knowledge and, on the other hand, a clear comprehension of the harmful potential of white medical care.

Only by looking closely at the everyday world of enslaved sufferers and healers can we understand the remarkable legacy they imparted. And only by shifting the framework of analysis from medical therapies to the social relations of healing can we begin to grasp the political and cultural importance of black doctoring traditions. Expressive African American culture arising from the antebellum rural South testifies to the collective genius of individuals, families, and communities, who created something of beauty in the midst of extreme subjugation. Songs, quilts, oratory, foodways, dance, and music have received deserved attention for their sophistication and vitality as well as for the history they represent.[4] This book is written with the conviction that African American doctoring arts belong equally to the list of complex and compelling cultural work produced by African descendants under slavery. In the hands of ordinary, but extraordinary, black men and women, acts of healing became arts of resistance, inscribing the vital link between personal health and collective freedom.

Acknowledgments

If anything, the study of African American history has taught me that we accomplish nothing solely on our individual merits. To the people and institutions who have ushered this book along toward publication, I owe a great debt. Rutgers University, the Albert J. Beveridge Fund of the American Historical Association, and the Virginia Historical Society's Mellon Fellowship Program all contributed to research funding. The National Endowment for the Humanities provided crucial support for writing the dissertation.

Several archivists and libraries offered gracious assistance: Henry Fulmer and his coworkers at the South Caroliniana Library; E. Lee Shepard, Frances Pollard, and the staff at the Virginia Historical Society; and the fine archivists of Duke University Special Collections, the Georgia Historical Society, the Southern Historical Collection, the Virginia State Library, and the Waring Historical Library. The South Carolina Historical Society staff who compiled the finding aid for slave lists provided a valuable tool for research on enslaved women and health work. Tera Hunter, Jill Snider, and Bryan Dalton generously shared their homes during early research trips.

Many people contributed to this project by reading all or part of the manuscript. Suzanne Lebsock patiently read numerous early drafts and supplied the best combination of encouragement and honest criticism. Her continued interest has offered a model of mentorship that few can match. I am also deeply grateful to Deborah White, whose first book contributes to the historiographic foundation of this one and whose suggestions were always on the mark. Gerald Grob offered congenial support and timely advice. Jerma Jackson and Elizabeth Rose gave me superb critiques of the early manuscript; their interest in the project fueled my own. Two anonymous readers for the University of North Carolina Press offered excellent criticism, saved me from many errors, and helped me finally to understand the manuscript as a book.

For conference collaborations, comments on working papers, and fruitful suggestions, I want to recognize Emily Abel, Elsa Barkley Brown,

Stephanie Camp, Yvonne Chireau, Vennie Deas-Moore, Leland Ferguson, Ariela Gross, Leslie Harris, Joel Howell, Tera Hunter, Walter Johnson, Philip Morgan, Martin Pernick, Leigh Pruneau, Leslie Rowland, Todd Savitt, Stephanie Shaw, Theresa Singleton, Brenda Stevenson, Daina Ramey, and Linda Sturtz. John Michael Vlach, Paul Von Blum, and Kym Rice also generously shared from their own knowledge of material culture and visual evidence to help with illustrations. Members of the history department and other scholars at Emory University helped me to rethink arguments about the sacred basis of African American health culture. Kate Douglas Torrey of the University of North Carolina Press consistently offered clearheaded advice while remaining unruffled by the manuscript's lengthy path toward completion. My thanks also go to Stephanie Wenzel for her marvelous editing skills.

Colleagues at the University of Arizona history department pushed the book forward with their enthusiasm and advice. In particular Karen Anderson read the entire manuscript with a keen eye and a generous heart. Katherine Morrissey, Bert Barickman, and Laura Briggs added their unique voices to the intellectual community that nourished my revisions. The U.S. Women's History Dissertator Group including Cathleen Dooley, Deborah Marlow, Mike Rembis, and Megan Taylor Shockley critiqued all or parts of the manuscript at crucial points in my writing. The women's studies department provided a forum in which to rethink arguments about African American herbalism. Each of these and many more contributors in some way strengthened this book; for any errors, I alone take responsibility.

Two unique communities deserve recognition for their indirect but vital inspiration in the last stages of this project. First, Ms. Barba's first grade class of 2000–2001 shared with me some of their first written stories and inspired me each week to go back to the computer and finish. Second, Mestre Amen Santo and Amy Santo allowed me to observe the work of Capoeira Batuque and to think in fresh ways about slave healing as an art.

Finally, I pay respect to those who have sustained my daily work. Many thanks to the skilled and dedicated childcare providers in several different states on whom I have depended. Bob Bonner first introduced me to the idea of a community of scholars; to him and equally to Barbara, Jenny, and Tim Bonner I owe much more than my choice of profession. My parents, James and Betty Fett, gave me a spiritual and intellectual foundation I will always cherish. Sheryl Fett-Mekaru and Debra Ahmed offered consistent support and lent me their strength. Ella Rogers-Fett and Jacob Rogers-Fett drained my work hours, kept me sane, and brought joy into each day. Finally, I thank John Rogers, my true companion, not only for superior editorial skills and practical support, but for much good humor along the way.

Working Cures

Introduction

[handwritten note: Tuskeegee Syphilis Study was not my first time]

The harrowing history of the medical abuse and neglect of African Americans reaches from enslavement to the present. For many people the U.S. Public Health Service's study from 1932 to 1972 of untreated syphilis in black Alabama men remains the most concrete symbol of scientific and medical injustice, but precedents for the infamous Tuskegee study litter the preceding three centuries. Before slaving vessels ever left the barracoons of the African coast, Europeans closely inspected the bodies of captive Africans, even tasting their sweat for signs of illness.[1] Domestic slave markets of the United States further subsumed all dimensions of black health under the rubric of soundness for sale. The institution of slavery defined enslaved men and women as "objects of property," enmeshing even intimate relations of sexuality and childbearing in a web of property interests.[2] In millions of daily interactions with enslaved laborers, slaveholders sought, in the words of Ida B. Wells, to "dwarf the soul and preserve the body."[3] When slaves resisted, whites also employed medicine, not to preserve the body but to discipline and torture.

[handwritten note in left margin: this was pseudoscience + me. I was endorsed]

Formal scientific endeavors also contributed to the exploitative dimension of medicine in African American history. From North America to Europe, learned white men put science to the service of proslavery ideology and white supremacy. Nineteenth-century white scientists and physicians advanced models of civilization informed by elaborately intersecting hierarchies of gender, race, and class. They posited differential capacities to feel pain as well as divergent sexualities and moralities, and polygenecists built their reputations arguing for the separate origins of distinct races. White physicians and medical students subjected enslaved men and women to experimentation and humiliating display as medical specimens. By the late nineteenth century, white pundits and scientists alike employed evolutionary theory and population statistics to project the extinction of the "Negro race."[4] Twentieth-century eugenics, forced sterilization of poor women, nonconsensual experimentation, and massive discrimination complete a history of medical abuse built on the legacies of slavery and racism.[5] It is a historical accounting that clearly renders African American distrust of white medical institutions, to borrow sociologist Kirk Johnson's phrase, "a sensible, rational act."[6]

The history of medical abuse is a grim but only partial account of the legacy of antebellum medical relations. Simply put, enslaved African Americans were not passive victims of medical malice, nor were they helpless dependents on white health care. Instead, communities in slavery nurtured a rich health culture, a constellation of ideas and practices related to well-being, illness, healing, and death, that worked to counter the onslaught of daily medical abuse and racist scientific theories.[7] At each historical juncture, enslaved communities cultivated their own practitioners and therapies, and they influenced southern rural health practices in the process.[8] Slave insurrectionists deployed protective medicine to shield themselves from white patrollers and pursuing hounds. Black midwives visited slave dwellings and white households to attend mothers and catch babies. Elderly root doctors built regional reputations among a multiethnic clientele. Skilled herbalists cultivated local botanical expertise that significantly influenced southern domestic medicine. Any serious exploration of African American health culture in the antebellum South quickly puts to rest the myth of slave dependency on white health care.

A close examination of African American doctoring traditions similarly reinforces the case for the African cultural impact on North American enslaved communities. This work situates the history of African American slave healing within the larger context of an Atlantic world and the African diaspora.[9] The maelstrom of the Atlantic slave trade hurled together a dazzling array of healing systems. Forcibly transported into the brutal Atlantic plantation complex, Igbo, Yoruba, Bambara, Kongo, and many other captives transformed their distinct traditions of healing to survive in the New World. African philosophies and therapies thus proved central to the development of African American doctoring traditions. Native American medicine also figured significantly in slave doctoring, as both European and African newcomers drew on indigenous botanical knowledge in the Americas. Finally, European popular and elite doctoring influenced slave health culture as Europeans and Africans borrowed from each other in colonial cities, farms, and plantations.

Africans in the Atlantic world forged cultures of healing as varied as they were geographically specific. From Haitian Vodou to Brazilian Candomblé to North American hoodoo, Black Atlantic religions of healing, still thriving today, reflect their particular place within the history of enslavement and forced migration.[10] African American healing traditions, while deeply embedded in the regional history of the American South, must also be understood in this context of the African diaspora. My primary goal in the following pages is not, however, to trace the ethnic origins and transformations of specific African healing practices across the Atlantic. Instead, this work explores the social relations of slave health and healing as they emerged in daily interactions among residents of nineteenth-century southern plantations.

what

↳ not to race origins but to illustrate what
↳ not social relations of slave health looked
like

African American doctoring has an Old South as well as a diasporic context. In large part, plantation health relations owed their politically charged character to the fact that fluid cross-cultural exchanges in medicine took place within a slave society characterized by a sharply defined social order. The antebellum years saw both an upheaval in the relations between professional and popular medicine and an elaboration of the mechanisms of control over the enslaved population. Plantation health practices drew on interlocking gender, race, and class ideologies that informed the actions and identities of practitioners and patients alike. In this setting, slave doctoring became simultaneously a valuable form of knowledge, a subjugated form of labor, and a challenge to the existing social order.

The history of slavery and the making of race strongly influenced the dynamics of southern plantation medicine. The years between the arrival of the first Africans and the birth of the new nation gave rise to a racial ideology that sustained the ideal of liberty in a republic heavily dependent on slave labor. As plantation production moved to the center of the southern economy, the idea of "race" itself congealed to support the exploitation of African labor in the southern plantation economy. Relatively fluid "societies with slaves" became heavily racialized "slave societies" that defined freedom as a prerogative of whiteness. What was new in these emerging North American slave societies was not the exploitation of unfree labor but the forging of a common notion of white freedom premised on the enslavement of Africans.[11]

Sex/gender systems played a key role in this transformation as English colonists reified notions of racial difference "by connecting them to other power relations defined as natural, like those of gender."[12] The earliest racial distinctions made by Virginia statutes, for example, distinguished

African women, who were expected to labor in the fields and were therefore counted as taxable laborers, from English women, who were exempted, at least in the ideal, from field labor. Likewise, colonial law departed from English patriarchal precedents in fashioning legislation designating slavery as a condition inheritable through the mother, regardless of the father's status. Gendered divisions of labor and laws exerting control over black women's children thus contributed to the racialization of social relations.[13] By the early nineteenth century an interlocking set of social hierarchies reinforced planter dominance, subordinated enslaved and free blacks, and recruited white yeoman support within the antebellum social order.[14]

In contrast to the established hierarchies of southern slave society, antebellum medicine and health care was a veritable free-for-all, characterized by experimentalism, skepticism, and contesting claims to scientific legitimacy. In the first half of the nineteenth century, orthodox (or "regular") medical doctors underwent a crisis in professional identity prompted by "therapeutic confusion" within the profession.[15] Compounding the effects of internal dissent, orthodox doctors also confronted a "medical counter-culture" composed of health reform movements often linked to other social and political causes of the day. Overwhelmingly white and male in profile, orthodox medical practitioners sought to carve out a more secure foundation of professional identity by establishing exclusive medical legitimacy.[16] In the antebellum South, white doctors' search for new grounds of scientific and social legitimacy merged with the sectional conflict over slavery. Professional southern doctors defended the merits of southern medical science by proclaiming a new domain of race- and region-specific medicine that reinforced emergent proslavery ideology.[17]

Heated sectarian battles had a limited direct impact on most antebellum Americans, but the contest over medical knowledge and authority prompted an even more significant realignment in the relationship between professional and lay practitioners. Throughout early American history, particularly in rural areas, sick care occurred primarily in households rather than hospitals or clinics. Preventative measures and nursing of the sick fell generally, though not exclusively, to women. As domestic healers women provided the foundation of popular health care, which was supplemented by the work of medical practitioners in private homes.[18]

The accepted relationship between domestic medical authority and professional medical authority began to change, however, with the advent of health reform and professional conflicts.[19] Although professional practitioners did not view domestic practitioners as their direct competitors, the domestic realm provided a convenient label with which to discredit newcomers vying for professional legitimacy. Seeking to secure their own professional place, male orthodox physicians and male "irregulars" alike sought to denigrate their competition by associating them with socially less powerful domestic practitioners. Professional practitioners painted their competition as purveyors of superstition and ignorance by associating them with "old women, root doctors, and quacks of all sorts."[20] Equating their rivals with the least powerful of domestic healers — older women, the rural, the illiterate, and the enslaved — competing white, male practitioners extended their exclusive claims to medical authority.

The combination of medical ferment with the planter-dominated social order of antebellum slave society produced a remarkable blend of cross-cultural experimentalism and dangerous social divisions. On one hand, antebellum southerners adopted an experimental attitude toward medical knowledge, seeking effective medicines and skilled practitioners across lines of social division. Therapies circulated with surprising fluidity as health seekers turned to Thomsonianism, homeopathy, water cure, Indian remedies, and hoodoo.[21] Southerners from all walks of life consulted peddlers and seers, scripture and almanacs, and above all, the acquired wisdom of their families, social circles, and local neighborhoods. Yet the rigid socioracial structure of southern slave society often put medical experimentalism on volatile ground and produced seemingly contradictory results. White southerners wrote slave remedies into their private recipe books even as they wrote laws curtailing the practice of enslaved doctors. Enslaved mothers learned cough remedies from planter women even as they bitterly condemned slaveholders who forced them to attend white infants at the cost of their own children's well-being. While therapies appeared to flow across social divides, enslaved practitioners and health seekers often struggled against racial, gendered, and class-based constructions of who was fit to claim the privileges of medical authority.

As laborers, mothers, and healers, bondswomen stood at the center of this struggle. Enslaved women grew herbs, made medicines, cared for the sick, prepared the dead for burial, and attended births in black and white households across the South. Unlike the proscriptions on white women's field labor, black and white women's duties as domestic healers partially overlapped. Yet white society denied enslaved women the prerogatives of womanhood and motherhood that undergirded white women's moral authority as domestic caregivers. Whereas privileged white women of the period could counter medical doctors' authority with the authority of home and maternal instinct, the institutions of southern slave society offered no such ideological reinforcement to the claims of slave women in the care of their own families.[22] Furthermore, distinctions between private and public arenas of healing failed to describe the realities of enslaved women workers, whose healing work enriched the southern plantation economy. Barred from both male professional and white maternal authority, enslaved women, along with enslaved men, nevertheless created an original definition of healing authority that did not depend on the gender norms of white slaveholders. Slave women's doctoring thus formed a critical part of southern domestic healing that until now has not received its due in the literature on gender and antebellum medicine.

Black healers drew their authority from a collective understanding of health and healing integral to African American culture under slavery. Plantation slave communities, I argue, maintained a relational vision of health that fundamentally diverged from slaveholder notions of slave soundness. This relational vision connected individual health to broader community relationships; it insisted on a collective context for both affliction and healing; it honored kinship relations by bridging the worlds of ancestors and living generations; it located a healer's authority in the wisdom of elders and divine revelation. In these respects the relational vision of health carried forward important dimensions of West and West Central African religions and worldviews. The relational vision of health was, at the same time, a concept forged in the crucible of North American enslavement. Incorporating Christianity into African holistic concepts of well-being, African American philosophies of health articulated important critiques of both slaveholder Christianity and planter definitions of humane medical care.

There were also certain things that the relational vision of health did not do. First, it did not reflect among enslaved African Americans a romanticized ideal of communal harmony. The relational vision of health assumed that conflict would be present in community life and in relations with slaveholders. As illustrated by African American conjuring, black doctoring traditions addressed bodily ills in the context of a broad spectrum of human relationships. Equally important, the relational vision of health did not win for slave communities a strictly autonomous space for black health practices. Rather, the evidence indicates that slaveholders intruded frequently on the health practices of the enslaved. Black men and women thus wrestled continuously, and sometimes unsuccessfully, with slaveholders, overseers, and white doctors for their chance to pursue their own visions of health. Accordingly, readers will find here an emphasis on the dynamics of struggle rather than an argument for the autonomous character of slave health practices.[23]

While my argument highlights the importance of African American doctoring to slave community, I am cognizant of the conceptual difficulties implicit in the term. "The slave community," as a homogenous and predictable social unit, has never existed, except in some historical scholarship. Slave communities, however, did prevail with rich variation throughout the antebellum South.[24] In this book the plural term is used to indicate both residential groups of enslaved families bound by geography and particular sets of relationships among the enslaved, influenced by but separate from master-slave relations.[25] Of necessity the boundaries of many enslaved communities reached beyond the property lines of individual plantations, extending to include friends, kin, and colaborers on other farms and plantations.[26] Furthermore, the term as it appears in this book does not apply only to the sundown-to-sunup hours within slave quarters, though these hours were indeed important to the cultural and social fabric of enslaved communities. Of equal concern in these pages, however, are fields, yards, workshops, and sickhouses where enslaved men and women built their communities as they labored.[27]

Acknowledging the many variations among antebellum slave communities, this study nonetheless argues for certain continuities in African American health experiences across the plantations of the southeastern United States. Certainly by some measures, such as the degree to which slaveowners intruded directly on slave healing practices or the extent of labor specialization among plantation health workers, size of plantation and region created important differences. Herbal practices, for example, changed with varying ecosystems. Certain regions, such as the Georgia and South Carolina Sea Islands, offered more concentrated evidence of African cultural retentions. At the same time, however, several broad themes, such as the objectifying concept of slave "soundness," the impact of the institution of slavery on the white medical profession, and the sacred foundation of African American doctoring, created similarities of experience throughout many slave communities. From the moderate holdings of the upper South to the great plantations of the Lowcountry, enslaved men and women critiqued the contradictions between their own vision of humanity and the slaveholders' valuation of their bodies.[28] Smaller holdings and more intimate relations with slaveholders could not shield enslaved families from the forces of sale and commodification, nor could lesser planters avoid the influence of property concerns on their health care decisions.[29] Sharing certain common experiences of white medical care, enslaved sufferers sought out (and were able to find) African American practitioners not only in the black majority areas of Georgia and South Carolina but in North Carolina towns and upper South farms as well.[30]

Plantations in four southeastern coastal states — Virginia, North Carolina, South Carolina, and Georgia — comprise the main focus of this study.[31] Representing both upper and lower South regions, these states varied widely in demography, geography, and main crops, including wheat, tobacco, rice, and cotton. Their diversity makes possible an investigation into slave health and healing across a large and varied portion of the South. Certain shared characteristics also facilitate a cohesive analysis of the southeastern Atlantic states. With their history of early and continuous British colonization, these states all contained regions where African American and Anglo-American traditions of medicines had developed for many decades in relation to the institution of slavery. In contrast to the newly cultivated areas of the cotton belt to the west, all four states featured regions with mature plantation economies and multigenerational slave communities. Established southern medical schools and a segment of white doctors who practiced on plantations meant that enslaved African Americans negotiated medical encounters with white doctors as well as with slaveholders and overseers. Their interactions produced a remarkable store of evidence on the social relations of plantation health and the content of African American healing.

The four states covered in this study are significant, too, for the ethnic distribution of the antebellum slave population's African-born ancestors. Historian Michael Gomez has proposed the existence of "African ethnic enclaves" in North America that laid the social and cultural foundations of later African American communities. Two of the three regions proposed by Gomez are represented in the geographical boundaries of this study. In Georgia and South Carolina, West Central Africans comprised the majority of the African-born population, while captives from the Bight of Biafra, namely the Igbo, made up the largest group in the upper South, including Virginia. Gold Coast Akan speakers, Senegambians, and later Sierra Leonians, contributed in smaller numbers to both upper and lower South regions as well. In addition to detailing the multiethnic base of African American healing practices, Gomez's analysis illuminates my interpretations at two other significant junctures. First, his model of ethnic enclaves suggests the possible cultural derivation for a heavy concentration of Kongo-based hoodoo in the Georgia and South Carolina Lowcountry. Though hoodoo (or conjure), which will be discussed at length in Chapter 4, appeared throughout the antebellum South, much of the evidence in this volume is drawn from the coastal regions of the lower South. Second, Gomez confirms my rationale for a separate consideration of African American healing in the lower Mississippi and in particular Louisiana. Here the stronger Fon-Ewe-Yoruba impact from the Bight of Benin contributed to voodoo (as opposed to hoodoo) religious practices distinctive to the lower Mississippi region.[32]

Evidence for the history of slave doctoring in the southeastern states lies scattered across the historical landscape. African Americans contributed heavily to the picture of their own health and healing. Both antebellum slave narratives and hundreds of interviews with former slaves conducted between 1920 and 1940 comment on the quality of slave health, relationships with white and black practitioners, and regional healing practices. Herbal remedies, illness narratives, and folklore collections drawn from southern African Americans make up the core of this book's evidence concerning the relational view of health and the doctoring practices embraced by enslaved communities. Supplementing this verbal evidence are the physical artifacts of healing practices—medicine bowls, birthing beads, and conjure kits—that remained in the earth long after their users passed on.

White residents of southern plantations also provided extensive evidence on the politics of black health and healing. From the diaries of southern mistresses to the weekly reports of white overseers, the written words of white men and women furnish evidence of the physical health of enslaved men, women, and children. Slave lists, family letters, and plantation journals document the importance of slave health to the economic success of every plantation. Even more important for this study, observations by white plantation residents and visitors reveal the tensions inherent in conflicting views of appropriate medicine held by slaves and slaveholders. Complaints raised against enslaved practitioners and patients exposed white assumptions about African American health practices and unintentionally confirmed postbellum accounts of slave reliance on African American healers.

White southern medical doctors make an important contribution to the story as well. Although white doctors only visited occasionally on many southern plantations, they made a considerable impression on slave health experiences. Intertwined with the slave trade and southern legal procedures, the southern medical profession depended on slavery for a patient base and on their slaveholding clientele for a living. In the southern Atlantic coastal states, medical schools such as the Medical College of South Carolina and Atlanta Medical College trained generations of antebellum practitioners keenly interested in the South's peculiar institution.[33] Medical school theses, case studies in medical journals, letters to colleagues, and notes from slaveholders requesting attention to enslaved patients all reveal not just the medical theory of the time but the texture of everyday medical practice.

Concerned primarily with the daily relations of plantation medicine, this book is a medical history in which human interactions, not diseases or treatments, occupy center stage. In many respects this study begins where medical historian Todd Savitt's important work *Medicine and Slavery* ends. Savitt paired the insights of public health models with social history to provide a detailed analysis of the diseases and health environment of Virginia slave quarters and the families who lived in them.[34] Combing the records of antebellum Virginia, Savitt richly documented a "dual system" of black and white health practices in which enslaved practitioners and popular remedies remained largely hidden from slaveholders.[35] Equally important, *Medicine and Slavery* placed plantation medicine in the context of southern social relations by arguing that slaves who sought their own remedies were not, as whites often charged, being "irresponsible" but were instead asserting "some independence" in determining the fate of their bodies.[36] While *Medicine and Slavery* convincingly demonstrated the existence of slave health practices, however, the book's biomedical framework does not permit a full exploration of their meaning.

Biomedical frameworks, grounded in the knowledge claims of modern, Western medical science, have in fact provided the basis for the bulk of historical scholarship on medicine and slavery throughout the Americas. Using the tools of twentieth-century medical theory, historians have learned quite a bit about antebellum southern disease environments and the health of black and white southerners.[37] Drawing from the fields of physical anthropology, nutrition, genetics, epidemiology, and modern medical diagnosis, Todd Savitt, Richard Steckel, Kenneth Kiple, and Virginia Himmelsteib King, among others, have etched the contours of slave health, highlighting horrific child mortality, compromised diets, and poor prenatal conditions. In these studies medical science provides a strong lens through which to peer into the antebellum South and understand the physical bodies of the individuals who inhabited the past. The result has been an increasingly nuanced view of regional southern health environments and a valuable analysis of the physical conditions faced by enslaved laborers.[38]

Notwithstanding their merits, biomedical approaches are not well equipped to analyze the experiential or political dimensions of health. Nor are they conducive to serious analysis of popular or indigenous healing knowledge embedded in alternative epistemologies. Despite their insights biomedical frameworks often obscure as much as they reveal about enslaved African American healing practices. Seeking a more appropriate approach, this study rejects a framework that posits some African American healing beliefs as "superstition" and others as "medicine." I have instead undertaken a meaning-centered and critical analysis rooted in the social, cultural, and political significance of healing. Accordingly, the interpretations that follow are concerned with the social reality of illness and healing, the ideological contexts in which illness and healing occur, and the hierarchies of power that inform health-related encounters. Viewed through this critical lens, the importance of healing to religion, labor, and community in the lives of enslaved African Americans comes sharply into focus.[39]

This book's topical organization reflects its emphasis on meaning and social relations. Part I begins by establishing the tensions between the slaveholder concept of "soundness" and the African American relational vision of health. Subsequent chapters delve into the sacred basis of African American doctoring practices, placing them in the context of community relationships, spiritual power, and African heritage. From the colonial period to the nineteenth century the African-based North American slave population underwent a wrenching cultural transformation. Between roughly 1780 and 1830 the African-born proportion of the enslaved population dropped from around 20 percent to less than 10 percent, with a large majority of African Americans being several generations removed from the direct memory of Africa.[40] Yet the African cultural presence in nineteenth-century slave doctoring remained strong. The Bambara use of protective amulets, the Kongo arts of *minkisi* and herbalism, and the Igbo and Akan concerns with the land and the ancestors met and merged on North American soil, furnishing the cultural underpinnings for an African American relational view of health.[41] This work's initial chapters delineate how enslaved communities invested this relational vision in a wide spectrum of healing practices, including sickbed attendance, herbalism, and conjure.

Though social conflict is apparent even in the initial chapters, the second half of the book turns more explicitly to questions of medicine and power relations on southern plantations. Franz Fanon, in a study of Algerian colonial medicine, argued that anyone who wants to understand how colonized peoples have viewed Western medicine must look to the histories of oppression underlying cross-cultural medical encounters.[42] Borrowing from this insight, Part II examines the many ways in which health and healing became arenas of struggle between slaveholders and the enslaved. As the latter chapters demonstrate, plantation health conflicts were far more than disagreements around the sickbed. So intertwined was slave health with other issues of plantation control that field labor, slave insurrections, and activities such as nighttime visiting among the enslaved also became venues of health-related conflict. Furthermore, the extensive involvement of enslaved women in plantation health work meant that plantation health conflicts involved childcare, childbearing, and slave women's skilled labor. Contention over alternative definitions of medical authority, particularly of slave women's authority, forms an important theme running through the second section.

Finally, the word "conflict" is used broadly throughout to indicate tensions, negotiations, outright opposition, and long-term, subtle contests for power. Wherever these conflicts occurred, slaves and slaveholders did not fight their battles on equal ground. Slave masters possessed the weapons of law, state-sanctioned violence, and legal ownership of the bodies of the enslaved. Enslaved African Americans countered with their own medical knowledge, confidence in their moral view of the universe, and a repertoire of survival techniques passed down across generations. As James Scott has pointed out, resistance of a subordinate class of people under extreme disparities of power is rarely carried out directly in the face of the dominant power.[43] To do so on the sickbed, as in the fields, was often simply too dangerous. Yet enslaved men and women nevertheless asserted their relational definition of health in daily acts aimed at maintaining self and community. The sum of their efforts provided a powerful counterweight to the systematic objectification of African Americans under slavery.

I Visions of Health

I am infirm and burdened with the influence of slavery,
whose impress will ever remain on my mind and body.
—*Mattie J. Jackson,*
   The Story of Mattie J. Jackson, *1866*

The up-country planter's wealth consists chiefly in his negroes,
and in proportion to their thrift and healthiness, just in such ratio
does he prosper. The principal value of the negro with us is his
increase, consequently [slave health] addresses itself to the interest
as well as the humanity of the slave-holder.
—*W. Fletcher Homes, M.D.,*
   Charleston Medical Journal and Review, *1852*

CHAPTER 1
Soundness

[handwritten: doesn't matter how kind the master is]

"The being of slavery, its soul and body, lives and moves in the chattel principle," wrote Presbyterian minister James W. C. Pennington in 1849. A fugitive from slavery and an active abolitionist, Pennington insisted that "kind and Christian masters" could never ameliorate the injustice of slavery. Without the destruction of the detested "bill of sale principle," warned Pennington, even persons enslaved in relatively milder conditions could at any moment face "the cart-whip, starvation, and nakedness."[1] The principle of human property, as James Pennington well knew, permeated southern society, extending not least of all to slave health. In southern fields, auction yards, and plantation sickhouses enslaved men and women confronted a political economy that cast the shadow of the marketplace over the most intimate events of birth, sickness, and death. While abolitionists and proslavery advocates argued over the moral fate of a society that held human beings as property, the system of slavery daily and concretely continued to mark African American lives and bodies.

Historians have for some time debated the influence of the property principle on the health of slaves. The topic of slave health, Todd Savitt notes, has served many historians as a barometer for the "benignity or harshness of 'the peculiar institution.'"[2] In the early twentieth century,

...storians U. B. Phillips and Carter G. Woodson disagreed markedly over whether slaveholders were generally "solicitous" or neglectful of slave health. Since that time some scholars have argued that economic interest motivated planters to provide a relatively high level of health care to their enslaved laborers. Others have disagreed, observing that property interest no more protected slaves against abuse than it did the land, tools, and livestock of the slaveholder.[3] Yet the debate over plantation health conditions, for the most part, casts slave health care as a problem only for slaveholders. It treats the property principle as a force that either did or did not motivate slaveholders to provide health care for their enslaved laborers. Missing from either side of the debate is any sustained discussion of how enslaved African Americans themselves understood the chattel principle and slaveholders' interests.

How did enslaved women and men analyze slave ownership and its impact on plantation health and healing? Approaching the history of plantation health from this perspective quickly brings into focus a struggle to define the very meaning of health and the terms of healing. This struggle gave rise to two competing visions of health and healing. The medicine of white slaveholders, on one hand, was deeply implicated in southern legal and economic institutions, which translated slave health into slaveholder wealth. In contrast, enslaved African Americans developed a powerful countervision of personal and collective endurance and, when possible, transcendence. The stories, songs, and testimony of enslaved African Americans reflect a shrewd critique of the influence of the property principle on slave health within the plantation economy.

The fusion of southern health and property concerns had immediate and life-changing consequences for an enslaved but defiant man named Harry living in South Carolina's Lowcountry. Less than a year before John Brown led the raid on Harpers Ferry, Harry struck his own blow against slavery. On a December Monday in 1858, physician John A. Warren of Colleton District wrote an urgent letter to his cousin John D. Warren, who was also Harry's legal owner. John A. complained that Harry had set fire to a rotting sill under the portico of the house that morning. He believed that Harry acted in collusion with another man, Jeffry, a runaway who had tried before "to burn me and my Family up." The fire was quickly contained, but it scarcely set John A. at ease. "I will be compelled to have an armed Guard at all times," he complained, "until the old demon can be caught & sent to Jail for I swear I would not have such a wretch about me for the world."[4]

Fett's intervention is to reveal how enslaved people actively understood and responded to the chattel principle w/ regard to slave healing

Harry had distinguished himself as a threat to the Warrens long before the morning of the fire. John A. identified Harry as "July's son, chip of [sic] the old block," perhaps indicating a family tradition of resistance. Some time earlier Harry had started another fire inside a table drawer in the Warren home. In 1857 he had been confined in the Charleston Work House, where he received one "correction," charged to John D. Warren's account for $1.50. Harry might also have had a history of escape that led to his incarceration, as the workhouse bill itemized four "Advertisements," which were often used to indicate the capture of a runaway slave or to advertise the inmate for sale. Now, with past trouble culminating in arson and conspiracy, John A. Warren vowed that "such an act must be crushed and the actors made an example of."[5]

John D. quickly made plans to ship Harry to Charleston for immediate sale, but Harry was determined not to be sold off so easily. Within a fortnight the Charleston slave merchant and auctioneer establishment of Capers and Heyward indicated it would be sending for Harry at Walterboro the following week.[6] Although exact events are not recorded, Harry most likely attempted an escape that led to violent confrontation. By early February Harry had been jailed in Walterboro, "shot with small shot" in his back. A search of his baggage revealed a pistol and ammunition, although it is unclear whether he had had an opportunity to use them.[7]

Harry's rebellious acts and subsequent injuries brought his status as chattel sharply into view. In the early days after his capture Harry was feverish, hemorrhaging, and coughing blood. For the next month his medical condition became the subject of frequent correspondence between the Warren cousins and Charleston physician Charles Pinckney. Their primary concerns were whether and when Harry would recover enough to be sold at the high prices of the booming 1850s slave market. When Pinckney visited Harry the following week, the physician reported hopefully that the sale would not long be delayed. "He is still improving and will soon be ready for *your purposes*," Pinckney wrote to John D. Warren.[8]

During this early period of convalescence John D. Warren sent an enslaved woman named Judy to nurse Harry in jail. In delegating Harry's round-the-clock care to Judy, Warren simply transferred a familiar pattern of slave women's health work from the plantation to the jailhouse. Enslaved women commonly served the daily health needs of the slave quarters, yet Judy had been sent to the isolation of a Charleston jail specifically to restore Harry's body for the market. Her relationship to Harry was unclear, but her objection to her assignment was unmistakable. Within days Pinckney sent Judy back to Warren's household, commenting that Judy "had great scruples about being in jail under any circumstances."[9]

As the immediate danger to Harry's life subsided, Harry's captors raised a new concern. John A. Warren warned his cousin that scar tissue around the wounds might in time irritate and inflame the lungs. If Harry had a "predisposition to Consumption," he warned, the irritation might eventually "excite that disease." For the present, however, the physicians decided they had nothing to fear. To support this contention they noted with satisfaction that Harry had not "lost any flesh" from his ordeal.[10]

Despite the doctors' optimism, Harry's wounds continued to present a barrier to his sale. The auctioneers, Thomas Capers and T. Savage Heyward, indicated in March 1859 that they had lodged Harry at the workhouse (where he had previously been incarcerated and whipped) but as yet had received no offer for him. "The objection is the marks of the shot in his back," they explained. "His teeth are also slightly defective. We hope to sell him soon but will not we fear get $1700."[11] Capers and Heyward's prediction proved true. On 23 March the slave traders sold Harry at a private sale on the Charleston docks "with distinct understanding that he be removed from and beyond the limits of the State [of] So Ca." John D. Warren received $1,100, the designated value of Harry's scarred and "defective" body.[12] Harry's harsh passage through the hands of slaveholders, physicians, and auctioneers vividly illustrated the dynamics of white southern medicine practiced in the interest of the planter class.

White Perceptions of Slave Health as Soundness

With the commodification of black bodies came the objectification of African American health. The intersection of medicine with the southern political economy produced a narrow definition of slave health permeated by concerns of slaveholder status and wealth. Questions concerning slaves' mental and physical health influenced the very nature of economic transactions in slave property. In turn, the principle of human property profoundly shaped the practice and theory of southern white medicine. Even the more mundane aspects of plantation health, such as the care of injuries and illnesses, reflected the fact that human property constituted the central form of southern wealth.[13] The Warrens' concern for Harry's health and sale value thus emerged from a context not peculiar to Harry alone. Although Harry's arson and rebellion may have been memorable events, both John A. Warren and his cousin routinely acted on matters

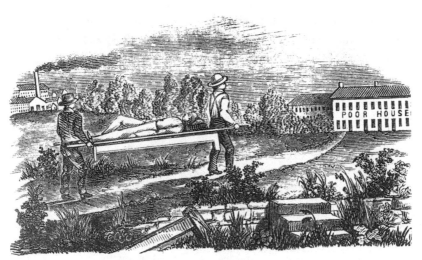

ATTENTION PAID A POOR SICK WHITE MAN.

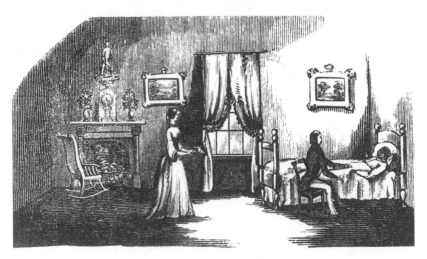

ATTENTION PAID A POOR SICK NEGRO.

Attention Paid a Poor Sick White Man *and* Attention Paid a Poor Sick
Negro. *This illustration from an antebellum proslavery treatise contrasts the
slaveholder's superior care of enslaved laborers against the callousness of
northern wage labor. Solicitous whites administer to a sick slave in the spacious
comfort of the planter's house. The actual conditions of slave health care were far
different from the scene depicted. (Josiah Priest,* Bible Defence of Slavery *[1853])*

of slave health as part of the daily business of running their plantations. In a thousand daily interactions the marriage of professional medicine and slavery put a price on black health. It shaped the terms of the medical attention slaveholders directed at enslaved men and women and deployed medical knowledge not only to heal but to preserve the status quo in a slave society.

The vision of slave health embraced widely by slaveholders and white medical professionals crystallized in the concept of "soundness." In 1858 Juriah Harriss, a physician and medical professor at the Savannah Medical College, deemed the evaluation of slave soundness "a question of great import to the southern physician and slave owner." [14] Frequently employed in both slave sales and medical jurisprudence, the term indicated an enslaved person's overall state of health and, by extension, his or her worth in the marketplace. [15] Harriss's lengthy discussion revealed the legal complexities of the concept of soundness. Soundness in its most basic sense concerned the health of a slave, measured in his or her capacity to labor, at the time of sale. Yet the definition of soundness included not only the present health of the individual but past and future health as well. In Harry's case, for example, John A. Warren worried that Harry's shotgun wounds would later dispose him toward consumption. [16] Soundness in enslaved women also described their future capacity to bear children. Juriah Harriss operated on an enslaved woman to remove a large tumor on her labia and afterward pronounced her sound. He further cautioned his professional readers that any "permanent cause of abortion, like [uterine tumors] would materially diminish the value," even if there was "no general disturbance of the system." [17]

Not limited to the physical body, the concept of soundness extended to mental and moral dimensions of slave health as well. Slave buyers frequently subsumed considerations of "character" under the general rubric of soundness guarantees. Buyers interpreted marks on enslaved men's and women's bodies as signs of past and future defiant behavior. The objectification of black health under slavery was thus not simply a matter of persons reduced to physical bodies but also of minds and personalities subjected to market assessments. [18] Through the concept of soundness, slaveholders — and physicians in their employment — defined slave health as the capacity to labor, reproduce, obey, and submit.

As medical practitioners and appraisers of slave soundness, white doctors participated actively in the business of the domestic slave trade. As early as the seventeenth century, European surgeons practiced their profession in the barracoons of coastal Africa, on slaving ships, and in the market-places of the colonial Americas. Late-eighteenth-century British law linked the medical profession formally to the Atlantic slave trade by requiring British slave merchants to hire physicians to oversee sick and dying captives on Middle Passage vessels.[19] After the legal closure of the Atlantic trade, the southern medical profession continued its close connections with the domestic slave trade. White doctors examined the bodies of men, women, and children in urban slave markets and issued certificates of soundness intended to protect buyers' purchases and sellers' liability.[20]

Though ordinary buyers in southern slave markets lacked the physician's claim to medical expertise, they shared a remarkably similar view of slave bodies. Buyers engaged in an intimate inspection of a slave's potential for labor, compliance, and for enslaved women, the ability to bear children. Probing for signs of chronic diseases and clues to character, prospective buyers closely examined slaves' scars and other marks that indicated past medical treatment.[21] Physicians Warren and Pinckney anticipated the buyers' gaze in their discussions of Harry's wounds, knowing well that Harry's injuries could raise questions about his medical and moral soundness.

Slaveholders were also concerned with issues of soundness in facets of the domestic slave trade beyond the actual sale transaction. Slave traders and slaveholders often viewed slave illness before and after sale as an encumbrance and a possible cause for litigation. John A. Warren reported his dismay over a young girl he had bought as "sound" but whom he quickly discovered to be quite ill with fever. The girl, Sarah, had seemed to have only an "Ephemeral" fever at the time of sale in early February 1859. "She went sound to the salesroom of Capers and Heyward," Warren recounted, because she had been able "to stand up & move about." Warren soon found out she had actually been fitful and feverish for several nights before. He feared she had contracted typhoid fever during her crowded confinement before the sale. On the way to the Warren plantation the girl became so ill that her mother, who had been "attending on her," had to carry her on her back. Eventually the illness forced Warren to make special arrangements to transport Sarah to her new quarters.[22]

The chattel principle at work in the marketplace translated human needs of men, women, and children awaiting sale into expenses for slaveholders. Soon after Sarah's illness, John D. Warren wrote the auction house in Charleston to inquire about the high lodging fee charged by the company compared with that of the Charleston Work House. Capers and Heyward replied that their higher boarding rates compared favorably to the workhouse's, since inmates had little recourse to medical attention at the workhouse. "The loss of one Prime Negro to you would have been more than the extra expense," they concluded.[23] This view of slave health as a logistical problem of the slave market was reflected as well by Samuel Browning, the man hired to trade Archibald Boyd's slaves in Mississippi. He wrote his employer that his return to North Carolina would be delayed because a "Girl that I have along . . . had a Child yesterday," and he would be forced to wait several days if he could not "make some disposition of her."[24] In each of these exchanges, whites calculated African American sickness primarily in terms of expense and inconvenience to slaveholders participating in the slave market.

The objectification of slave health by slaveholders and white doctors extended from the slave market into the courtroom. Unexpected illness, death, or even unruly behavior in a newly purchased slave prompted buyers to bring warranty suits against sellers. Warranty law varied from state to state. In Georgia the buyer was expected to obtain a warranty of soundness from the seller at the time of sale or forfeit rights to later suits. South Carolina buyers, on the other hand, presumed that, unless otherwise stated, the person being purchased was sound of body.[25] Across the South physicians provided expert court testimony on the possible fraudulence of soundness certificates. A Georgia court case in 1854 featured a dispute over a slave woman who had died from "pulmonary consumption" that developed three months after her sale. Although the new owner had purchased her without a warranty of health, he nevertheless brought suit. During the court hearing a physician offered evidence of the woman's illness at the time of sale, saying that upon examination of the woman, he had observed "marks of blistering and cupping on her breast," a likely sign that she had been previously treated for pulmonary illness.[26] Medical testimony in the courtroom provided an opportunity for white doctors to claim expertise and to advance racialized medical theories.[27] In this vein Savannah doctor Juriah Harriss argued the need for greater medical training in "medico-legal" questions "in their application to the negro slave." He lamented the lack of confidence of lawyers and juries in medical testimony and advocated only "intelligent and reliable medical men" in the witness box.[28]

As potential litigants, slaveholders often sought to avoid the trouble and expense of lawsuits in conflicts over warranties of soundness. During the months of Harry's recovery, John D. Warren relied on his brokers to arrive at an out-of-court settlement concerning another slave sale. Capers and Heyward informed Warren that in one family they had sold for him, "one of the boys by the name of Beverly and his sister had some defect." To avoid litigation, the auction house had deducted thirty dollars from the original purchase price because of an ulcer on the boy's leg.[29] Similarly, slave trader Samuel Browning informed a North Carolina slaveholder in 1849 that a sale agreement in Louisiana had run into complications. To avoid a lawsuit, Browning explained, he had had to exchange two women, Burline and Louisa, for "Candis unsound and Rose an Ediot."[30] In these examples slave traders and slaveowners shared with physicians the confidence that they could place a specific price on the pain and sickness of enslaved individuals.[31]

Slave life insurance likewise relied on measurements of slave soundness. Insurance policies on human property never became commonplace, but rising cotton and slave prices in the 1850s led to the increasing popularity of slave insurance. Numerous life insurance companies offered policies to slaveholders to protect against losses in the event of slave deaths. Slaveholders who hired out slaves to dangerous public works projects and industrial companies that owned enslaved laborers were most likely to buy insurance.[32] They paid premiums more than twice the rate for free persons and sometimes even more when the policy covered persons engaged in extremely dangerous labor, such as digging canals or laying railroad tracks. The Greensborough Mutual Life Insurance and Trust of North Carolina, for example, issued a policy in 1855 for the life of bondsman Felix Miner. For $21.36 per year the company agreed to cover Miner for the amount of $800, in keeping with the tendency of companies to insure slaves at two-thirds to three-fourths of their market valuation. The policy restricted Miner from traveling beyond state boundaries without the company's consent and voided its coverage if Miner died "for want of proper medical or personal attendance" or by riot, insurrection, or war.[33] Northern companies, too, offered slave policies. For a premium of $13.50 Connecticut's Aetna Life Insurance Company issued a twelve-month policy in 1856 on the life of Selina, a twenty-four-year-old washerwoman in Charleston. Based on Selina's market value of $800, her death would result in the payment of $600 to her South Carolina owner's trustee.[34]

Like southern courts and auction houses, the insurance business drew on white doctors to evaluate the health of enslaved men and women prior to issuing a policy. The enslaved woman Selina underwent a medical examination for which the insurance company charged a physician's fee of one dollar. Many insurance firms stipulated that practitioners employed for

policy examinations should be "regularly" trained, rather than the proponents of "irregular" medical sects.[35] In Virginia, insurance agent Archibald
Alexander Little attempted to recruit physician Andrew Grinnan for this
task, promising that collaboration could "benefit both of us." Little offered
to pay Grinnan two dollars for each slave he examined. Grinnan was to forward the insurance application, collect the premium, and deduct his fee.
Little encouraged the physician to join his venture by suggesting he could
make between fifty and one hundred dollars a year.[36] Certification of insurance policies created yet another instance in which white doctors directed
medical attention at enslaved men and women for nonhealing purposes.

A final arena in which law and medicine intersected with an objectified
definition of slave health involved the annual hiring of slaves. Slaveholders
who hired out slaves to urban households, industries, or other plantations
had an obvious economic interest in seeing the hired slave return in good
health. Hiring contracts often did not explicitly cover responsibility for
medical care, although both custom and law addressed the issue.[37] In Virginia the owner was expected to reimburse the hirer for medical expenses,
a custom confirmed by Virginia's higher courts in 1847. This practice was
apparently intended to protect slaveholders against the medical neglect of
hired slaves by hirers who did not want to shoulder the cost of medical
bills.[38] South Carolina, on the other hand, stipulated that medical expenses
were the responsibility of the hirer. A Charleston medical journal cited an
1848 legal decision for its readers: "Where a person, who hires a slave,
sends for a physician to attend him while sick, the person so employing
the doctor and not the *owner* of the slave is liable to the physician."[39] Yet
as was frequently the case with laws concerning enslaved African Americans, statutes governing hiring agreements did not accurately reflect actual
slaveholder practice. Thus the question of who should assume the cost of
medical bills fueled bitter disputes between owners and hirers.

Two years after Harry's sale, John D. Warren became embroiled in just
such a disagreement with Charleston businessman and printer Benjamin
Evans of Evans and Cogswell. Evans penned an angry letter concerning a
woman accompanied by her four children whom he had hired from Warren. The woman had fallen ill and, according to Evans, had turned out to
be "but a delicate servant." Evans wanted to send her home, but Warren
refused, insisting that Evans retain her for the entire year in keeping with
their original agreement. "As a matter of humanity I would have sent her
a Physician during the sickness of herself and children even had I known
that you would have refused to pay for his services," protested Evans, who

had clearly expected Warren to show more flexibility regarding the arrangement. After investigating his legal responsibilities, Evans concluded that *"we are so bound* [and] we are *ready* to pay both yours and the Drs. bill." He remained, nevertheless, intensely unhappy about the outcome of the dispute. When slave health expenses were involved, matters of "humanity" were inseparably joined to property concerns for both owner and hirer.[40]

The fusion of slave health and property concerns carried just as forcefully into daily plantation labor. Doctors and lawyers in the legal arena equated slave sickness with lower market prices; whites overseeing plantation labor equated slave illness with specific amounts of labor lost. During harvest time on the Hermitage Plantation near Savannah, manager K. Washington Skinner wrote owner Charles Manigault, "The indisposition of the negroes retards the progress of the work very much. Jimmy, Ben, William, Lilly & Phillis are the sick today, and some of them have been sick several days."[41] William Cain of North Carolina reported in a letter to his daughter Minerva Caldwell that "poor Jinny Kirkland is grunting [complaining] and will be of no possible use for months but to consume good."[42] South Carolina planter Thomas Chaplin expressed the same frustrations with poor slave health in numerous journal entries, including the following:

> *January 13, 1849:* Moll taken to her bed with fever. This sickness is bad for me in getting out my crop.
> *Feb. 18, 1850:* Isaac & Moll still sick. God knows when I will get all of my small force at work. So many mouths to feed & so few to work that it is *impossible* for me to get along.
> *January 9, 1856:* Sancho sick, therefore one gin stopped.[43]

The direct relationship between sickness and its significance for the crop was clear: Sancho's illness meant one less gin; Moll's fever impeded planting. Chaplin's remarks may have been uncharacteristically pointed, but the record he left reflects the general manner in which planters and overseers greeted slave illness as an obstacle to agricultural production. Paternalist ideology invoked the familial image of planters caring tirelessly for their sick slaves.[44] Yet when it came to the business of the plantation, slaveholders and overseers filtered their attitudes toward slave sickness through the screen of progress and profit in the fields.

The equation of slave health with the ability to perform daily plantation labor had important implications for the enslaved elderly and disabled. Advanced years, chronic ailments, or maimed limbs invariably compromised the soundness of aged and infirm slaves in the eyes of slaveholders. Elderly and disabled slaves continued to perform many plantation tasks, such as childcare, nursing, and basket making, but their bodies were nevertheless appraised at lower market values.[45] Just days prior to the beginning of Harry's ordeal, John D. Warren attempted to include three old and apparently ailing men in a large group sent to auction in Charleston. His broker appraised the group, found two of them "worthless," and advised him to retain the three, as they would only "depreciate the Gang" and endanger Warren's prospects for a healthy bid.[46] Across the South, estate inventories routinely listed the low values of the aged and those judged incapacitated. An 1855 appraisal for the estate of Virginian James McLurg included valuations ranging from $900 for seventeen-year-old Hannah to $0 for Phillis, "aged and infirm." Other younger adults, such as a herniated man listed as "badly ruptured" and a young girl declared "Idiotic," received lower appraisals as well.[47] Hiring contracts also reflected the devaluation of enslaved elders. In Camden, South Carolina, John Chesnutt attempted to renegotiate terms for hiring a group of slaves. He protested that several old women in the group were worth only half-wages. "Galbo's Wife in particular," he claimed, "has the Rheumatism so very bad in her Wrists, arms & legs that she is not worth more than her Victuals and cloths."[48]

Low property appraisals translated into increased instability and uncertainty for the enslaved elderly. Conditions for aged slaves formed a common theme in the rhetoric of both proslavery and abolition advocates. Proponents of slavery painted a reassuring picture of old men and women living their last years in comfort provided by southern planters. In actuality younger adults in slave communities cared for many of the elderly. Some elders, however, found themselves at the mercy of slaveholders who, despite legal proscriptions in some states, attempted to shed the financial burden of weakened laborers by abandonment, manumission, or hire.[49] In 1824 Virginia lawmakers took moderate steps to discourage the practice of abandonment by passing an act stipulating a fine of up to fifty dollars for slaveowners who permitted slaves of "unsound mind, or aged or infirm" to "go at large" without support.[50] The devaluation of aging slaves by slaveholders, as I will discuss in later chapters, posed a stark contrast to the veneration of the elderly in communities of enslaved African Americans.

The chattel principle objectified the health of younger slave women differently from that of their elders. Slaveholders measured the soundness of slave women on a dual scale of both productive and reproductive labor.[51]

In other words, the market value of slave women of childbearing age rested in their ability not only to work the fields but to bear new generations of wealth. A South Carolina physician put it frankly: "The principal value of the negro with us is his increase," he wrote, and consequently the question of health "addresses itself to the interest as well as the humanity of the slave-holder."[52] Again slaveowners' concerns about humanity, when articulated, coexisted comfortably with their property interests.[53]

Nevertheless, the collision of slaveholders' interests in plantation production and slave reproduction produced real and terrible consequences for slave women's well-being. Despite the advantages gained from enslaved women's childbearing, slaveholders fretted about the impact of pregnancy on field work. The overseer of a Georgia rice plantation, for example, reported that slave health was tolerable that month, but "the worst is P[r]egnant women[.] there is now five which weakens the force very much."[54] Another South Carolina planter wrote of the "time lost by laying up, *Five Women* in a family way have done little or nothing this season."[55] Even planters who advocated less strenuous field work for pregnant women nevertheless pushed slave women to the limits of physical exertion during harvest.[56] Conflicts inherent in the dual definitions of slave women's soundness may help to explain why enslaved women became particular targets of hostility in conflicts over health and healing. William Massie penned this indictment of Betsy, a thirty-two-year-old mother of five children: "This worthless lazy thing, after being good for nothing from the time I bought her—From pure fear of being put to work run mad on 4th July 1850 & died on the 9th July 1850."[57] In later chapters I will explore the suspicions slaveowners held about enslaved women as incompetent mothers, surreptitious abortioners, ignorant nurses, feigners of pregnancy, and transmitters of venereal disease.

Questions of soundness and value in turn carried important implications for the degree and quality of medical attention slaveholders directed at slaves. As enslaved African Americans themselves recognized, slaves with high market value often received more intensive medical care from slaveholders. Two notes requesting attention from a Virginia physician illustrated the character of treatment based on the value of slaves. John Peter Mettauer, widely known in Virginia for his work with diseases of the eye, practiced extensively with enslaved patients. In 1835 Alfred Eggleston sent an enslaved man, George, to Mettauer bearing a request for an operation on a "stricture" (an obstruction of the urinary passage). "You will please take the case in hand," Eggleston wrote. "He is a very valuable slave and I feel great solicitude about him."[58] In contrast an 1839 note from a second man, James Neal, bore instructions concerning the treatment of an older slave: "I have [sent] old Bob to come and see if you can do him any good[.] if you can without too much expence you will please afford him relief if you can."[59] In these two cases the wealth of the slaveholders may also have influenced the differences in their appeals; nevertheless, their notes provide an explicit contrast between a special plea for George's high value and a request for limited treatment for the elderly Bob.

Slaveholders also interpreted the death of a slave in terms of the value of the deceased. In 1849 a white Virginian reported the death of an enslaved man. "Capt. Bondurant's Henry died about three weeks ago," he commented; "he was the most valuable negro he owned."[60] Similarly, another Virginian wrote to Thomas Massie about the death of three young slave women, noting regretfully, "If they had been exposed to sale, I suppose the three would have commanded more than two thousand dollars."[61] David Gavin, a lawyer and planter in South Carolina, observed the deaths of several persons enslaved in his neighborhood: "Mr. C. Rumph has also been unfortunate with regard to the loss of property within the last 12 months, he had a woman and child burnt up in their house, and last summer lost six prime hands with typhoid fever, which makes eight negroes within a year and seven of them working hands."[62] Gavin felt the sting of a slave's death in his own pocket as well. When a small child he owned died several years later, he observed, "Celia's child, about four months old died Saturday the 12th. This is two negroes and three horses I have lost this year."[63]

The property value of a slave had the potential to shape greatly his or her fortunes with white medical practitioners as well. A physician reporting on a number of surgical cases for a South Carolina medical journal cited the example of an enslaved miller who suffered a crushed leg in a pounding mill. Describing the subsequent amputation of the miller's leg, the author commented that he "saw no reason why [he] should not attempt to save the knee joint as the limb appeared perfectly healthy at point of election, and the negro was very valuable to his owners."[64] A skilled slave mechanic in his prime, implied the doctor, was well worth the effort and expense of the operation.

Race, class, and property status played an alarming role in the medical decisions of some southern doctors. Georgian W. H. Robert presented his professional peers with the case of an enslaved fifteen-year-old whose injured leg had been amputated above the knee without any less-drastic attempts to save the limb. The surgeon's decision stemmed in part, Robert maintained, from a conviction that the significance of amputation "should be very differently estimated in the different classes of society." Amputation threatened a rich man with "horrid deformity and destruction of enjoyment," and it robbed a free laborer of his means of subsistence. However, argued Robert, amputation to the slave was "a matter of comparatively little importance. Idleness being his greatest enjoyment, and having but few wants, and the certainty that these will always be met by his master, the negro dreads nothing from the operation but the pain it may occasion." Having less anxiety than free patients, argued Robert, a slave could more easily recover from the operation. Furthermore, as in the case of the young man, he could be put to productive work that did not require full mobility. Thus, Robert concluded, a surgeon should "hesitate much less to remove a limb, whose affection endangers the life of the patient, if he be a slave, than if he be a free man, and especially a white man."[65]

In the legal and popular idea of soundness, slaveholding southerners created a definition of health that was both remarkably supple and severely limiting. No simplistic measure of bodily strength, the definition of soundness incorporated subtle variations of age, skill, gender, fecundity, physical strength, mental acuity, and character. Flexible enough to coexist with slaveholders' emotional investment in individual slaves, the concept of soundness fit comfortably with the definitions of "humane" treatment expressed by white southerners interested in preserving their peculiar institution through reform. Furthermore, its subtlety allowed white practitioners to adapt notions of soundness to changing antebellum theories of racial medicine.

Despite its flexibility, the concept of soundness irrevocably bound the health of enslaved African Americans to the chattel principle. Like a pair of blinders, prevailing concerns of soundness and value constrained slaveholder perceptions of slave health to a narrow range of bodily suffering and well-being. The idea of soundness required white doctors to fill nonhealing roles as medical experts in slave markets and courtrooms. In the fields slaveholders and overseers equated healthy bodies with rows hoed and ditches dug. In response enslaved men and women recognized the limitations of slaveholder definitions of slave health. As one facet of their health culture, enslaved African Americans identified and indicted the impact of the chattel principle on their bodies and souls.

"Just Like the Hogs": The Slave Indictment
of a Chattel Definition of Health

Men and women in the slave quarters viewed plantation medicine in light of the broader experience of being defined as property. Looking back on slavery, many African Americans underscored their objectification by comparing their treatment to that of domestic animals. This theme also figured strongly in abolitionist narratives of fugitive slaves. James Pennington wrote forcefully of the humiliation of the slave who "finds his name on a catalogue with the horses, cows, hogs and dogs."[66] Another figure in a late-nineteenth-century collection of slave narratives bitterly testified, "The white people thought in slave-time we poor darkies had no soul, and they separated us like dogs."[67] Likewise, in the twentieth-century Federal Writers' Project interviews, Alabama freedwoman Jenny Proctor gave a scathing rendition of the white preacher who admonished his enslaved audience, "You just like the hogs and other animals—when you dies you ain't no more, after you been throwed in that hole."[68] In their use of these animal metaphors, enslaved men and women condemned the chattel principle and asserted their basic humanity.[69]

African American oral literature, or orature, also addressed the indignity of being defined and treated as chattel.[70] Reflecting both the realism and the humor of slave trickster tales, one Virginia story concerned an old man, Uncle Abraham, who was trying to find a palatable way of confessing to his preacher that the roast pig and potatoes being served at his table had been taken from the master. Abraham offered the following prayer, to the satisfaction of the black preacher: "A Lord, dou . . . taught dy sarvents dat it want no harm fur ter take de corn out er de barril and put it into de kag. De barril 'longs to de marster and de kag 'longs ter de marster, dar-forth it aint no diffunce when de darkie take de marster's pig out er de pen an put it into de darkie, case de darkie 'longs ter de marster, an de pig pen 'longs ter de marster."[71] The story of Abraham's stolen meal resembled other tales that distinguished between stealing from enslaved neighbors and rightfully appropriating goods from the slaveowner. After all, many former slaves pointed out, in stealing Africans away from their kin and homelands, whites had committed the ultimate act of theft.[72] Abraham's analogy also served as a penetrating commentary on the contradictions of planter ideology that justified the possession of human beings as property but condemned slaves as immoral for acting on human needs and

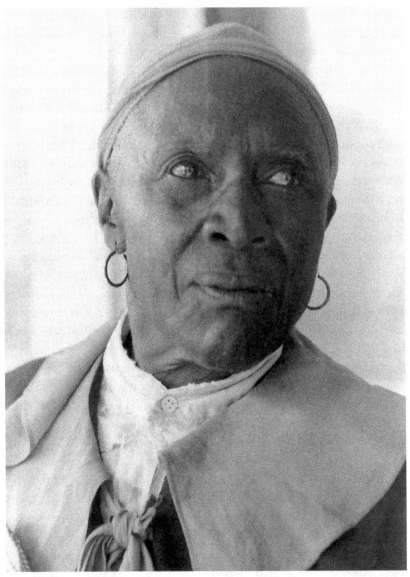

Fannie Moore, Asheville, North Carolina, ca. 1937. Born in 1849 on a large and brutal plantation in South Carolina, Mrs. Moore recalled that her brother George died of a fever and her mother was unable to leave the cotton fields to attend him. Mrs. Moore's African-born grandmother doctored her family aggressively with medicines made from leaves, roots, and bark. (WPA Ex-Slave Narrative Collection, LC)

desires. As part of African American orature such tales pointedly demonstrate the analysis and condemnation of the chattel principle embedded in the culture of the slave quarters.

Nineteenth-century African Americans keenly dissected the concept of soundness and found the chattel principle at its heart. Authors of antebellum slave narratives described how the pressures on the seller to present as sound a specimen as possible produced a situation ripe for fraud and added abuse. According to John Brown, an escaped fugitive from Georgia, dealers in the New Orleans slave pens flogged both adults and children for not looking "bright" on the action block. The men doing the beating, related John Brown, used a leather paddle designed especially not to cut the skin and "depreciate the value of the 'Property.'" In addition Brown described the many tricks dealers developed for what they termed "'shoving off a used up nigger.'"[73] Another abolitionist fugitive and medical practitioner, William Wells Brown, described the "blacking process," in which the graying hair and whiskers of elderly slave men were either plucked or colored to make them appear younger.[74] In the macabre theater of the slave sale, enslaved African Americans were forced to present themselves as fit and able-bodied.

Seeking to determine the soundness of their prospective purchases, buyers inspected the bodies of enslaved women and men, as John Brown put it, "with the most elaborate and disgusting minuteness." For both men and women, he claimed, "What passes behind the screen in the auction room, or in the room where the dealer is left alone with the 'chattels' offered to him to buy, only those who have gone through the ordeal can tell."[75] Couched in the terms of abolitionist rhetoric, the narratives of John Brown and William Wells Brown powerfully critiqued the objectification of slave health and linked the concept of soundness to their fellow slaves' experiences of pain, diminishment, and violation.

Even the records of slave traders revealed that enslaved men and women understood and attempted to exploit the concept of soundness to temper their utter vulnerability within the slave market. In their conversations with buyers, some slaves used the topics of illness and infirmity to divert a particular sale.[76] Upcountry South Carolina trader A. J. McElveen wrote to a Charleston broker concerning difficulties in his attempt to sell a man named James. "I could sell him like hot cakes if he would talk Right," McElveen protested, but "the Boy is trying to make himself *unsound.*" Apparently James warded off prospective buyers by claiming, against the word of McElveen and other traders, that he had worn a truss in the past. To wary buyers this piece of personal history implied the possibility of hernia, a serious "defect" in the parlance of the marketplace. James only managed to delay, not prevent, the eventual sale that separated him from his wife and home.[77] The record of his resistance, left in McElveen's letters, indicate James's manipulation of the cold calculus of soundness in the domestic slave trade.

From the auction yard to southern plantations, enslaved men and women had ample opportunity to observe how their value as property shaped the medical decisions of planters. Many concluded that the threat to property remained the chief motivation for a planter to summon a white doctor. When a slave became sick, one former slave remarked, "they put a messenger boy on a mule and sent him for Dr. Hudson quick, 'cause to lost a Negro was losing a good piece of property."[78] Solomon Northup, kidnapped from the North into slavery and dangerously weakened by fever and chills, received medical attention only when "Master Epps, unwilling to bear the loss, which the death of an animal worth a thousand dollars would bring upon him," agreed to pay for a physician.[79] As a small boy, however, James Smith was worth little to his Virginia owner. When James Smith's mother begged for medical care for her son's injured knee, the slaveowner replied that he had plenty of property and "did not care if I did die."[80]

According to the testimony of former slaves, slaveholding women were no less inclined to calculate slave health in terms of their ledgers. Jenny Proctor reported that despite meager provisions everyone on her plantation received red flannel underclothes for the winter. "Old Miss she say a sick nigger cost more than the flannel," she recalled bitterly.[81] Born and enslaved in Georgia, Tines Kendrick spoke of a "mighty stingy" mistress who would call a physician for sick slaves only when the illness became serious enough to threaten the loss of life.[82] John Brown likewise described a white mistress who encouraged the enslaved children to take a daily dose of garlic and rue, saying that it would make them "grow likely for market."[83] Long-held memories clearly articulated links between the domestic duties of white slaveholding women and the objectifying effects of the chattel principle.

Many enslaved men and women found the explicit economic motivations of slaveholders cause for distrusting the medical attention of white practitioners.[84] Their critique extended to both neglect and unwanted medical attention from whites. On one hand, enslaved men and women charged that slaveholders hesitated to call for white doctors when they would have readily done so for white family members. At the same time, however, bondsmen and -women held great misgivings concerning the attention they did receive from slaveholders and white doctors. Elisha Cain, overseer for the Telfair family of Georgia, found his task of investigating and treating several cases of venereal disease in the slave quarters difficult because enslaved men and women resisted his inquiries.[85] In this case slaves greeted the overseer's medical attention, which was directed not only at treatment but at sexual control, as an intrusion. Many ailing slaves also distrusted the white doctors called in by planters and sought to avoid their prescriptions. Whether neglect or intrusive treatment, the core criticism of enslaved men and women remained the same: the inability of whites to see African American health apart from principles of property and subjugated labor.

The political economy of antebellum slavery married questions of slave illness and health to slaveholder property interests and plantation labor goals. The Warren cousins' attempts to heal Harry for the Charleston slave market vividly illustrated the fusion of slave health and the chattel principle. Imprisonment magnified the opportunities for medical control over Harry by white physicians and slaveholders. Except for temporary attendance by the enslaved woman Judy, who protested her role as prison nurse, Harry remained isolated from the realm of African American healing that would have been available to him on the Warren plantation. We have no words from Harry himself about his ordeal, but evidence from African American sources suggests a widespread indictment of market value and soundness as guiding concerns in slaveholder medical decisions.

Within the slave quarters of southern plantations, a culture of healing that was not organized around the market value of slave bodies provided a powerful resource for survival, resistance, and community building. Enslaved sufferers pursued a vision of health that valued personal and community integrity over the maintenance of productive and reproductive labor. Black healers grounded their work in notions of spiritual power, human relationships, and community resourcefulness, thus addressing a much wider range of healing needs than slaveholders considered legitimate. In short, two views of health operated on antebellum plantations. These competing visions of health indicated more than simple disagreements over diagnosis and remedy. Instead they spoke profoundly to how black and white southerners perceived the boundaries of their communities. The following chapters explore how, under a system of slavery that isolated and objectified black bodies, African Americans pursued a broader relational vision of health.

Ike di na awaja na awaja—*Power runs in many channels.*
—*Igbo saying, translated by Chinua Achebe in* Igbo Arts, *1984*

Negro folklore, evolving within a larger culture which regarded it as
inferior, was an especially courageous expression. It announced the
Negro's willingness to trust his own experience, his own sensibilities
as to the definition of reality, rather than allow his masters to define
crucial matters for him.
—*Ralph Ellison,* Writers at Work, *1963*

The screaming baboon lived under their own white skin; the red gums
were their own.
—*Toni Morrison,* Beloved, *1987*

CHAPTER 2

Spirit and Power

Whereas the concept of soundness was used to appraise slaves
as individual units in relation to slaveholder wealth, African Americans
in slavery treated illness and well-being in markedly different terms. The
relational vision of health held that collective relationships influenced an
individual's well-being. Furthermore, collective relationships extended beyond human interactions to encompass what scholar Yvonne Chireau has
termed "an enchanted universe."[1] Illness or affliction could arise from
abraded relationships within a broadly defined community of living kin and
neighbors, ancestors, and spirits. Enslaved healers, working in relation to
this spiritually empowered world, often described their skills as "gifts" and
attributed their knowledge to divine intervention. The midwife's touch,
the conjurer's roots, and the herb doctor's pungent teas addressed the sufferer's pain as well as her or his standing within an extensive web of relationships. Seen in this light, slave doctoring, far from being a quaint and
marginal folk practice, formed an integral part of the "invisible institution"
of slave religion.[2]

Black healing practices were not always hidden from slaveholders, however, and visibility could be dangerous. In the mid-1840s Virginian E. G.

Crumpe wrote to planter William Jerdone advising him on the state of Jerdone's plantation. "All the servants are well," Crumpe wrote, "with the exception of Patience to who Dr Carter has been twice. He says that she has the rheumatism. But she thinks that she is tricked and desires a negro Doctor. My advice is to apply Hickory oil to the back frequently as I have found that to be an infallible remedy and the only one to remove that notion from the head."[3] Read in context, Crumpe's reference to "Hickory oil" indicated not a family remedy but a euphemism for whipping. Southern planters did not use hickory in rheumatism remedies, but they did use the word routinely as a metonym for corporal punishment — an interpretation reinforced by the recommended application of the remedy to the patient's back.[4] Furthermore, Patience's request for a "negro Doctor" may have been prompted by a previous experience in 1838 when she had gone to live with an "Old Doctress," a bondswoman from another plantation who treated Patience's sore foot.[5] If Crumpe was aware of this history, he may have been encouraging Jerdone to take more aggressive control of Patience's complaints.

Crumpe's advice to "cure" Patience by force illustrated the collision of two conflicting views of illness and healing. For Patience, healing required an appropriate practitioner's attention to communal relationships. Claiming that someone had "tricked" or conjured her, Patience understood her illness in terms of spiritual forces unleashed against her. Only someone able to contain and counter those forces could cure her. Patience's outlook clearly angered Crumpe, who seemed to have encountered "that notion" previously. He maintained that Patience suffered from rheumatism, a disease whose origins lay in interactions between the physical body and the natural environment. Medicines prescribed by Carter for rheumatism would have been directed at the individual body in the form of infusions, tonics, or rubbing solutions.[6] Each diagnosis, conjuration versus rheumatism, implied a unique understanding of bodily affliction and a different course of healing.

The threat to "apply Hickory oil" graphically illustrated contrasting notions of power underlying conflicts over slave illness. Crumpe, Jerdone, and the white doctor possessed the social power to name Patience's illness and treat her accordingly. Patience's owner possessed legal power to remedy her claims of illness with violence and force her compliance. His power to define her experience of illness remained incomplete, however, for Patience acknowledged sources of affliction that lay beyond the realm of slaveholder authority.[7] The rituals employed to "trick" Patience did not erase the slaveholder's power, but they existed outside his understanding. In addition they rendered white medical doctors impotent; only a "negro Doctor" trained in spiritual intercession could cure Patience. In this conflict over slave illness and healing, the participants claimed and exercised power on several fronts. Their disagreements reflected tensions between the several cultures of healing coexisting uneasily on antebellum plantations.

Contention between slave and slaveholder also reflected more broadly the changing boundaries of antebellum medicine, religion, and science. The nineteenth century is often portrayed as a period of secularization in which science gradually replaced religion as the discourse of authority within the dominant society. Nineteenth-century medical history, it has been argued, reflected this process of secularization as public understandings of illness shifted from fears of divine affliction to a focus on public health.[8] Yet the secularization of health was an uneven and highly contentious process. Throughout the nineteenth century large segments of the U.S. population, including large numbers of evangelical Christians, continued to understand illness and practice healing as an extension of their faith.[9] Thus slaves and slaveholders disagreed not so much over sacred versus secular worldviews as over the very terms in which spirit mattered to health. Shifting alignments of religious experience, scientific knowledge, and medical authority critically shaped the responses of slaveholding whites to slaves who enlisted spiritual power for healing.

North American Slavery and the African American Pharmocosm

Enslaved healers practiced mundane arts laden with cosmic significance. If historians have failed to recognize the religious importance of a wide range of slave doctoring traditions, the fault surely lies with a combination of scattered evidence, a tendency to discount enslaved women as spiritual leaders, and a focus on the institutional aspects of slave religion. Yet the picture is slowly shifting. Recent scholarship broadening the perception of "black sacred culture," conjoined with existing scholarship on the folk religion of plantation slave quarters, provides the critical framework for reassessing African American healing as spiritual praxis.[10]

The reassessment begins with a new look at the concept of the cosmology forged by Africans and their descendants in the crucible of North American slavery. Religion scholar Theophus Smith has coined the word "pharmocosm" to describe the biblical worldview of enslaved African Americans. A contraction of the phrase "pharmacopeic cosmos," the term "pharmocosm" emphasizes the healing and harming capacities of spiritual power. In advancing this formulation Smith has built on important earlier work by historians as varied in approach as Sterling Stuckey, Eugene Genovese, Lawrence Levine, and Margaret Washington Creel, who describe a "sacred world" fostered among the enslaved communities of the antebellum South.[11] According to these scholars, enslaved African Americans made no distinctions between secular and religious spheres but, instead, merged African cultural legacies with Christianity to create a world wholly imbued with sacred meaning. Spirituals rang out in the fields as in worship services. The ring shout, originating from African sacred dance, became the template for slave worship and celebration.[12] African American storytelling depicted a universe in which animals and inanimate objects, as well as human beings, had a voice.[13] This sacred worldview prevented "legal slavery from becoming spiritual slavery."[14] It formed a foundation for an "ethos" of resistance and inspired the expressive culture African Americans created under enslavement.[15] In this sense African American spirituality was transformational, creating an internal world that could endure against the master's will to power.

Delving more deeply, Theophus Smith argues that African American sacred culture contains a curative as well as a transformational dimension. The "black American conjurer," Smith points out, acts not only as "a magician but also as a kind of doctor."[16] In this sense the concept of the pharmocosm adds dimension and momentum to the idea of the sacred world. First, the pharmocosm describes spiritual power in action. The pharmocosm, explains Smith, "designates a world capable of hosting myriad performances of healing and harming."[17] As an ongoing creation the cosmos is "constituted and reconstituted by healing and harming processes and practices."[18] Moreover, Smith asserts that healing and harming, rather than being dichotomous expressions of good and evil, are instead dual aspects of an African American conjuring culture. Within the conjunctive modes of the "wisdom tradition of Black North American folk culture," Smith argues, "ambiguity and multivocity are taken for granted."[19]

Applied to the context of slave doctoring, the concept of the pharmocosm illuminates how both healing and harming might be involved in a single transformational process. A conjurer's trick could afflict a person such as Patience terribly while working simultaneously as a curative measure for a broken relationship. Beyond Crumpe's brief allusion to conjure, we know almost nothing about the human relationships that gave rise to Patience's affliction. Yet she clearly insisted on the services of a "negro Doctor" who understood the duality of healing and harming powers. In the pharmocosm, harming could be employed toward curative purposes, and destruction could sometimes serve the purposes of creation. In other words, there were tonic as well as toxic sides to conjuration, and both could work for the broader purpose of curing.

Two accounts from African American orature further elucidate the dynamics of healing and harming in the pharmocosm. These stories, collected in the twentieth century about nineteenth-century events, demonstrate an interpretation of illness as God's visitation on whites for the sin of slavery. South Carolinian Isom Roberts told of his parents' wealthy master, who died mysteriously of smallpox. During the Civil War this planter had threatened to kill his slaves before he would allow them to see freedom at Yankee hands. But, Roberts related, "Providence, or some kind of mercy spirit, was sure walking round that plantation that night. Sometime in the night it was whispered round amongst the slaves that Old Master done took the smallpoxes and was mighty sick." Two days later they buried him.[20]

Reflecting a similar view of epidemic illness as divine intervention, Virginia Hayes Shepherd remembered the account of her mother and grandmother about "the pestilence Days," an 1869 smallpox epidemic in Norfolk, Virginia. They told her that God "made up his mind to punish [the white folks], Killeen' off the cruelest." Smallpox struck whites on many plantations, and many died; "but not a single slave" was afflicted. "Everywhere you went, the slaves was sittin' on the front porches jes' a rockin' and the white folks stretched out inside, all dead. Was good times after that for the Negroes. Wouldn't any white folks dare treat 'em mean no more."[21] Apocryphal as this family story may have been in relating the extent of "good times" for black Virginians, it carried an important message about sickness as a divine instrument of justice and a transformer of established relations of power. In both of these accounts smallpox served as a righteous "medicine" sent by God to root out the injustices of the slaveholders.[22]

An emphasis on the duality of healing and harming linked the African American pharmocosm to numerous precolonial African cosmologies. Despite their striking diversity, many African religions acknowledged dual aspects of spiritual power, directed toward both creation and destruction. Many African deities could intervene either positively or negatively in the lives of human beings.[23] In 1915 Kongo nationalist Simon Kavuna eloquently described the power of *minkisi*, sacred medicines and spiritual entities widely employed across West Central Africa: "These are the properties of *minkisi*, to cause sickness in a man, and also to remove it. To destroy, to kill, to benefit. To impose taboos on things and to remove them. To look after their owners and to visit retribution upon them."[24] African captives transported to North America brought with them a conviction that intercession for spiritual power involved both healing and harming.

Nineteenth-century African Americans recognized a similar duality in the spiritual work of black healers. Conjurers, for example, possessed the ability both to harm and to heal; in fact, the act of healing one person might entail harming the person who originated the "fix." As an elderly Georgia woman phrased it, "I wouldn't trust dem sort of folks 'cause if dey can cyore you dey can kill you too."[25] Throughout more than two centuries of enslavement, African American concepts of illness and healing continued to reflect, in Albert Raboteau's words, a "refusal to dichotomize power into good and evil."[26] The persistence of a dualistic notion of spiritual power well into the nineteenth century owes much to the distance that the colonial slave population kept from Christianity.

Until the first evangelical awakenings of the eighteenth century, few enslaved Africans or their children had embraced Christian conversion on the British colonial mainland. Indifferent or wary slaveholders made few efforts toward Christian proselytizing among their slaves. Although some Africans had encountered Christianity before they left the African coast, Protestant Christianity figured "scarcely at all" in North American slave culture prior to the mid-eighteenth century.[27] Even after that, Christianity spread slowly and unevenly for the next several decades. Within the constraints of New World enslavement, Africans continued to hold to their religions of birth, while they and their children slowly identified and incorporated aspects of ritual and worldview from other West and West Central African ethnic groups.[28]

Integral to African religions, African healing practices persisted as well. Several recent historical studies reveal an active presence of African healers among North American slave populations. Possessing a limited vocabulary for describing what they observed, European colonists used the words "obi" or "ober" (related to West Indian "obeah") to indicate men and women who employed their power to poison and to cure. Sylvia Frey and Betty Wood suggest that necessity forced African "sacred specialists" in the Americas to subsume under one person several originally separate roles, such as diviner, herbalist, and spirit medium. Evidence from white colonists indicates that African practitioners sold charms, led insurrections, preached, and healed illnesses throughout the Americas. Their prominence among the enslaved was such that Europeans employed African ritual specialists (even those they suspected as "witches") to attend the sick on colonial plantations.[29] Islam, brought by Senegambians and other West African Muslims, also shaped the healing practices of early slave communities.[30] Furthermore, as Philip Morgan argues, African-born practitioners passed their knowledge to sons and daughters, creating a succeeding generation of Creole practitioners versed in the harmful and curative capacities of their medicines.[31]

By the time enslaved African Americans began adapting the Baptist and Methodist message to their own worldview, slave healing arts based in a dualistic vision of power had attained a secure place within the religious life of plantation slave quarters. The pharmocosm of nineteenth-century slave communities drew much more heavily on Christianity than it had in the past, but it maintained the "conjunctive" thinking that embraced both malevolent and beneficent uses of power. In the words of scholar Yvonne Chireau, "A kinship emerged between supernaturalism and slave Christianity."[32] This is not to argue that enslaved communities were of one mind about the morality of conjuring. Black Christian churchgoers, for example, at times censured members of their congregations who consulted conjure doctors.[33] Yet antebellum slave healing practices continued to partake of the older African dualities of power alongside the newer practices of black southern Christianity.

Evangelical Christianity as espoused by whites, however, countered the African dualistic view of power with the sharply opposed powers of heaven and hell, thus exacerbating tensions between slave and slaveholder medicine. During the same period in which Europeans became more hostile toward indigenous religions in Africa, whites in the American South increasingly disparaged black healers' claims to spiritual empowerment.[34] Emerging ideologies of colonialism and civilization further reinforced the association made by whites between black healers and grotesque distortions of African religions. In this way Africa played a second, vital role in plantation medicine, alongside its cultural legacy for black healers. More accurately, the image of Africa in the imagination of antebellum whites contributed to widespread assumptions about the "superstitious" basis of black healing practices.[35]

In 1858 Mary P. Randolph, a white woman of Virginia's planter class, wrote to her nephew in medical training urging him to consider "how much good, a christian physician has it in his power to do! ministering to the soul as well as the body of the poor sufferers he visits."[36] As Mary Randolph's remarks indicate, enslaved African Americans were not alone in embracing the spiritual dimensions of health. It would thus be misleading to characterize the difference between slave and slaveholder visions of health as a contrast between the sacred and the secular.[37] Distinctions in the dominant culture between science and religion, although slowly becoming more marked, remained blurred for much of the antebellum period. In this context southern slaveholders, like many white Americans of their time, employed both a religious and a scientific lexicon to pursue the question of mind-body-spirit relationships.[38]

Nineteenth-century white Americans believed generally that personal health depended on the mutual interaction of mind and body. An advocate of botanical medicine in 1839 summarized one version of this belief in the statement, "Body and mind are not two as separate and independent entities, without relationship, but one—and are only two by abstraction."[39] The degree to which antebellum whites separated mind from body varied, yet most white laypeople and trained practitioners believed that good health depended on physiological balance, which could be regulated through the body's systems of intake and output. Although symptoms of illness indicated a disruption of bodily equilibrium, disease was not an exclusively physical phenomenon. Moral and mental influences could alter physiological equilibrium as drastically as the natural environment.[40] As medical historian Charles Rosenberg observes, "Psychic and somatic ills were not rigidly demarcated: mental, moral, climatic, and hygienic factors all interacted continuously to vary the manifestations of disease." Physicians therefore perceived illness as "a changed state of being affecting the whole man and capable of being altered by any of his myriad activities."[41]

Within the health cultures of antebellum white America, the emotions, or "passions," exerted a strong effect on individual well-being. Careful regulation of emotions as a virtue has often been associated with the rise of the industrial bourgeoisie in the North.[42] The books and periodicals of the southern planter class, however, offered similar fare. Alongside descriptions of diseases and remedies, domestic medicine manuals cautioned southern readers to protect their bodily health by moderating their emotional lives. Excessive anger, fear, grief, and love were just a few of the "violent passions of the mind" that wreaked havoc upon the heart, digestive functions, liver, and brain.[43] An 1844 agricultural journal advocated the healthful effect of controlling one's emotions by including a remedy for "cross words and bloody deeds" in a list of cures for croup, ringworm, and headache.[44] Medical publications, both orthodox and reformist, educated their readers about the possibility of "extraordinary changes produced upon the body from passions of the mind or sudden emotions."[45]

White popular and professional medical literature urged emotional regulation for the sake of bodily health and Christian salvation. A writer in the *Botanico-Medical Recorder*, for example, cautioned that a diseased body impaired receptivity to the Holy Spirit and brought on bouts of melancholy.[46] At least two domestic medicine manuals, the nationally popular *Gunn's Domestic Medicine* and a South Carolina publication, *The Family Physician*, included a discussion of religion within longer sections on health and emotion. Alfred Folger, author of *The Family Physician*, wrote, "Though some persons may be astonished, that the subject of religion should be introduced in this place, I assure the reader that religion has a powerful effect upon the health of an individual."[47] Lydia Riddick, a white southern mother, heartily agreed with such advice. She wrote to her son after his conversion to evangelical Christianity hoping to find his "temporal, as well as spiritual health" improved.[48] A general consensus about the interrelationship between religious practice and personal health prevailed across the spectrum of white southern health beliefs.

Some white southerners eschewed an explicitly Christian framework for mind-body relationships, preferring instead the language of science and progress. In the pages of their journals, for example, medical doctors debated mesmerism and spiritualism as new frontiers of scientific knowledge.[49] Public exhibits of clairvoyance in southern cities such as Richmond drew curious spectators. Southern families also consulted mesmerists for serious medical problems, hoping that these new practitioners could accomplish what professional physicians could not.[50] In short, white southerners adopted a broad array of ideas about the relationship between spirit, mind, and body expressed in health reform, religiosity, and popular science. At the same time, however, many southern slaveholders drew a line of essential difference between themselves and the persons they enslaved. In particular, middle-class, wealthy, and formally educated whites distin-

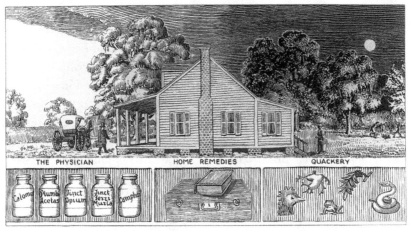

THE PHYSICIAN   HOME REMEDIES   QUACKERY

The Physician, Home Remedies, Quackery. *Portrayals of African American healing as superstition persisted long after the demise of slavery. This image in a 1950s volume on plantation medicine pits the rationality of the white doctor's medicine and the respectability of the white family's domestic medicine chest against the exoticism and "quackery" of slave medicines. (Reprinted by permission of Louisiana State University Press from* The Health of Slaves on Southern Plantations, *by William Dosite Postell; copyright © 1951 by Louisiana State University Press)*

guished their own beliefs about religious, moral, and mental influences on health from so-called "negro superstition."[51]

What white southerners meant by "superstition" revealed a great deal about the social relations of slaveholding society. The frequent pejorative use of the word directed at the enslaved and lower classes points to its importance in maintaining boundaries central to middle- and upper-class identity. Formally educated Americans often employed the concept of superstition to distinguish between enlightenment and ignorance, progress and primitivism, reason and irrationality, and medicine and quackery. Moreover, these familiar dichotomies subsumed constructions of race and gender that closely linked "women" and "negroes" to "superstition."[52] The idea of superstition thus operated as a racial currency that inflated the value of certain knowledge holders while devaluing others.

Throughout orthodox medical journals the phrase "old women" served as a metonym for the ignorance of popular remedies. North Carolina physician Alfred Folger railed in his domestic medicine manual against vain, old midwives who endangered the lives of mothers and infants: "How many mothers are doomed to drag out a miserable existence, from an injury sustained by the conduct of some ignorant old lady!"[53] A medical school thesis propounded the dangers of "old women's teas" in the treatment of childhood diseases and lamented the frequent use of herbs and roots prescribed by "a dear old Grandmother somebody."[54] Orthodox medical journals embroiled in conflicts over professionalism and licensure decried the public's reliance on "old women, root doctors, and quacks of all sorts."[55] Even Thomsonian practitioners, reviled as quacks by orthodox physicians, sought to identify Thomsonianism as a "system" and to distance their botanical practice from "old women's conjurations."[56] On the surface, references to "old women" merely reflected women's primary role as domestic healers within antebellum families.[57] Yet the ubiquity of this phrase as a metonym for ignorance and bad medicine in professional journals signaled something more. The denunciation of old women's remedies pointed to deep-seated gender and racial hierarchies in antebellum thinking about science and medicine.

Middle- and upper-class white southerners sought to place themselves on the upward side of hierarchies of scientific and medicinal knowledge. Embattled professionally, white doctors strove to set their understanding of the human body apart from the notions of persons without formal medical school training. In one telling example, a North Carolina doctor described an unusual case of lactation in an older woman serving as foster mother to a small child. He contrasted the professional and popular views of this event as follows: "The illiterate of the neighborhood, look upon the whole thing with superstitious wonder, and believe that a miracle was performed for the preservation of the life of the child." He quickly offered his own interpretation, which reconciled both divine purpose and scientific explanation: "It is but another proof, however, of the wonderful adaptability of nature to every possible emergency, and an additional evidence of the power and goodness of that Providence which 'orders all things for the best.'"[58] Although the doctor and the town's citizens shared some assumptions about God's hand in the old woman's sudden supply of milk, class and professional distinctions shaped their separate understandings of this startling event.

Positioning themselves as warriors of reason against a "dense cloud of ignorance and superstition," orthodox white doctors explicitly asserted the legitimacy of their training over the popular knowledge of old women and black practitioners.[59] As an example of popular ignorance, physician W. H. Robert of Georgia complained that sufferers of gonorrhea tended to consult "quacks [and] old negroes" instead of men of science.[60] Early-nineteenth-century domestic medicine manuals authored by physicians began to question popular wisdom and to urge the public to rely on the advice of regular doctors.[61] Savannah doctor James Ewell endorsed popular education in orthodox medicine in order to thwart the advances of "empirics" who sold patent medicines for specific diseases.[62] Antebellum medical journals called for the education of the public in medical matters. "Such a general knowledge of medicine, diffused throughout the community," asserted Virginia physician James McCaw in 1853, "would make men more wary in their encouragement of old women, root doctors, and quacks of all sorts."[63]

Along with their condemnation of specific therapies, professional doctors employed the rhetoric of superstition to ridicule entire traditions of learning. Most antebellum white doctors acquired their expertise through an idiosyncratic patchwork of lectures and practical training. They nevertheless looked upon books, medical school instruction, and mentored training as the legitimate path to medical knowledge. As James Ewell argued in *The Planter's and Mariner's Medical Companion,* "medicine is not intuitive" but requires instead "a slow, toilsome and ardous [*sic*] probation."[64] Many popular practitioners, in contrast, relied on claims of divine revelation or employed remedies acquired by oral training alone—paths that physicians considered "intuitive" and ignorant. Such was a Virginia doctor's complaint when he condemned the city of Richmond for allowing an enslaved man to practice medicine "upon the same footing with the man who has spent time, wealth, and talents" in medical training.[65] By attacking the training of their competitors, antebellum professional medical men hoped to rally public support for their embattled profession.

If the discourse of superstition had been limited to professional debates alone, its impact on plantation medicine would have been more limited. This was not the case, however. Assumptions about whose knowledge constituted superstition extended broadly through white southern perceptions of health, the human body, and the natural world. To be sure, southern slaveholders differed among themselves in their views on medicine, science, and religion. Yet slaveholders consistently distinguished their own knowledge of the world, of which their health beliefs were a part, from the "superstition" of the poor and enslaved.

Unsettling dreams often prompted privileged whites to distance themselves from persons they perceived as superstitious. Some sought the reassurance of Christian faith to offset their anxieties. Keziah Hopkins Brevard, disturbed by an unpleasant dream, pondered in her diary, "I don't wish to be superstitious. I want all my faith to be strengthened in God through his Son, my blessed Savior."[66] Quoting a Presbyterian clergyman whose writings she admired, Brevard reminded herself, "Superstition is only for faltered minds—for those who believe in man instead of God."[67] An unsettling dream about a rattlesnake elicited a similar comment from David Gavin, who wrote in his journal, "I do not like such dreams, but do not think I am superstitious."[68] In these private musings on identity and faith, slaveholding Christians spent the currency of superstition to purchase whiteness, reason, civilization, and knowledge.

Unexplainable occurrences in nature raised similar anxieties among the planter class. Southerners of privileged backgrounds attempted to explain in rational terms phenomena that in previous centuries would have been viewed as "divine wonders." In the seventeenth and early eighteenth centuries unusual cures, monstrous births, ghastly diseases, and rare animals evinced the marvels of God's will in the universe.[69] By the nineteenth century, however, the middle and upper classes looked for opportunities to associate themselves with what they believed were enlightened views of the body and nature.[70]

The brilliant meteor shower of 1833 provided just such an occasion. For individuals who understood the meteor shower as a manifestation of divine power, the illuminated night skies evoked both wonder and terror. Sarah Gudger, a freedwoman born into slavery in North Carolina, remembered a night when the stars fell "jes' lak rain." Her mother told her that each falling star was a sign of an impending death. To such observers the 1833 meteor shower of falling stars portended apocalyptic events.[71]

The Towneses, a slaveholding family of the lower South, thought differently. In November 1833 Henry H. Townes wrote to his mother, Rachael Townes, reassuring her that the unusual celestial display was not a sign of the Judgment Day, as "many negroes and some silly white persons" seemed to believe. "It is a natural phenomena, produced by natural causes," he declared, "& not a particular act of divine Providence to warn us of impending danger."[72] Just days later Henry wrote again congratulating his mother for her calm response to the nocturnal display, and he returned to the theme of popular ignorance: "At Abbeville C[ourt] House, many were desperately frightened. They pushed and shovled [*sic*] & called on their God to forgive all their sins—The church was opened at night & the Methodist preacher had a great many in the house & they had a terrible time of it.—One negro woman was howling up & down the streets & shaking her hands & crying Jesus Jesus, how I do love my Jesus!!—You ought to calm the negroes fears & assure them, that nothing unusual is agoing to happen. They are ignorant & require to have fears quieted."[73] Contrasting his own interpretations against the "ignorance" of slaves and the "silliness" of some whites, Henry Townes, a practicing doctor, found confirmation of his view of the universe.

Many antebellum whites assumed, like Townes, that Africans and their descendants in America were by nature superstitious and suggestible. Whereas many whites commonly associated moderated emotions with good health, they perceived in enslaved African Americans an excessive and unhealthy emotionalism. The notion of mental suggestibility as inherent in the black body flourished in the proslavery scientific racism of the 1850s and appeared regularly in medical journals. Physician A. P. Merrill agreed with this general assessment of "superstitious fear" as a characteristic of the "negro race." In 1856 he wrote, "No people can be more completely under the influence of the mind in sickness, than the negro race." Furthermore, Merrill argued, "his mind is continually exercised upon supernatural agencies, is easily depressed by his confidence in witchcraft, and much of his unhappiness, as well as many of his diseases, proceeds from purely imaginary causes."[74] Medical student William McCaa even characterized superstition itself as a sickness. Citing the example of an enslaved man who, like Patience, believed that his "rheumatism" was caused by conjuration, McCaa opined that black "credulity and superstition" could be understood only as *diseases* of the mind."[75] White doctors echoed the general opinion among planters that the influence of mind on body was different and more exaggerated among enslaved African Americans. Conflating biology and culture, they defined "superstition" as an inheritable racial trait.[76]

Representations of Africa figured heavily in white constructs of black superstition. The idea of benighted Africans intensified in the nineteenth century and replaced seventeenth- and eighteenth-century portrayals of the partially "noble savage."[77] A London bishop's sermon on the Anglican mission in the South reflected the view shared by many Americans that slavery delivered Africans "from the Pagan Darkness & the Superstition in which they were Bred."[78] The Reverend Charles C. Jones, arguing for Christian instruction among the enslaved, claimed, "They believe in second-sight, in apparitions, charms, witchcraft, and in a kind of irresistible Satanic influence. The superstitions brought from Africa have not been wholly laid aside."[79] Charleston investigators likewise reported that conjurer Gullah Jack, a leader in the 1822 Vesey conspiracy, held influence over "his own countrymen, who are distinguished both for their credulous superstition and clannish sympathies."[80] Most white southerners simply and uncritically believed that "fearful superstition" among slaves was a "heritage of their African origin."[81]

To the extent that they were willing to acknowledge some element of power within the practices of African American healers, however, southern whites could not wholly deny their abilities. Despite the ubiquitous references to black superstition, some white southerners nevertheless sought the services of African American conjurers and diviners. One North Carolina man, mentioned in an 1822 court decision, consulted frequently with a "negro conjurer" and "negro doctor" about illness, when to sell his corn, and how to deal with property disputes. Another South Carolina slaveholder engaged an enslaved conjure man to doctor his slaves and kill his own wife.[82] In the urban South, men and women crossed racial lines to consult African American diviners on matters of courtship and sexuality. The fortune-teller whom William Wells Brown consulted before his escape drew an interracial clientele from the white and black "young ladies" of St. Louis.[83] When need and opportunity coincided, white southerners proved themselves willing to diverge from their rhetoric and consult African American healers.

White thinking, speaking, and writing on superstition nevertheless had far reaching consequences for both slaveholders and enslaved African Americans. Although the prejudices of whites were most damaging to their enslaved targets, it is also worthwhile to examine, as writer Toni Morrison has argued, "what racial ideology does to the mind, imagination, and behavior of masters."[84] The frequent appearance of the term "superstition" in the writings of antebellum slaveholders suggests the usefulness of the idea in shoring up the elaborate scaffolding of civilization and whiteness. Among white slaveholders who depended on black labor, art, and skill, the idea of African superstition secured a sense of confidence in Euro-American traditions of learning and claims to knowledge. Among southern white doctors, the idea of superstition lent credence to orthodox therapies and conviction in the superiority of white medical training. It allowed slaveholders to depend on the labor of enslaved healers and to imagine holding moral and intellectual mastery over them at the same time. The discourse on superstition, which served as a shorthand code for several overlapping hierarchies of race, creed, gender, and class, thus comprised an important ingredient in the recipe for nineteenth-century white identity.

As an ideological weapon in the continued subjugation of African Americans, the idea of superstition also had a powerful effect on the way enslaved communities created and sustained their relational vision of health. For the sake of self-preservation, enslaved healers and sufferers had to take into account slaveholders' hostile and patronizing view of black doctoring. Lessons in the white discourse of superstition were readily available. Harriet Jacobs, for example, recounted a sermon aimed specifically at the Edenton, North Carolina, slave population. "You are rebellious sinners," the minister intoned. "Instead of being engaged in worshipping him [God], you are hidden away somewhere, feasting on your master's substance; tossing coffee-grounds with some wicked fortuneteller, or cutting cards with another old hag. . . . You are quarreling, and tying up little bags of roots to bury under the door-steps to poison each other with."[85] Though the sermon "highly amused" the enslaved congregation, the minister's admonishment also instructed listeners that certain rituals and remedies could be safely carried out only in secret.

White doctors could be equally transparent in their racial ideology. Mildred Graves told of a hostile encounter in the midst of her work as a plantation nurse and midwife. Called to a white woman's bedside to assist a complicated birth, Graves arrived only to find two white doctors already attending the woman. "I tol' dem I could bring her 'roun'," she recalled, "but dey laugh at me an' say, 'Get back darkie, we mean business an' don' won't any witch doctors or hoodoo stuff.'"[86] The two men attempted to discredit Graves as a competing practitioner by dismissing her skills as African superstition. They deployed a racialized arsenal against her that they could not have used against a white midwife. Further illustrating the complexities of antebellum medical relations, the laboring woman soon sent the white doctors away and retained Graves, who successfully delivered the baby. Though Graves persevered in this encounter, the incident suggests that black practitioners could rarely practice without an awareness of white attitudes toward their work. In this context of white suspicion and condescension, enslaved African Americans forged their sacred doctoring practices.

"The Lord's Laws": Spiritual Empowerment in Slave Doctoring

Black doctoring traditions reflected a rich complexity, volition, and creativity that defied the flat caricature of superstition. Rarely does the written evidence contain such a direct refutation of the white doctrine of "negro superstition" as the sentiment expressed in an interview with

William Adams, a healer born into slavery in Texas in 1844. "There am lots of folks, and educated ones, too, what says we-uns believes in superstition," Adams told his interviewer. "Well, it's cause they don't understand. . . . Now, just 'cause you don't know 'bout some of the Lord's laws, 'tain't superstition if some other person understands and believes in such."[87] In explaining his work as a healer, Adams asserted the primacy of his own experience. "What am seen," he argued, "can't be doubted." "The power," according to Adams, connected him to a series of divine revelations reaching back through his mother and the old folks who knew "the working of the signs" to Africans in "they native lands."[88] While he directly addressed how slavery and racism robbed him of institutional schooling, Adams was also quick to point out that while education was one thing, understanding was another.

According to Adams, the confidence of southern whites in their own racial superiority blinded them to a sophisticated and spiritually empowered body of knowledge claimed by African Americans. Slaveholders exercised power in a social, legal, economic, and political sense. To the extent that they were able to define reality according to their worldview, slaveholders also exercised cultural power. Nevertheless, their mastery on all fronts remained incomplete. Enslaved men and women consistently refused, as Ralph Ellison put it, to allow slave masters to define crucial matters for them. Bondsmen and -women exercised their healing knowledge in a world that attempted to define slaves as powerless and dependent. Since slave health was intimately bound to the economic health of plantations, the struggle to carry out the relational view of healing was never easy and often costly. As William Adams implied, struggles over slave doctoring exposed conflicts over the very nature and meaning of power on southern plantations.

African American healing under slavery reflected a definition of power as the capacity not only to control but also to create and transform. The insights of anthropologists W. Arens and Ivan Karp regarding African conceptions of power provide a useful model for the deployment of power in African American healing. In their work on power and ritual throughout Africa, Arens and Karp seek to "consider power in [an] ideational capacity," rather than perceiving it as a purely rational and mechanistic concept. The Weberian notion of power in Western culture, Ivan Karp contends, defines it in terms of "access to and control over people and resources." However, another dimension of power emerges from the spiritual realm in African cultures. Here humans interact with ancestors and spirits, and power is created through ritual. Karp concludes, "The stress in Africa is not on the elements of control but on the more dynamic aspect of energy and the capacity to use it. . . . African ideas of power . . . have to do with engaging power and creating or at least containing the world."[89] Persons engaging in ritual thus become agents of transformation for renewing and creating social life. In parallel ways, enslaved healers became agents of transformation, altering the very terms of slaveholder medical attention and creating new claims to healing authority.

Speaking a language of spiritual empowerment, African American healers described their occupation as vocation, their knowledge as revelation, and their expertise as holy gift. In a 1938 interview, for example, Alabama midwife Lula Russeau stated that she could foretell the future and see spirits. The caul covering her face at birth, she explained, was a sign of her second sight and her gift of healing. "I was born one [a midwife]," she declared; "God made me dat way." Moreover, Russeau's spiritual calling linked her generationally to other gifted women in her family. Her mother, an enslaved woman with Chickasaw ancestry, had worked as a laundress, a midwife, and a spinner, and she made medicines from local plants as well.[90] Lula Russeau learned much about herbs, charms, and birthing under her mother's instruction. The maternal lineage of healing abilities merged with special birth signs and the sense of divine calling to form the foundations for her legitimacy as a healer.

Just as nineteenth-century white male doctors cited medical schools or reputable mentors to authorize their practice, African American healers pointed to spiritual insight as a legitimating source of their abilities. They did so in a language that reflected African American Christianity's transformation of both African religions and European Protestantism. Insight included guidance from God or "Doctor Jesus," lessons passed on from previous generations, dreams, signs, and visions. Whether they worked as conjure doctors, midwives, herbalists, or sickbed nurses, African American healers described a universe alive with revelations for persons called to heal. Some healers referred to their knowledge as a birthright. A Georgia root woman explained, "Seems lak yuh jes' hab tuh be born wid duh knowledge. I jes allus seemed tuh know how tuh work cures and make medicines."[91]

Many women, as well as some men, used a distinctly Christian language to describe the spiritual significance of their work. "When the Lord gives such power to a person," claimed healer William Adams, "it just come to 'em."[92] In another early-twentieth-century interview a Tennessee woman described a lifetime of reliance on God as she doctored her family. "I don't remember ever paying out but three dollars for doctor's bills in my life for myself, my children, or my grandchildren," she declared. "Doctor Jesus tells me what to do."[93] Another woman who had nursed numerous patients described herself as "an instrument in God's hand." She testified, "I always take Doctor Jesus with me and put him in front, and if there is any hope he lets me know."[94] The metaphor of serving as God's instrument enabled the healer to speak of her skills in terms of Christian humility while at the same time claiming her own authority and efficacy.[95]

Black southern healers, like white evangelicals generally, often emphasized God as the ultimate source of healing. A Georgia revival song emphasized the healing power invested in a Christian God.

Sin sick or soul sick, hallelujah, (3x)
Glory hallelujah!

Send for de doctor, hallelujah, (3x)
Glory hallelujah!

He kin cure, hallelujah, (3x)
Glory hallelujah!

Doctor Jesus, hallelujah, (3x)
Glory hallelujah!

He kin save, hallelujah, (3x)
Glory hallelujah![96]

In these stanzas God's power to heal was not simply a metaphor for redemption but, quite literally, the power to cure body and soul. The emphasis on Doctor Jesus and the curative dimensions of salvation echo Theophus Smith's portrayal of the African American biblical world as a pharmocosm, a world in which healing is central to the working of spiritual power.

Evidence from the early twentieth century, however, shows that southern African Americans during and after slavery did not limit revelations to a Christian God alone. Knowledge from past generations was as much a part of spiritual empowerment as revelations directly from God. Healing knowledge from God often passed through the dead in dreams and visions. One elderly woman near Tuskegee described the encouragement she received when her sick baby granddaughter did not seem to be recovering. A friend who had passed on came to her in a dream and reassured her that the child would not die. The dream restored the grandmother's confidence in her treatments, and the child lived. It was "a miracle sent from God," concluded the woman.[97] Justine Singleton of Georgia also received a remedy though revelation. When her dead sister came to her, she recalled, "I knowd dat it wuz huh." Singleton's sister told her to boil weeping willow and make a wash for her sore feet.[98] Similarly, midwife Marie Campbell described how Aunt Jeanie, her late mentor, came to her "in the spirit" during a difficult labor to guide her hands "to do the right thing."[99]

In the antebellum South, enslaved communities attributed wisdom to black healers in ways that ran counter to white slaveholders' standards of knowledge and education. A northern teacher in the South Carolina coastal islands in 1862 remarked, "'Learning' with these people I find means a knowledge of medicine, and a person is valued accordingly."[100] African American healers established their knowledge and reputations through intergenerational instruction, spiritual calling, accumulated expertise, and dramatic recoveries from their own illness. Yet while slaveholders and white doctors showed interest in the practical skills of black healers, they often viewed the intellectual basis of their work with skepticism and condescension. To physicians such as James Ewell, who protested that "medicine is not intuitive," African American claims to healing authority spelled quackery and ignorance. Their assumptions about superstitious slaves and their investment in existing social relations frequently prevented southern whites from acknowledging the legitimacy of black healers' knowledge.

For one, enslaved communities differed from those of slaveholders in the value placed on black elders. While age devalued a slave in the marketplace and the fields, it provided a significant foundation of authority for black healers within slave communities. The elderly, though a small proportion of the southern enslaved population, were honored for their learning and the services they continued to provide to slave communities. Enslaved children soon learned that sassy words to an older person brought swift discipline from parents or neighbors.[101] For some, elders represented the closest link to Africa. Their spiritual potency increased as the approach to death brought them closer to the ancestors.[102] Slave healers, many of whom were women, came from the ranks of the elderly, and age contributed to their authority in the community. The active engagement of respected older women with the health of slave communities directly contradicted the scorn for ignorant "old women" so prevalent in antebellum medical journals.[103]

Equally important to African American doctoring as old age and revelation was its communal context. As they did with music, storytelling, and rituals of worship, enslaved African Americans approached healing as a collective enterprise. The relational vision of health placed healing in the context of a broadly conceived community that included living persons, ancestors, spirits, and God.[104] A vivid illustration of this concept of community was the cosmogram, a West Central African sign of the universe consisting of intersecting horizontal and vertical lines inside a circle: ⊕. Art historian Robert Farris Thompson argues that the Kongo cosmogram and its transatlantic variations in Cuba, Brazil, and the United States symbolized the relationship of the worlds of the living and the dead. The basic form of the cosmogram mirrored the structure of the universe, with God above, the ancestors below, and the earth between. In African American lore the cosmogram signified power created through connections to one's ancestors. More than a symbol, a cosmogram drawn on the ground or embodied in the form of a forked stick or crossroads drew spiritual power to a particular point on earth.[105] Crossroads and cosmograms traced in the ground marked points of contact between the world of the living and the world of gods and ancestors.

The sickbeds of enslaved sufferers became a kind of crossroads in the context of the collective care that enslaved men and women attempted to provide one another. Plantation architecture obviously contributed to the communal setting of sickcare. The small size of one- and two-room slave housing with single fireplaces inevitably brought the sick, injured, and whipped into the social life of evening gatherings.[106] Despite the existence of sickhouses or hospitals on some large plantations, most enslaved families did what they could for the sick within their dwellings.

Gathering at the sickbed became an integral social and religious ritual within the practice of black doctoring. Though they have received far less attention than burial ceremonies in studies of slave religion, sickbed gatherings were religious rituals in their own right. Particularly as death approached, enslaved men and women placed great emphasis on surrounding the sick person with songs and prayers that anticipated the sufferer's "crossing over."[107] A South Carolina spiritual emphasized the fear of isolation and the need for spiritual support around the sickbed:

When my health is weakening,
Never leave me alone;
When I am dying,
Never leave me alone;

If you see me failing,
Never leave me alone;

My Jesus promised,
Never leave me alone.[108]

Although the song called on Jesus to walk with the sufferer, the lyrics also appealed to the human community. At the intersection of human pain and spiritual transcendence, sickbed gatherings became a crossroads between the world of the living and the realm of the dead.

Slaveholder violence increased the chance of isolation and amplified the importance of African American sickbed rituals. In several antebellum slave narratives, care for one another in the face of slaveholder neglect served as a metaphor for the humanity of enslaved African Americans as contrasted with the callousness of slaveowners. In his narrative of abduction from the North into slavery in the Deep South, Solomon Northup described the comfort of such a community gathering. After a beating, Northup lay in his cabin bleeding and unable to move. As the workday ended, men and women came in from the fields and gathered around him. Two women boiled bacon, made him scorched-corn coffee, and tried to console him as they recounted the day's events.[109] Because of the overt violence underpinning the southern labor system, this scene was replicated in plantation quarters across the South, where after a day's labor, enslaved women applied medicines to the gashes, welts, and bruises of those who had been whipped and beaten.[110]

Twentieth-century sources also linked sickbed practices to community values. The Reverend William J. Faulkner recorded South Carolina freedman Simon Brown's description of neighbors at the sickbed in the slave quarters. Brown explained that "if a slave became ill, he wasn't left alone to suffer unattended. . . . In time of illness or other trouble, fellow slaves would 'turn in and help out.'" Men and women aided the afflicted person through different types of work. Men cut firewood, and women came to the cabin to cook, tend children, and wash clothes. The spirit in which men and women performed these chores was important to Brown's story: "Women would come over just to sit a spell and sing and pray around the sickbed. Nobody was left to suffer alone. Sometimes a man or woman with a healing touch would brew an herb tea, mix a poultice or apply peach tree leaves to a fevered brow, to help the sick get well. And all this loving care cheered up the troubled soul, whether he got well or died."[111] Margaret

Charles Smith, a twentieth-century midwife of Greene County, Alabama, described a similar gathering around the sick. Smith's grandmother, whom she described as "a slavery time lady," had been sold into the Deep South at age thirteen. In her grandmother's time, Smith recalled, "people would sit all night long, but they don't do that no more. They sit right there till they die, [or] get better. . . . If somebody was lying up in front of death, if she needed anything, they would be there."[112] Both of these descriptions of southern African American sickbed attendance, it is important to note, come from twentieth-century oral historians intent on communicating lessons from the past to younger listeners. As distillations of rural slave community values, both descriptions paint a remarkable portrait in which neighbors offered their presence as a healing balm to both the body and the "troubled soul."

The image of the community at the bedside described in retrospective accounts represented an ideal that, in the dangerous circumstances of slavery, was difficult to attain. Indeed, as I will show in later chapters, many slaves encountered great difficulties when their desire to nurse sick family members conflicted with planter labor priorities or measures of control. Yet the fact that both Simon Brown and Margaret Smith emphasized neighbors gathered around sickbeds suggests that the social context was a vital component of slave healing experiences. Through their presence at the pallet of a sick or injured person, African American women and men reaffirmed their collective relationship with God and acknowledged the connection between life and death.[113] Prayer and song worked as medicine alongside the teas and poultices.

Enslaved African Americans engaged power through healing rituals by defining health as a community enterprise and healing knowledge as spiritual empowerment. Within the slave quarters, neighbors and kin struggled to ensure that the sick did not suffer alone. Slave doctoring was transformative, first, in the sense that it redefined black health in terms of a relational vision that emphasized the importance of the community to individual well-being, rather than in terms of soundness. In the midst of an institutional assault on enslaved families, slave doctors and their clients envisioned intricate relationships between generations of the living and the world of the ancestors. To some extent communal sickbed attendance was possible because of the dependence of slaveholders on slave healing work. At other times enslaved men and women pursued the collective meanings of slave health in secret and at great risk.

African American doctoring also proved transformative in its engagement of realms of power beyond the slaveholder's control or understanding, and thus it provided an arena in which enslaved men and women asserted the primacy of their experiences and sensibilities. The confrontation between the visiting planter and the afflicted woman Patience, to return to the opening vignette, evinced both the slaveholder's coercive power and its limitations. Within the pharmocosm of Afro-Christianity, enslaved men and women looked for guidance in healing from their elders, their ancestors, signs of nature, and ultimately, a healing God. Furthermore, the influence of African religions infused the pharmocosm of enslaved African Americans with a dualistic notion of power that encompassed both healing and harming. Healing and harming were not envisioned as two opposing moral forces; rather, both contributed to the dimensions of spiritual power. This dualistic view of power informed African American health culture in ways incomprehensible to the planter class. While privileged white southerners avidly investigated the relationship between body, mind, and soul and even sought the services of black practitioners, they persisted in their belief that African Americans possessed an essentially superstitious nature, a "trait" they vaguely located in an African ancestry. Conflicts over health on antebellum plantations thus revealed a politics of knowledge in which white slaveholders, doctors, and overseers trivialized or disparaged the spiritual basis of black healing expertise.

Yet southern medical practices never fully followed the neat ideological divisions implicit in pronouncements against superstition. Slaves and slaveholders borrowed considerably from one another as they searched for effective medicines to add to their household repertoire of remedies. The experimental bent of southern domestic practitioners and the dependence of planters on slave healing labor also ensured a measure of contact between black and white members of plantation communities. Throughout these interactions enslaved men and women continued to locate their doctoring practices in a sacred pharmocosm that enlivened even the roots and leaves of the southern forests.

There is a balm in Gilead,
To make the wounded whole.
There is a balm in Gilead,
To heal the sin-sick soul.
— African American spiritual

Without leaves, no orixá.
— *Candomblé proverb,*
   Zeca Ligièro, Divine Inspiration, *1993*

CHAPTER 3

Sacred Plants

If the sacred foundation of African American doctoring was a battleground, antebellum herbalism proved instead to be a local market in which remedies were tested and traded. Plant medicines, whether in the form of food, teas, or poultices, formed the core of rural American household health care. Yet antebellum herbalism in any region of the country was comprised of more than a body of specific remedies. Herbal practice involved a dynamic set of social relations and distinctive relationships to the natural environment. American herbal recipes and the oral and written descriptions that surround them carry long histories of cultural transformation fueled by both colonial expansion and the desire of ordinary people for effective remedies. In the antebellum South both the social relations of slavery and the cultural heritage of African herbal practitioners shaped the contours of herbal practice. As healers and sufferers, enslaved African Americans significantly influenced the herbal repertoire of southern white households and cultivated a distinctive tradition grounded in a sacred view of the land.[1]

An episode from the journal of Virginia planter John Walker suggests both the experimental nature of southern herbalism and the prominent role of African Americans in it. In the summer of 1833 Walker penned several entries about Jack, an ailing enslaved man. Confined to his house for several weeks and steadily losing his eyesight, Jack feared that he had been poisoned. Walker also suspected poisoning, though "poisoning" may have had different meanings for each man. Both, however, agreed that special measures should be taken. When treatments by a local white doctor failed, Walker sent Jack to stay under the care of "Old Man Docr. Lewis," a slave in nearby King William County. How Walker heard about Doctor Lewis is unclear, but the planter noted in his journal that Doctor Lewis "says he can cure him." Indeed, after six weeks the practitioner returned with Jack, whose sight now seemed "as good as ever." Instructing Jack to continue taking a "decoction of herbs," Doctor Lewis collected his fee of ten dollars from the planter and returned home.[2]

Doctor Lewis's visit to the Walker plantation indicates that at least some white southerners willingly searched for medical remedies and services across lines of social division in the antebellum South. John Walker hired Doctor Lewis in the course of an active search for better household health. When it came to the efficacy of orthodox white doctors, John shared with his wife, Margaret, a skepticism painfully gained from the deaths of five of their seven children. The year after Jack's recovery, John Walker rejected the practice of "Calomel doctors" altogether and adopted the Thomsonian system of botanical medicine, immersing his family in rounds of lobelia emetics and steam baths. In the Walkers' case, experimentation with botanical medicine reached easily from Doctor Lewis's "decoctions" to the contents of a Thomsonian medicine chest.[3] While the planter's hiring of an enslaved doctor makes this story somewhat unusual, planter interest in slave medicines was not unique to the Walker household. As we shall see, enslaved African Americans significantly influenced the repertoire of southern herbal practice, while at the same time they adopted some of the remedies employed by slaveholders.

Despite some overlap, the streams of slave and slaveholder herbalism also diverged in important ways. As John Walker's account reveals, class strongly influenced a practitioner's relationship to the southern landscape and its wealth of medicinal plants. By the 1830s many members of the planter class participated in a wider consumer market for botanical medicine that distanced them from local herbal expertise.[4] John Walker, for example, was a moderately wealthy cotton and wheat planter and master of his household. In his search for domestic medicines Walker consistently paid large bills for medical supplies and white doctors. When his faith in orthodox physicians failed, he entered the national market in self-help remedies, paying $23.87 for his Thomsonian guide and medicines.[5] Doctor Lewis, active in the local economy but constrained by his bondage, drew on readily available materials such as soot and pine tree roots to make his teas. African American expertise with local medicinal plants marked important differences between slaves and slaveholders in their views of the land.[6]

A spiritual relationship to the land characterized African American medicinal plant practices. Nineteenth-century southerners, white and black, subscribed to the general idea that God supplied medicinal plants for curing human ills, yet most elite whites did not view herbal medicine through a spiritual lens. Hence John Walker, a devout Methodist who saw the hand of God in every illness, did not describe plants as spiritually potent, nor did he consider his knowledge of herbal remedies as divinely given. In contrast, principles of spiritual empowerment occupied a central place in African American herbalism. From the gathering of plants to the transmission of herbal knowledge through the generations, southern black herbalism reflected the sacred relational view of health and healing. In this respect black herbalism in North America shared similarities with herbal practices arising under slavery throughout the Black Atlantic.

The Cross-Cultural Context for African American Herbal Medicine

Southern herbal medicine was characterized by a high degree of exchange across lines of race, ethnicity, class, and region. Consider the letter written by South Carolina planter William Berly in 1855. Berly wrote to his brother with a new remedy for the intestinal troubles afflicting their father. A "little weed" called opossum ear boiled in port wine had revived Berly's hope for his father's recovery. According to Berly, opossum ear was an Indian remedy passed on to him by a white neighbor, Mr. Wingard: "Mr. Wingard learned it from his old negro Sam who set himself up as a Doctor. Sam learned this mystery from a man from New Orleans, who had learned it directly from the Indian Doctor."[7] For later readers, the much-traveled opossum ear recipe is a warning against the search for static and separate ethnic herbal traditions in the American South. Berly's cure beckons instead toward a complex history where remedies were borrowed, purchased, and stolen to create overlapping traditions of southern herbalism.

The eclectic character of antebellum remedies had its roots in the colonial period, when European newcomers, African captives, and indigenous Americans avidly sought medicines to survive in their changing worlds.[8] Indeed, the colonization of the Americas initiated a global movement of plants as well as of peoples and diseases. Early European colonists set out to document and collect new plant species from the Americas, hoping to find new commodities and make their American colonies less dependent on European medicines.[9] The Enlightenment project of European botanical classification emerged in part from the collection of exotic plants that accompanied colonization of Native American lands and the forced transportation of Africans to plantation labor.[10] At the same time colonists transplanted European flora such as apple, dandelion, and mullein that became quickly naturalized to the North American landscape.[11] In South America as well, where sugar planters and Jesuits brought pennyroyal, basil, and English plantain, the "frenetic" rate of "floristic exchange" led to an astonishing revision of the indigenous biotic inventory.[12]

The Atlantic slave trade also fostered an exchange of Old World and New World plants. Some West African captives undergoing the terror of the transatlantic crossing may have worn strings of red and black wild licorice seeds and thus brought the licorice plant to the Caribbean. The roots of the licorice plant served as a common medicine aboard slaving vessels, and West African descendants in the Caribbean continued to use wild licorice medicinally for coughs and fevers.[13] African grasses crossed the Atlantic with slavers who discarded on American shores the straw used to line the putrid holds of slave ships. In addition, benne (sesame), yams, okra, and black-eyed peas originated in Africa and were later grown by enslaved Africans for food. Some of these cultivated foods served medicinal purposes in the New World as well. Africans in the Americas employed okra leaves as poultices, Jamaican senna as a laxative, "Surinam poison" as a cure for chronic sores, and kola seeds for belly pains.[14] By the eighteenth century the herbal medicines of enslaved Africans included not only native African plants but also indigenous American plants, such as Jerusalem oak and capsicum (red pepper), which had circulated in the Atlantic world for over a century.[15] This colonial exchange of plants across the Atlantic reorganized the pharmacopoeia that both European and African descendants drew on for medicines in North America.

Native American knowledge of medicinal plants no doubt influenced African American (and European) herbal medicine, though the exact historical processes of this exchange are difficult to identify.[16] Africans and Native Americans enslaved alongside one another under the harsh conditions of early English and French colonization would have had ample opportunity to blend their botanical traditions. Native American towns that offered refuge for fugitive slaves and fostered intermarriage between Africans and Indians also provided a context for exchange of herbal knowledge.[17] An elderly Texas woman alluded to this dual heritage when she described how her mother taught her "a lot of doctorin' what she learned from old folks from Africa, and some the Indians learned her."[18] Some enslaved Africans encountered indigenous American medicines when their European masters hired Native American practitioners. Clergyman botanist John Clayton recorded the case of a slaveholder in seventeenth-century Virginia who paid an Indian healer two quarts of rum to treat an enslaved black man suffering from an eye disease. The native practitioner collected plants from the woods, performed a cure, and refused all offers of payment from the planter to reveal his medicines.[19]

Enslaved black practitioners also carefully guarded their herbal recipes, occasionally exchanging a cure for precious freedom. Significantly, this avenue to manumission was offered only to enslaved men. In 1729 Virginia authorities freed the aging Papan in return for a venereal disease remedy that he had kept "as a most Profound secrett" until that time. The Virginia burgesses judged the exchange a good bargain. They hoped that Papan's recipe of "Roots and Barks" would save "the lives of a great number of Slaves" afflicted with yaws and other venereal diseases.[20] In 1749 the South Carolina Assembly manumitted Caesar in exchange for snakebite and poison cures that would become popular in antebellum remedy books.[21] Six years later the South Carolina Assembly made a similar proposal to Sampson, a healer known for his fearless handling of rattlesnakes. He received his freedom and a fifty-pound annuity as payment for his rattlesnake bite medicine made from heart snakeroot, polypody, avens root, and rum.[22] English colonists clearly saw something of value in eighteenth-century slave herbalism and did not hesitate to appropriate African cures.

The exchange of herbal remedies between slaveholders and the enslaved carried into the nineteenth-century, even as the institution of slavery became more rigid and racial ideology congealed. Deep social divisions in a slave society, however, did not deter the continued experimentation of domestic practitioners in either white or black households. Herbalism among plantation residents continued to be a pragmatic, cross-cultural affair, with planters and enslaved African Americans adopting one another's medicines when they seemed to promise results.

Antebellum slaveholders maintained their interest in black practitioners who performed effective cures. As John Walker's hiring of Doctor Lewis indicates, planters sometimes chose black practitioners over white doctors or yielded to the persistent suggestions of enslaved patients. George White, an herbal healer himself, spoke of his father as a man who was "a kinda doctor too like his master" and who "knowed all de roots" for any kind of sickness. On one occasion when his master, a physician, "said a woman couldn't live," White recalled, "papa went to see her an' gave her some medicine an' in a day's time she was up eatin' ev'ything she could get."[23] Slaveholders took notice when enslaved practitioners on their plantations developed regional reputations. Lowcountry planter Thomas Chaplin grudgingly observed free African Americans traveling to his plantation seeking help from Old Sancho, a "Negro doctor."[24]

Botanical science motivated some elite whites to investigate what they termed "negro remedies." Francis Peyre Porcher, a South Carolina surgeon and botanist, often alluded to herbal medicines used by enslaved men and women in his publications on southern botany. Reflecting the common prejudice of white physicians who viewed their own systems of training as superior, Porcher saw his research as elevating to a scientific level the plant lore of "charlatans and herb doctors" who "know only by *memory* the name of the plant and the disease which it is said to suit."[25] Nonetheless, this member of a wealthy plantation family displayed a keen interest in the herbal medicines of enslaved practitioners. In his Civil War–era *Resources of the Southern Fields and Forests* Porcher documented numerous medicinal plants "extensively employed" in South Carolina slave quarters and described their uses "according to the negroes." With this book Porcher aimed to disseminate this local botanical expertise for the benefit of Confederate soldiers and civilians cut off from commercial medicines.[26]

Porcher's publication also revealed that slaveholders investigated herbal medicines in order to counter their clandestine use by slaves. Rumors that enslaved women used the cotton root as an abortifacient, for example, greatly concerned southern planters. Quoting an 1868 Atlanta medical journal, in his postwar edition of *Resources of Southern Fields and Forests* Porcher advised readers that witch hazel effectively counteracted the effects of cotton root in an attempted abortion. Another article in an 1860 medical journal reported on enslaved women's use of tansy, rue, pennyroyal, and cedar berries to end a pregnancy. In these cases white doctors attempted not only to appropriate but also to control use of medicinal plants by African Americans.[27]

Daily interactions among plantation women, however, produced the most fertile ground for exchange between planter and slave herbal medicine. Slaveholding women who viewed the oversight of children's health

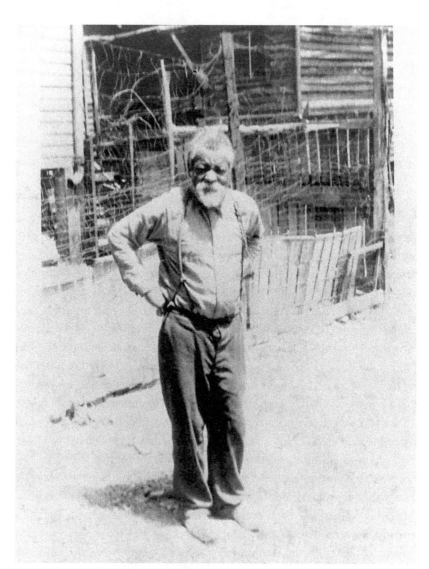

George White, Lynchburg, Virginia, ca. 1937. Mr. White was born into slavery in 1847 near Danville. His father, the slave of a white medical doctor, was known as a root doctor. Mr. White continued this family tradition with his own divinely inspired knowledge of roots and herbal medicines. (Courtesy of Hampton University Archives, Hampton, Virginia)

as part of their domestic duties frequently dosed slave children with herbal remedies.[28] Indeed, many elderly African Americans speaking to interviewers in the 1930s mentioned the herbal preparations given to them during their childhood. Emoline Glasgow from South Carolina remembered the bitter "mackaroot tea," a worm medicine dispensed by the mistress before breakfast.[29] Another South Carolina mistress dosed the children every morning with a spoonful of "worm cure," a "black lookin seed mixed up in molasses."[30] Mary Henderson, a North Carolina slaveholder who had lost several of her own children to sickness, remarked in her diary on a young enslaved girl, Viney, stricken with dysentery: "I told her mother to give the tea made of the inner bark of Pine, Sweet Gum, and Dogwood."[31] While we have no evidence as to whether Viney's mother actually adopted Henderson's recipe, the entry suggests how remedies might have been exchanged between women in the daily care of children.

The demands of nursing the sick and supplying the plantation with medicine sometimes brought together slave women and slaveholding women in common tasks. A former slave from South Carolina remembered that instead of a doctor, "our Missus an' one of de slave' would 'tend to the sick."[32] Household health work, while in no way erasing structural divisions between women, did provide a venue for exchange of herbal remedies.[33] Louisa Collier, for example, swore by the cough remedy her enslaved mother learned to make while working with the mistress.[34] When slaveholder Mary Bethell's young daughter was terribly burned in a yard fire, an enslaved woman, Abi, worked with Mary during the girl's last hours to soothe her burns with linseed oil and wheat dough.[35] In such moments of crisis, white and black women used whatever available medicine they thought would work, in the process learning new remedies from each other for future use.

Though the herbal repertoires of slaves and slaveholders were by no means identical, the remedies themselves sometimes circulated with surprising fluidity. Despite a widespread assumption of black intellectual inferiority, the planter class willingly absorbed reputed cures from African American practitioners. In their turn, despite distrust of white medical interference as a whole, African Americans also borrowed from the stock of planter remedies. White and black herbalism on antebellum plantations thus formed two related but distinct spheres of knowledge; necessity and circumstance led to some overlap, while class and race divisions created important differences.

Several historical developments contributed to the differences between the herbalism of elite white planters and of enslaved blacks. Literacy, direct access to white physicians, and participation in distant markets marked the herbal practices of southern white elites in ways not seen among slaves (or poorer whites, for that matter). In turn, enslaved African Americans, by virtue of their labor and subsistence patterns, maintained an intimate knowledge of the surrounding landscape. The herbal repertoire of the slave quarters as a result drew heavily from African American local botanical expertise.

Among the influences on the herbalism of elite whites was the growing antebellum print culture. By the early nineteenth century several authors of domestic medicine manuals were marketing their advice to southern slaveholding families. These manuals, such as James Ewell's *The Planter's and Mariner's Medical Companion,* recommended treatment with imported botanical medicines, such as "Peruvian bark," as well as locally grown remedies, including dogwood bark and carrot juice tonic.[36] Authors of domestic medicine manuals sought to provide middle- and upper-class households with the knowledge to treat and prevent basic illness, all the while impressing upon their readers the limits of lay practitioner knowledge.[37]

In addition to published domestic medicine guides, many white planter households kept homemade remedy books into which planter women copied instructions for cough syrup and cancer cures next to their recipes for cakes and puddings. Washington Dozier, a former slave in South Carolina, described these volumes as "doctor books" that slaveholders would peruse in times of sickness.[38] While some remedies relied heavily on the heroic effects of calomel and castor oil, other planter prescriptions revealed continued use of local medicinal plants by whites. For example, a Georgia remedy from the late eighteenth century titled "A Powder to cure a Rupture" called for scurvy grass, comfrey root, fern root, juniper berries, and Solomon's seal.[39] Likewise, a dropsy remedy from a late antebellum remedy book required juniper berries, mustard seed, ginger root, horseradish, parsley root, and hard cider.[40]

Some planter remedy books reflected appropriation of African American remedies by whites. One of the most commonly cited herbal remedies in the recipe books of white families was Caesar's prescription for snakebite and poisoning, consisting of plantain root and wild horehound.

In North Carolina the Lenoir family's 1830s scrapbook of remedies included Caesar's antidote copied from an 1816 almanac as well as an "African Cure" for the "watery gripes in children" cut from the *Raleigh Star* in 1821. More than one hundred years after Caesar's manumission the agricultural journal *Southern Cultivator* carried the African doctor's remedy for snakebite.[41] Family recipe books, almanacs, and newspapers revealed the influence of African American herbal knowledge on the planter-class pharmacopoeia and provided evidence of the translation between oral and written herbal knowledge. Nevertheless, they also illustrated distinctive attributes of slaveholder domestic medicine, with its greater reliance on orthodox physicians and distant authors of popular medical advice.

Household remedy books also revealed southern planters' participation in expanding commercial markets. Throughout the eighteenth century, wealthy southern whites had routinely employed medicines imported from Europe through the seaport cities or produced domestically in the North.[42] The market revolution of the antebellum period further increased slaveholders' access to imported botanical products. Plantation medicine chests were filled with ipecac from South America, jalap from Mexico, opium from the Far East, quinine from the Andes, and chamomile from Europe.[43] Consumption of internationally marketed botanicals reflected the increase in medical consumerism in middling to wealthy white households. Though they did not abandon homegrown medicines, many slaveholders grew less knowledgeable about local medicinal plants even as they expanded their purchase of commercially marketed medicines. To Silvia King, a former Texas slave stolen from Africa as a young woman, whites seemed oblivious to the sacred power of forest plants. "White folks just go through de woods and don't know nothin'," she declared.[44]

In contrast, as King implied, the slave quarters of southern plantations harbored many botanical experts. Mart Stewart has argued in his environmental history of the Georgia coast that enslaved African Americans who worked the fields developed a "keen awareness and precise knowledge of the environment" not available to planter families.[45] While slaveholders might experience the landscape from a cleared road or a shaded veranda, enslaved men and women moved through the fields and forests at eye level.[46] Agricultural labor, subsistence hunting and gardening, and the domestic economy all oriented enslaved African Americans toward a working knowledge of the local flora. The complex repertoire of North American black herbalism grew out of this particular relationship to the natural environment.

Enslaved African Americans put their extensive botanical knowledge to every imaginable use. Whether for clothing, games, visual arts, food, or medicines, they found in local plants the answer to a broad spectrum of human needs. Children fashioned stick games out of twigs and whistles out of cane.[47] Young women perfumed their bodies with honeysuckle and rose petals hidden in their bosoms. When courting, they adorned themselves with strings of dried chinaberries painted with dye. Men and women used the strong "skin" (bark) of fresh mulberry saplings for belts and tying up loose clothing while they worked.[48] It is not surprising that enslaved and poor white families sometimes used local plants similarly. Francis Peyre Porcher's botanical guide included a reference to the leaves of the calico bush "used by negroes, and the poor white people, as a cure for itch, and for the mange in the dogs."[49] Slaves and lower-class whites whose subsistence economies drew far more on local materials than those of elite whites gained a closer view of potentially useful plants.

Female domestic labor, in particular, fostered enslaved women's intimate knowledge of local botanical resources. Although plantation mistresses participated in domestic production, they were more likely to order bondswomen into the woods and gardens for necessary supplies than to make the excursion themselves. Virginia healer George White recalled that when the mistress wanted a certain kind of moss to dye fabric, she sent his mother to collect it.[50] Centenarian Tempie Herndon Durham still remembered vividly the older woman named "Mammy Rachel" in charge of dyeing homespun wool and cotton on a Chatham County plantation. "Dey wuzn' nothin' she didn' know 'bout dyein'," marveled Durham. "She knew every kind of root, bark, leaf an' bery dat made red, blue, green, or whatever color she wanted." Evidence of intimate knowledge of the North Carolina piedmont terrain, Mammy Rachel's dyed cloth strung on the line in the sun was "every color of de rainbow."[51]

In the course of their productive plantation work, enslaved women learned several uses for any given plant. Hominy, for example, was not only eaten but also used in laundering. Annie Wallace remembered the crackling sounds of her mother's petticoats, heavily starched in hominy water, as her mother moved swiftly down the path to her house ahead of pursuing patrollers.[52] Similarly, a turn-of-the-century portrait by North Carolina painter Mary Lyde Hicks Williams showed another southern staple, the collard leaf, bound to a black woman's head as a headache cure. Responsibility for a wide range of domestic tasks requiring plant knowledge

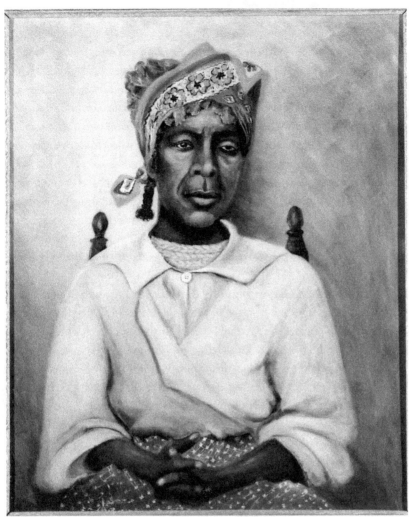

Woman with Collard Leaf to Cure Headache, *by Mary Lyde Hicks Williams,*
ca. 1890–1910. This oil painting by a white North Carolina artist illustrates the
medical use of greens commonly found in southern cooking. The woman shown,
Victoria Brown, grew up under slavery on the plantation belonging to the
artist's family and continued to work there after emancipation. Enslaved women
also used wraps of cabbage or ginseng leaves to cure a fever. (Reprinted with
permission; copyright © North Carolina Museum of History)

contributed to the prominence of enslaved women as herbalists for their families and the larger community.

Enslaved women cultivated some common medicinal herbs, such as sage, garlic, and calamus root, in their small garden "patches."[53] Della Barksdale remembered the patch of flag root planted by her mother and grandmother during slavery in Virginia. As an adult she continued to grow the tall grasslike plant whose root was chewed or made into a tea for stomach trouble. Another elderly woman grew jimsonweed in her garden that was used, among other purposes, for headache and dropsy.[54] Other stock remedies grew in larger plantation fields but were prepared and administered by slave women. On one St. Helena Island plantation in the 1850s a nurse and midwife named Judy laboriously ground and processed the arrowroot crop into gruel for babies and invalids.[55] Cultivation, however, supplied only a small portion of the herbal repertoire of enslaved communities.

Forests and wetlands surrounding the cultivated plantation fields comprised an even larger storehouse of possible remedies. The sheer volume of herbs listed in the vernacular by African American elders born into slavery suggests a detailed knowledge of wild-growing medicines, even from the distance of several decades. Rhodus Walton, for example, recalled that Queensy's light root, butterfly root, scurry root, red shank root, and bull tongue root all grew in the Georgia woods and made useful teas.[56] Sarah Gudger remembered very few white doctors during her enslavement in North Carolina. Instead, she recalled, people gathered their medicine from the woods, using bark of all kinds for making teas that would "bring yo' around."[57] Whether it provided pepper and dogwood tea for fever or snakeroot for stomachache, the forest served as a veritable pharmacy for those with the right training.[58]

The keenest knowledge of the woods resided among the oldest members of slave communities. A former slave from Maryland recalled, "The old people could read the woods just like a book. Whenever you were sick, they could go out and pick something, and you'd get well."[59] From the son of a South Carolina planter family comes a valuable description of one such "reader" of the woods, an enslaved elder named Eliza Nelson. L. G. Miller recalled that on his father's plantation in the Spartanburg district Eliza Nelson gained a reputation as a maker of efficacious herbal remedies. She spent many hours searching the woods with her mattock, a short-bladed pickax used for loosening the soil and digging up roots. Over her shoulder Nelson carried a bag, which she called her "lap," designed to hold the

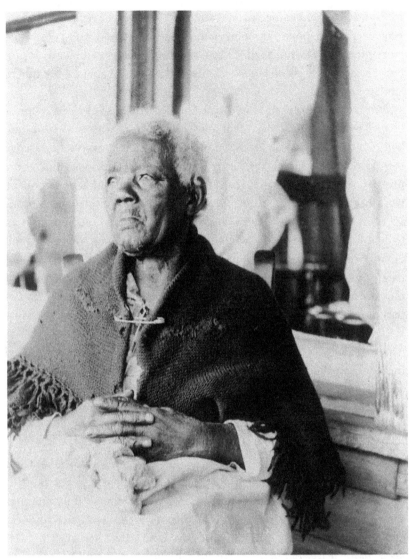

Sarah Gudger, Asheville, North Carolina, ca. 1937. Believed to have been born in 1816, Sarah Gudger remembered a life of unending work under slavery. On the large North Carolina plantation of her youth, ailing slaves were assigned to the sickhouse, where an enslaved nurse attended them. Recalling few white doctors, Mrs. Gudger described the effective poultices and teas she and her neighbors made from plants gathered in the woods. (WPA Ex-Slave Narrative Collection, LC)

roots and plants she gathered. After the day's harvest, she returned home to make medicines, pounding some of the herbs with a hardwood pestle and mortar made by her husband.[60] From rituals of picking to methods of processing, Nelson drew on her storehouse of knowledge about the southern landscape.

It bears repeating that African American herbalism was indeed a sophisticated body of knowledge. Though white doctors with elite education believed that black herbalists were mere "empiricists" whose knowledge consisted of crude remedies learned by rote memory, a close look at the process of making medicines shows otherwise.[61] The herbal practitioner's work began with the ability to identify a wide range of plants at various stages of growth. In the dense woods or marshy lowlands an herbalist had to be able to identify specific plants and distinguish between poisonous and curative ones.[62] Next the herbalist considered several subtle factors about harvesting the plant. She or he needed to know when a plant was ready for picking, at what time of day or lunar cycle it would be most potent, what part of the plant to use for particular remedies, and how much could be safely given. The common southern herb pokeweed, or pokeberry, offers just one example of the complexity of herbal practice. The berries crushed in alcohol were given for rheumatism, a decoction of pokeweed tops made an external remedy for boils, and the new leaves were eaten as a spring tonic. Healing with pokeweed required a practiced hand, however, for the roots could be fatally poisonous and the tops also became toxic as the plant matured.[63]

Matching the correct tea, poultice, or ointment to a specific complaint, too, required a series of skilled decisions. Faith Mitchell, in her study of Sea Island herbalism, notes that compared with the more elaborate prescriptions written in the recipe books of literate whites, black practitioners tended to use only a few plants for each remedy.[64] Slave herbalists brewed tea from the leaves of the peach tree to calm upset stomachs. They heated sage and catnip leaves to make soothing poultices when babies broke out in hives.[65] Black women collected pine tops in the woods and soaked them in a steaming tub so that children with pneumonia could ease their labored breathing with the strong-smelling vapor.[66] These recipes may have been streamlined partly because of the limited time and materials available to enslaved practitioners. Mitchell also suggests that their simplicity may have been "indicative of a more exact knowledge of the nature and function of each plant."[67]

To their extensive knowledge of local plant life, African American herbal healers joined their understanding of the human body. Although evidence from the antebellum period is scarce, modern studies of southern black traditional healers suggest the outlines of the diagnostic system that enslaved herbalists may have embraced. First and foremost, enslaved herbalists located the body within the relational vision of health that acknowledged physical, moral, and supernatural causes of bodily affliction. For those "natural" illnesses not caused by conjuration or sent directly by God, black herbalists considered the condition of a person's blood as the most important factor in diagnosis. The view that balance in the blood's qualities was the key to good health reflected African therapeutic precedents as well as European diagnostic systems based in Greek humoral theory. Herbalists in consultation with their clients weighed a series of interrelated binary qualities of blood—high/low, thick/thin, fast/slow, hot/cold, pure/impure—and prescribed medicines to bring the blood back into equilibrium. In addition to these already complicated considerations, the herbalist further distinguished an illness by the location of symptoms in key regions of the body, including the head, stomach, lungs, and kidneys.[68]

The widespread practice of seasonal blood cleansing, common for both white and black antebellum southerners, illustrates the central importance of the blood to good health. Comparing the body itself to a plant, present-day African American herbal practitioners explain that the blood rises like a tree's sap in the spring. During the winter, however, the blood has thickened and acquired impurities.[69] To prevent colds and other sicknesses, the blood needs to be purged in anticipation of the summer's warmth. Enslaved herbalists on southern plantations used several remedies to clean the blood, but none was more popular than the locally available sassafras tree. Della Barksdale of Virginia reported that sassafras root tea "'searches de blood' and finds out what's wrong and goes to work on it."[70] Though the sassafras remedy was widely known, herbal specialists accumulated a far more extensive pharmacopoeia for regulating, purifying, and balancing the body.

Younger men and women in plantation communities learned this complex body of knowledge through an extended process of apprenticeship. John Jackson, an elderly man, recalled his boyhood in slavery: "You know, they lays a heap o' stress on edication these days. But edication is one thing an' fireside trainin' is another. We had fireside trainin'."[71] Jackson's apt phrase conveys the process of learning from enslaved elders after the sun had set on the day's work. William Edwards, a Georgia root doctor, began his education as a young boy learning from the "ole people bout herbs dat wuz good fuh diffunt ailments." With few white doctors around, Edwards told an interviewer, "we hab tuh fine remedies fuh our sickness an know how tuh cuo snake bite aw cuts and boils, eben female complaints."[72] Fireside training allowed older herbalists to pass on their knowledge of the local woods for the purpose of a community's survival.

African-born elders played an important role in the transmission of medicinal and herbal expertise, which was often passed on through kinship networks. The large numbers of African captives transported in the last decade of the Atlantic slave trade, as well as the subsequent illicit smuggling of captive Africans, ensured some continuing influence from African-born practitioners, especially in the Lowcountry.[73] One elderly Georgian recalled an "Igbo doctor" who cut and bled his patients.[74] Rosanna Williams's African-born father extracted teeth and made herbal medicines for the sick.[75] Jack Waldburg, who was also from coastal Georgia, acquired knowledge of how "tuh make medicine from root" from his African grandmother, a midwife.[76] Upon their forced arrival in the South, African healers would have found a strange countryside bearing perhaps some transplanted species from their native landscape. In teaching what they knew, they passed on their acquired knowledge of local plants as well as the cultural values by which these plants could be interpreted and used.

African American Herbalism as Sacred Art

A spiritual orientation toward the local landscape defined the herbal practice of enslaved communities. The herbalism of southern blacks, it can be argued, expressed a sacred worldview as clearly as singing, praying, or dancing. As they gathered, administered, and taught about botanical medicines, enslaved African Americans enacted a relationship with the land that was both practical and spiritual.[77] Antebellum black herbalism thus became not only a pragmatic resource for survival but also one of the sacred arts of slave doctoring in North America.

Although African Americans' historical reliance on herbal medicines is widely acknowledged, the religious dimension of these medicines has been neglected. Santeria scholar George Brandon argues that while the role of plants in African religions is well known, "little attention has been devoted to examining the use of plants in the context of the various Afro-American religions."[78] Brandon's argument is especially valid for North American black herbalism, where most of the scholarship on slave religion does not explore plant use and most of the scholarship on plant use does not substantially address religion. Instead, folklore, ethnobotany, and ethnopharmacology studies have tended to emphasize remedies, plants, and pharmaceutical properties at the expense of the religious context in which much of African American herb doctoring took place. Placing North American black herbalism in hemispheric perspective clarifies important continuities and differences between various sacred plant uses across the Black Atlantic world.

An emphasis on the spiritual significance of plants extends broadly across African-based religions in the Americas. Santeria and Candomblé, both strongly shaped by Yoruba cosmology, provide instructive examples of the integral ritual role of herbs. Within Yoruba religion, one's well-being ultimately depends on *ashé*, a "vital force" representing "power, energy, and strength," which "permeates the entire universe."[79] *Ashé*, residing in the liquid-bearing parts of plants, can be enlivened and directed by ritual specialists to secure health and well-being. Santeria, a Yoruba-based religion originating in the Caribbean and influenced by Spanish Catholicism and French Spiritualism, reflects this concept of spiritually enlivened medicinal plants. Santeria rituals employ specific herb combinations associated with particular deities. Priests or priestesses prepare herb mixtures during the first stages of initiation and use them to cleanse and purify both initiates and ritual objects. During an extended ritual of healing, for example, a *santero* might apply a plant mixture to "cool" and balance the sufferer's head.[80]

While *ashé* is found in cultivated plants and weeds as well, many Cuban herbalists look to the forests for spiritually powerful plants. Art historian Robert Farris Thompson points to the Cuban appropriation of Osanyin Elewe, the Yoruba god of herbalism. As the domain of Osanyin and the repository of curative plants, the forest possesses a spiritual life and power of its own. Cuban herbalists familiar with the lore of Osanyin acknowledge this power with libations of rum, tobacco, and chicken blood when they enter the forest to collect their materials. Those who honor Osanyin in this way, concludes Thompson, "also honor forests, teaching their impartial spirituality, teaching that the woods are grander than any document, teaching that man cannot assume the bush is his alone, or else be answerable to God."[81]

Candomblé, a religion instituted in Brazil by enslaved Yoruba and their descendants, similarly incorporated an elaborate array of ritual and medicinal plants. Candomblé adherents in Bahia, a region of rich botanical exchange during the colonial years, used local plants that had their origins around the globe. For example, the African kola nut employed in divination in West Africa became widely used by Candomblé practitioners for divination as well.[82] West African captives taken to Brazil adopted an indigenous tree and renamed it *iroko* to serve in place of the African *iroko*, home of the Yoruba deity of the same name.[83] Plants such as the European rue are still worn to ward off the "evil eye," while other leaf combinations are used to prepare ritual baths, called *abo*.[84]

Adherents of Haitian Vodou reflected a similar understanding of the sacred nature of the forest and its plants. Emerging fully after 1804 from a fusion of Kongo, Fon, and other West African religions with an overlay of Catholicism, Vodou in Haiti incorporated a strong sense of the "power of leaves" (*makaya* in Creole).[85] Among the *lwa*, or Vodou deities, Gran Bwa reigns over the mystery and impenetrability of the forest and is associated with healing and initiation. Members of secret societies associated with Gran Bwa gather at night for ceremonial leaf gathering.[86] Simbi, an important Central African water spirit, is also linked with healing in Haiti and is invoked with many titles, including "Simbi of the healing leaves (*makaya*)." Medicinal leaves also lend important symbolism to the construction of Vodou power objects, or *pakèt kongo*, which can be activated and enlivened by ritual experts. A well-known class of *pakèt kongo* called *Simbi Makaya* is called upon in rites of healing.[87] Clearly Vodou, like many other religions of the Black Atlantic, incorporates many complex associations between plants, spiritual power, and healing.

Compared with sacred plant use in Cuba, Brazil, or Haiti, North American traditions show less evidence of direct African retentions. The history of British colonization and the demography of North American slavery have made linguistic connections more difficult to establish. In addition, nineteenth-century African American religious practice in the antebellum southeastern states did not seem to emphasize the collective ritual use of plants or the honoring of African forest deities evident in other parts of the Atlantic world.[88] Nonetheless, the daily medicinal practices of enslaved communities in the United States rested on a notion of a spiritually enlivened landscape drawn from both African cosmologies and African American Christian theology. To find black sacred plant traditions in the southeastern states that are the focus of this study, we must look to the practice of African American herbalists for whom gathering and making medicines was holy work.[89]

Artifacts from the eighteenth century suggest that enslaved practitioners carried elements of African ritual into African American medicine making.

For years archaeologists working in the coastal Atlantic states have un-
earthed both pieces and intact samples of a slave-made pottery called
Colono Ware. Excavations in South Carolina, many of which are of under-
water sites, have uncovered pottery shards from Colono Ware bowls with
distinctive markings carved into their bases. Archaeologist Leland Ferguson argues that the crosslike marks are in fact cosmograms, concrete evidence of the continuity of Kongo ritual in colonial North America. The
Kongo influence on the South Carolina coast, the emphasis in Kongo religion on water spirits, and the manner in which the marks were made
support the case for the ritual significance of these slave-made artifacts.
Though the interpretation of these marks is still under way, Ferguson
furthermore suggests that the marked vessels may have served as bowls for
minkisi made by African colonial herbalists. As a sacred mark of Kongo
cosmology, the cosmogram on the clay bowl created a point of contact with
spiritual power on the exact spot where medicines were mixed and administered.[90]

By the mid-nineteenth century, enslaved herbalists had combined African sacred plant traditions with Christianity. The Exodus story, a central
theme in the theology of enslaved communities, contained a strong message
of God's provision for the oppressed that extended to herbal medicines.[91]
Just as God had supplied manna in the wilderness to the Israelites, so too
did God provide healing for the sick during slavery. Della Barksdale echoed
this widespread sentiment when she voiced her conviction that the Lord
had provided roots and herbs for every imaginable illness human beings
might face.[92] Similarly George White, the healer whose enslaved father had
also been an herb doctor, explained, "Dere's a root for ev'y disease an' I
can cure most anything, but you have got to talk wid God an' ask him to
help out."[93] A Tennessee woman who doctored her family through many
illnesses experienced divine intervention in one of her own ailments. "The
spirit directed me to get some peach-tree leaves and beat them up and put
them about my limbs," she recalled. "I did this, and in a day or two that
swelling left me, and I haven't been bothered since."[94]

When African American herbalists spoke of encountering a deity in the
swamps or woods, they often referred to the Christian God while reflecting an emphasis on the sacredness of the forest similar to that expressed
by Cuban devotees of Osanyin. Particularly in searching for wild-growing
medicines, southern black herbalists stressed their reliance on sacred revelation. A Georgia woman called "Aunt Darkas" by the interviewer established a reputation as a healer and a skillful gatherer of forest medicines

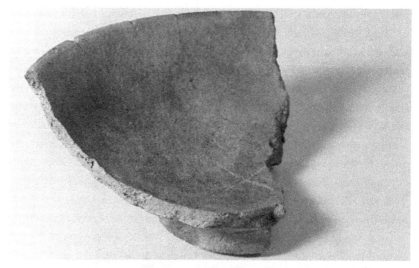

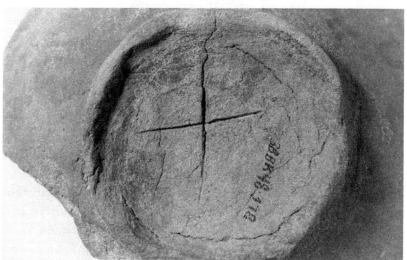

Marked Colono Ware bowls from South Carolina. Initially identified as food containers, eighteenth-century artifacts such as these have been reinterpreted by archaeologist Leland Ferguson as ritual medicine bowls incised with the Kongo cosmogram. Lower image: *Base of a bowl from the Cooper River.* (Photographs by Emily Short, courtesy of Leland Ferguson)

despite her blindness. A black woman previously cured by Aunt Darkas remembered, "She always said the Lord told her what roots to get, and always 'fore sunup, you would see her in the woods with a short-handled pick."[95] With one important difference, this description of Aunt Darkas bears a striking similarity to the portrait of herbalist Eliza Nelson. The latter account from an African American informant, however, goes beyond the physical description of herb gathering to an emphasis on the spiritual significance of Aunt Darkas's ability to "see" medicines in the forest. Many enslaved healers, such as Aunt Darkas, looked for God's hand in the southeastern forests.

Other herbal practitioners listened to the spirits of the plants themselves. Limited evidence suggests that some African American healers relied on spiritual force residing within plants, an idea that resonated with the Yoruba concept of *ashé*. Slave gardens in the Georgia and South Carolina Lowcountry, for example, featured benne, or sesame, at the ends of the rows. Sesame had West Indian associations with obeah, and its presence in these Lowcountry gardens may have been intended to repel thieves and other intruders.[96] Even more than cultivated flora, wild-growing plants were animated by spiritual power. Old Divinity, an elderly African American "tree-talker" from Mississippi, told his interviewer that the wind, trees, and birds had spirits, too. Human beings were just "a part uv de livin' souls, no mo' an' no less." The healing properties of plants resided in their spirit. Thus, explained Old Divinity, the spirit in the jimsonweed cured asthma and the spirit in the buckeye drove away rheumatism.[97]

In the woods and wetlands beyond plantation grounds, spiritual power intensified and the social power of slave society waned. Amidst the perils of North American enslavement, the wilderness held many layers of meaning for black men and women.[98] In Harriet Jacobs's narrative of escape from slavery in North Carolina, the "Snaky Swamp" provided a refuge whose dangers "were less dreadful to my imagination than the white men in that community called civilized."[99] Forests and swamps, though dangerous, offered encampments for runaway slaves, hiding places for appropriated goods, and retreats from punishment and overwork. Sanctuary and spirituality merged in the brush arbors of the deep forest, where enslaved congregations stole away to sing and pray.[100]

From this unique historical relationship to the land, African American herbal expertise emerged. Black herbal practitioners frequently described their skill as a God-given knowledge acquired in the hard school of bondage. According to healer George Briggs, no college could match the "gift of understanding" that he gained from a sacred encounter in the South Carolina woods. Briggs recalled, "Years ago I had de toothache; went to de woods in my misery. Something told me to git some rats-vein (wild Arsenic weed) and make some tea and drink it. It soon rid me of dat misery in my tooth."[101] Later in the twentieth century Janie Cameron Riley of North Carolina spoke with equal confidence of the herbal knowledge of her ancestors. "They knowed what they was doing back in those days," she declared. Emphasizing the interpretation of black herbalism as a revered form of sacred knowledge forged under slavery, she insisted, "I'm telling you right now, the black people had to have some kind of knowledge from God; they had to, 'cause they didn't have nothing else to dwell on."[102] The experience of enslavement, these informants tell us, uniquely shaped the religious significance of African American herbalism.

From forest spaces to garden patches, enslaved African Americans grounded their practice of herbal medicine in a historical relationship between the gods, human beings, and the environment. Several centuries of Atlantic exchange refigured the southern landscape that African American slave herbalists used so creatively. Drawing on plant traditions of Africans, Europeans, and Native Americans, enslaved men and women created an herbal practice marked by innovation and adaptation. As John Walker's hiring of Doctor Lewis and the long life of Caesar's colonial-era remedy for poison both illustrate, enslaved herbalists had a significant impact on white domestic medicine as well. Not an insular tradition by any measure, African American herbalism was nevertheless a distinctive practice embedded in particular historical and spiritual landscapes. Harsh agricultural labor and a rural subsistence economy fostered an intimate knowledge of the surrounding environment among enslaved men and women. Enslaved practitioners acting on their botanical expertise created African American herbal traditions that varied with the regional terrain.

A prized form of local knowledge, African American herbalism also became a sacred art. From the forest to the sickbed, enslaved herbalists described spiritual empowerment as necessary to their efficacy as healers. Herbal specialists sought to instill their sacred art in the younger generation through a process of oral instruction and extended apprenticeship. In placing such heavy emphasis on the spirituality of herbal doctoring, enslaved African Americans maintained a sacred orientation toward living plants evident in a broad array of African-based religions in the Americas. Moreover, herbalism formed the bedrock of a wide range of African American doctoring practices under slavery. Midwives, conjure doctors, and women in ordinary household sickcare all drew on herbal knowledge in their work. While these practitioners differed in their relationship to plantation production and slaveholder power, each used medicinal plants to pursue a vision of health with a strong social and spiritual basis.

Ef dey wants you to get 'em well, Hoo-doo
Dat is de han' at moves de spell, Hoo-doo
Take it out before der eyes,
An' you mus' be awful s'prised
And dey well think dat you is wise, Hoo-doo
—Kentucky Narratives, ca. 1937

Disease as represented in biomedicine is localized in the body, in
discrete sites or physiological processes. The narratives of those who
are subjects of suffering represent illness, by contrast as present in a
life. Illness is grounded in human historicity, in the temporality of
individuals and families and communities.
—Byron J. Good,
  Medicine, Rationality, and Experience, *1994*

CHAPTER 4
Conjuring Community

After suffering for months, the young slave woman Calia died in the spring of 1810. The black and the white residents of Roslin Plantation disagreed on the cause of her death. Overseer William McKean wrote to his employer, "Calia poor thing was taken ill about Christmas & died on the 19 April—the people say that she was poisoned, or *tricked* as they call it, by a young man who wished to marry her, & she would not have him—but I believe she died of a consumption."[1] These brief remarks begin and end the written record of Calia's illness. Slave deaths often received only terse mention in the letters of overseers; in a subsequent report McKean devoted more words to the death of the plantation's English bull than he had to Calia's passing.

The overseer's commentary nevertheless opened a valuable window onto the relational vision of health among enslaved families on the Roslin Plantation. Unlike the majority of Roslin's residents, McKean believed that Calia wasted away with consumption, a physical ailment compounded by weather and internal predisposition. The enslaved community of Roslin, on the other hand, held that Calia died because her rejected suitor "tricked," or conjured, her. According to this second theory, the roots of Calia's illness lay not within her body but in a publicly acknowledged and troubled courtship.[2] Whereas McKean sought to explain Calia's death by naming her disease, enslaved residents of the plantation looked instead to the social basis of her affliction.[3]

Among the arts of African American doctoring, conjuration most explicitly reflected the relational vision of health and healing. Conjuration, also called "hoodoo" or "rootwork," was (and is) an African American practice of healing, harming, and protection performed through the "ritual harnessing of spiritual forces."[4] Enslaved men and women frequently used conjuration in their struggles against slaveholders, yet conjuration also figured strongly in the internal conflicts of slave communities. Accounts of conjuring reveal that men and women frequently "worked roots" to resolve or escalate personal disagreements that had little to do with the immediate actions of whites. On their own and often with the assistance of a conjurer, enslaved men and women manipulated spiritual power to "trick," "fix," "poison," "witch," or "conjure" their antagonists.[5] Believing their distress was intentionally caused by another party, afflicted persons told stories of bodily misery replete with the details of human conflict. In other words, African American conjure stories are richly textured "illness narratives" that reveal the collective context for illness and healing in southern plantation communities.

The analysis of "illness narratives"—a term borrowed from literary theory and medical anthropology—aims to understand how human beings represent and interpret illness in particular times and places. Medical anthropologist Byron Good describes "narrativization," the act of telling about an experience of illness and pain, as "a process of locating suffering in history, of placing events in meaningful order in time."[6] Rather than describing illness through the eyes of the practitioner or an outside observer, illness narratives delineate the world of the sufferer. Persons afflicted with sickness and pain, Good argues, represent their illness "as present in a life."[7] The many African American conjure narratives contain exactly this sense of illness as a social and spiritual phenomenon unfolding in the context of specific historical communities.

First-person accounts of conjuring abound in southern black oral histories and collected folklore from the 1870s through the 1940s. As a "subgenre of African American oral literature," conjure stories frequently shared a common narrative structure.[8] Consider, for example, the following account by Fred Jones, an elderly Georgia man born in the 1850s.

I don't like to talk 'bout myself, but I can't never forget the time I had a dose put on me by a woman I didn't like. I was a good friend of her husband and she didn't like for us to go out together; so she told me not to come to her house no more. I ain't pay no 'tention. Well, suh, the next night soon as I laid down, I feel myself swoon. Every night it happen. This thing keep up till I get sick. I couldn't eat and just get to pining 'way. The doctor he can't help me none. Finally I went to a root man. He say right off somebody done give me a dose. He say, "I'll be round tonight. Get some money together cause I can't do you no good less you start off with some silver."

When he come that night and get the silver, he look all around the house and then dig a hole under the door step. There he find a bottle. He throw it in the fire and hollar, "Git gone, you devil." After that I get better, but I ain't never been to that woman's house since. And I don't like to talk about it.[9]

Jones's account of affliction and healing contained four stages common to southern African American narratives of conjuration. Though the structure and form of conjuring narratives displayed some flexibility and were, furthermore, shaped by the interviewers who recorded them, they typically proceeded in the manner of the above story. First, conjure accounts laid out a conflict, identifying a soured relationship with a well-known neighbor or family member as the source of the conjure spell. In this postemancipation story Jones found himself at odds with the wife of a good friend who perhaps saw Jones as a threat to her marriage. Next, the narrator described his or her affliction by mapping out the bodily effects of the hoodoo "dose." Often the suddenness or particular nature of physical symptoms, such as a "swoon" or a sharp pain, prompted the fearful victim to suspect an "unnatural illness." Third, the afflicted person searched for a conjure doctor, a healer with "second sight" into the workings of the spiritual world. Fourth and finally, the narrator recounted the steps taken by the conjurer to bring about a cure. The conjurer located the offending object, such as Fred Jones's buried bottle, identified the person who sought the fix in the first place, and either negated the trick or turned it back on the originator. The teller concluded with the results of the cure or an explanation of why the cure did not work. The following sections trace the four stages of African American conjure narratives and explore the relational vision of health in the course of the journey from affliction to healing.

Most illness caused by conjuration originated in conflicts over love, sex, economic resources, and interpersonal power.[10] Although troubles with love or money might be construed as concerns of any age, it would be a mistake to view African American hoodoo as a timeless folk practice.[11] Examined carefully, conjuring narratives clearly illustrate the historical contingency of hoodoo affliction. The phenomenon of socially based illness stretches across African American history, but the conflicts giving rise to each narrator's afflictions were bounded by the particulars of time and space. Early-twentieth-century conjuration accounts, for example, often revealed the impact of the postemancipation political economy on the personal relationships of black southerners. For example, when Ellen Dorsey fell ill, she immediately suspected her estranged husband of hiring a root doctor to cause her malady. The Georgia woman believed her husband had her conjured so that she would be fired by her white employers and forced to return to him.[12] Other conjure narratives from the early twentieth century involved African Americans using conjure doctors as the "poor man's lawyer" to combat Jim Crow courts and police of southern cities and towns.[13] Antebellum conjuration just as readily reflected the historical conditions of enslavement.

Many African Americans looking back on the period of slavery tended to focus on conjuration used against slaveholders, but antebellum evidence shows an active use of conjuration to mediate daily conflicts within enslaved communities as well.[14] Dissension and the ensuing need for revenge or protection emerged from constant interaction with a known group of people within a local neighborhood. Face-to-face interaction in plantation slave communities minimized the value of individual privacy and familiarized enslaved families with one another's affairs.[15] Detailed knowledge of Calia's courtship, for instance, would not have been hard to come by for the enslaved residents of Roslin Plantation. By 1816 the slave quarters consisted of three structures built by McKean to replace several deteriorating buildings. Two double-room houses, which probably shared a common center fireplace, each sheltered two families (including all the women) belonging to the estate. Another twenty-two-foot-square building housed "single" men and the "hirelings," slave men hired for the year from other slaveholders.[16]

Close living and the oppressive strictures of enslavement bred both mutual aid and reciprocal animosity. When a group of fugitives took shelter in the woods surrounding Roslin several years after Calia's death, McKean complained of the complicity of slaves who provided them with food from the plantation's stores. In a letter to his employer, McKean observed that "there is scarcely a runaway in any neighbourhood but a great portion of the servants about know of it & assist in supporting him."[17] In the same year McKean also recorded disputes stemming from "jealousy" between individuals permanently enslaved at Roslin and those hired for the year.[18] Whether the earlier trouble between Calia and her suitor emerged from these local patterns of conflict is uncertain. It is clear, however, that among the enslaved families of Roslin Plantation, explanations for Calia's fatal illness began with the social life of their neighborhood.

Hoodoo served an important juridical function within communities of the enslaved. Conjure — as well as stories about conjure — reinforced public standards of slave community behavior pertaining to property, sexuality, and relations between young and old.[19] Historically, violation of community norms has frequently been construed as an immediate cause of illness within African American health culture.[20] Conjure vividly illustrated the healing and harming dynamics of the African American pharmocosm by connecting an individual's well-being to his or her conduct within a community.

The moral lessons of conjuration narratives can perhaps best be seen in fearful stories about impudent children. Proper respect for one's elders figured powerfully within the behavioral code of enslaved African Americans, and individuals who transgressed that code walked on dangerous ground. Some question existed within African American conjuring lore as to whether children could be targets of hoodoo. Since the kinds of conflicts that led to conjuring fell largely in the domain of adult affairs, adults naturally comprised the majority of those afflicted. Some believed that small children and infants, in their innocence, could not be endangered by ill intent.[21] Other witnesses disagreed and described babies conjured in their cribs and children barking and running in circles like dogs.[22] Stories passed on from slavery promised fearful results for disrespectful youngsters. One account related the fate of a group of children who mocked and threw stones at an elderly man "hobbling" along a road. According to Ellen Betts, who had been enslaved in Louisiana, the man cursed a particularly bold boy, saying, "Go on, young-un, you'll be where dogs can't bark at you tomorrow." To the children's horror the boy dropped dead the next day. Ellen Betts concluded, "Nobody ever bother that old man no more, for he sure lay the evil finger on you."[23] Such cautionary tales dramatically impressed upon young children the necessity of respecting one's elders.

Conjuration also entered conflicts between adults over the scarce resources available to enslaved families. James Smith recalled from his boyhood how his father, Charles, had nearly died at the hands of a resentful woman named Cella. Cella had been displaced from housekeeper to field worker when Charles and his family were assigned by the slaveholder to occupy the plantation and house where Cella had lived. Stung by her new situation and perhaps worried for her young daughter's future, Cella disappeared overnight (presumably to seek a conjure doctor) and returned the next evening with a "poisoned" whiskey bottle, from which Charles drank. His resulting affliction only worsened under the white doctor's treatment. Finally Charles's owner, desperate to save his valuable slave, agreed to consult a black doctor, who divined the origin of the problem and provided the needed cure. Cella did not escape unharmed from this conflict, however. Charles's owner, informed of Cella's role in the matter by the black doctor, brutally beat and eventually sold her.[24]

Events on a Georgia plantation similarly revealed white authority and violence as a presence in slave community conflicts. In this case the growing internal economy of the nineteenth century set the stage for conflicts over petty property or access to cash-producing work.[25] Overseer A. H. Urquhart became the perhaps unwitting scribe of a conjuration account when he chronicled a series of clashes over access to domestic production at the Mills Plantation of Burke Country, Georgia, in 1839. In terms of utmost disdain, Urquhart related to employer Margaret Telfair his troubles with an enslaved woman he called "Darkey." Most likely a woman past her physical prime, "Darkey" worked in the plantation yard, milking cows, churning butter, and tending the poultry. Occasionally she was allowed to market the fruits of her labor. A previous overseer's notes concerning goods sent to and from Mills Plantation included evidence of her industry throughout the 1830s: "Darkey sends 8 chickens, 2 Ducks, 1 Doz of Eggs 1 small Gord of Butter, 1 small Bag of potatoes."[26] She also seemed to have greater mobility and more influence with the Telfairs than many of the other men and women enslaved at Mills Plantation. "Darkey says that she wants a straner," reported the overseer, and again, "Darkey says that you send word for her to come up there [to Augusta] with the Waggon."[27]

The opportunities "Darkey" had for raising her own produce became the subject of contention with plantation overseers and possibly with individuals enslaved beside her. By 1836, for reasons that are unclear, the overseer had informed "Darkey" that she "must not Rase Ducks & Turkeys for her self."[28] When Urquhart took up his position as the new overseer at Mills Plantation in the late 1830s, he began to report conflicts with the enterprising bondswoman. Although he declared hopefully in the fall of 1839 that "Darkey" would soon have twelve to thirteen cows to milk, by the next February he wrote in consternation that only two cows remained productive: "Since December she managed them so Badly they have nearly all gone dry." Considering the prolific store of dairy goods sent by "Darkey" from the plantation for sale in earlier years, it is reasonable to speculate that she deliberately sabotaged the plantation's dairy production in retaliation for the overseer's new restrictions.

The conflict soon escalated beyond the issues of domestic production when the overseer attempted to gain control of "Darkey" by force. Complaining of her "most troublesome" and "cruel" disposition, Urquhart reported that "Darkey" had made such "disturbances" and "interruptions" that few of the others working nearby "will Ever go near the yard." Finally, Urquhart wrote, "she got so high I went there and give her a moderate correction and that had a bad affect[.] she then threatened their Lives and said that she would poison them[.] they became alarmed and ask me permission to move to the Quarter."[29] Told from the overseer's perspective, this account demonstrates how intracommunity conflict could be exacerbated by white violence. Stung by Urquhart's whipping, "Darkey" intended to retaliate against her colaborers in the plantation yard.

The request to move to the plantation quarters strongly suggests that the enslaved workers near "Darkey" understood her warning as a conjuring threat. Fearing their food and the very ground itself, they viewed the yard as a place of danger that lay beyond the overseer's power. After all, one did not have to ingest or even touch the conjurer's roots; merely walking over something "put down" for an intended victim would be enough to cause grave affliction. A Georgia planter and amateur white folklorist in 1896 made a strikingly similar complaint concerning an argument between two women who worked in the kitchen and dairy, both outbuildings in the plantation yard. He reported, "It was with great difficulty, while all this 'cunjer' was going on, that I could get any one to enter the yard in order to perform the slightest offices. . . . Some would not even pass through the yard."[30] In both the later account and the Mills Plantation incidents, the pharmocosm entered the very spaces in which men and women labored. Whether it was caused by jealousy for her small earnings, resentment of her authority, or confrontation with her thorny personality, the discord surrounding "Darkey" developed into direct threats against the health and lives of those with whom she lived.

By far the most common source of conflict leading to affliction, however, involved discord between men and women in the arena of love, sexuality, and marriage.[31] Efforts such as those of former slave Henry Bibb to attract an admired woman with love charms represented a relatively benign use of hoodoo. Much more was at stake when men and women sought relief from painful relationships and exacted revenge through conjuration. Calia's fatal illness, described at the beginning of this chapter, began with the resentment of an aspiring suitor. Although it carried its own risks, the use of conjuration offered a way to injure, drive off, or kill someone without assaulting him or her in person. Conjuration represented an arena in which men and women attempted to defend their sense of worth and protect what they regarded as their own, regardless of their physical strength.[32]

The institution of slavery immeasurably complicated the effort to defend and even define what was one's own. Gender conflicts were exacerbated by forced sexual relationships, slaveholder limitations on desired slave partnerships (such as "abroad marriages" across plantation boundaries or marriage to free partners), and separations due to sale and hiring out. Affliction arising from sexual conflicts was therefore deeply embedded in the attempts of a white slave society to control enslaved families, sexual partnerships, and reproduction.

One recurrent theme in conjure narratives involved the affliction of younger women who happened to cross older conjure men. Emmaline Heard's father told one such story about a conjure man from his Georgia boyhood in the early nineteenth century. Within the lore of the quarters, Ned, an older man, was said to have conjured a young woman because "she wouldn't pay him any attention." He attempted without success to gain her affection by staying close and helping her hoe in the fields. Field workers left their hoes in the field when they stopped to take their noon meals. As Emmaline related the story to her interviewer, "When that gal went back ter the field the minute she touches that hoe she fell dead. Some folks say they saw uncle Ned dressing that hoe with conjure."[33] Similarly, a North Carolina woman told Charles Chesnutt about her affliction by an old conjure man whom she had verbally insulted after he said some "rough, ugly things" to her.[34]

In the face-to-face communities of many slave quarters, sexual conflicts between men and women frequently drew in entire groups related by work, kinship, or household. A series of poisonings on the Butler family's Hampton Plantation in Georgia illustrated lines of fracture and mutual assistance within enslaved communities. Roswell King, the overseer at the time, recorded what he knew of the poisonings after investigations that revealed, in his words, "too much for my quiatude." In the summer of 1814 King reported trouble between Jacob, a mechanic, and his wife, Evander, who tended the Hampton poultry. The driver Elijah had "been thick" with Evander. In turn Evander protested to Jacob that "she could not help keeping with Elijah, for he had conjore Phisick and she could not help it." Roswell King believed that Elijah had made several nocturnal visits to an old conjure doctor on a neighboring plantation. "It appears that Mrs. Wright has an Old Negro that is a conjure Doctor," he wrote, "and it is said Elijah is one of his customers." Within several weeks Elijah and several other men and women were implicated in a spate of poisonings among slaves whom King considered the plantation's "best negroes." At least four other men, including Jacob, who had been in poor health all spring, "all had a dose" strong enough to make them ill. Supported by his mother, Betty, Jacob wished to take Evander out of Elijah's influence and was allowed by the overseer to move to another of the Butlers' holdings.[35] The effect of the affliction reached beyond the initial triangle of Elijah, Evander, and Jacob and rippled through several of the families enslaved at Hampton Plantation. Conflicts over family, sexuality, and marriage spread from Evander's first claims of being conjured to the poisoning of Jacob and several of his allies.

Conjuring narratives, from their beginning, identified disorder and affliction in human relationships, which were in turn grounded in the spiritual forces of the pharmocosm. Though enslaved men and women did not interpret all illness as the work of a conjurer, the possibility of conjuration was present when supporters attempted to determine the cause of a person's sudden pain or declining health. In considering a path toward healing, the afflicted person often scrutinized the character of past relationships and recent encounters with neighbors. The relational vision of health unfolded as narratives of conjuration moved from a description of social relations and personal relationships to an exploration of the nature of affliction itself.

Affliction and the Signs of Power

Illness that could not be cured by home remedies or a medical doctor's attention bore the mark of conjuration. What had begun as social conflict moved onto a metaphysical plane as the sufferer began to consider the meaning of her or his symptoms. Within conjuring narratives, detailed descriptions of the signs of affliction helped the teller elaborate illness as a spiritual crisis manifested through the body. Just as the Christian conversion narrative built up to the moment of salvation by detailing the convert's previous sin and anguish, conjure narratives anticipated the moment of healing with lengthy and vivid descriptions of bodily suffering.

Victims of hoodoo commonly pinpointed a moment of revelation when they realized with certainty that their pains had a supernatural origin. Alex Johnson was conjured while hoeing a field in Georgia. A sharp pain began in his feet, moved through his body, and came to rest in his head. "I went home," said Johnson, "and knew I was cunjered."[36] Swelling, bumps on the skin, and growing pain alerted sufferers of the presence of a hoodoo trick. A resident of Yamacraw, Georgia, told an interviewer, "I dohn know who done it, but all ub a sudden muh leg begin tuh swell an swell."[37] Another Georgia woman remembered stepping near a bottle that had been "fixed" for her. "Right den and deah I took sech a misery in muh lef side an den uh swell up al obuh," she recalled.[38] The elderly North Carolina freedwoman "Aunt Harriet," whose story was recorded by Charles Chesnutt, described the onset of affliction by a conjure man: "De ve'y minute I step' on de spot he tech', I felt a sha'p pain shoot thoo my right foot, it tu'n't under me, an' I fell down in de road. . . . I cried an' cried an' went on, fer I knowed I'd be'n trick' by dat ole man."[39]

Immobility and gradual wasting away also plagued conjure victims despite futile attempts to alleviate pain through home remedies and medical doctors. Sarah Fitzpatrick reported that "somebody tricked me in ma' left foot, an' I couldn't walk no mo' dan a baby."[40] A Georgia woman who suffered for six months from something another woman had put in her drinking water recalled, "When de spell come on me de meat would jump on my bones an' I could'nt sit still."[41] The immediacy of a person's suffering testified to the manifestation of spiritual forces in human flesh.

Among the signs of affliction, hoodoo sufferers frequently related the horror of reptiles or insects moving under their skin. Victims of hoodoo understood that hoodoo charms contained parts of scorpions, spiders, or snakes, which reproduced inside the body. A Georgia freedwoman remembered the fear inspired in her neighborhood by a conjure woman who afflicted her victims with snakes and scorpions.[42] In the final moments before either the victim's death or cure, these creatures often emerged from the victim's body, confirming the supernatural nature of the affliction. Mrs.

Rush, a Georgia midwife, told how her daughter had been conjured by sitting on a chair that had been "dressed" for her. Shortly before the daughter died, the skin on her hip split, revealing a snake.[43]

Not limited to physical suffering, the signs of affliction also included mental confusion, impeded judgment, and outright insanity. Evidence suggests that antebellum African Americans often attributed mental affliction to conjuration and sought black doctors for a cure. According to Thomas Chaplin, for example, Free Billy and his "deranged" sister Nancy visited Chaplin's coastal plantation seeking the services of Old Sancho, a "Negro doctor" enslaved by Chaplin. Nancy, Chaplin noted, "has been sick for 2 years & will not speak to anyone."[44] Although he allowed the visit, Chaplin judged Free Billy "an infernal fool" for this expedition. His skeptical journal entry suggests that white and black southerners sometimes understood the nature and origin of mental ailments quite differently.[45]

Likewise, the conjured body was not the medical body understood by nineteenth-century white doctors and scientists. White physicians assumed that the body was subject to both external and internal forces; a person could be sickened by poisonous air or unbalanced by extreme emotion. Their medical training did not, however, allow for physical affliction by the spiritual power of conjuration. Though their training in anatomy was frequently spotty, antebellum white doctors envisioned the body as a skeletal frame with specific organs inside predictable body cavities held together by connecting ligaments and mesenteries.[46] In contrast, conjure stories portrayed the afflicted body as a porous entity, permeable to graveyard dirt, snakeskin powder, and the spiritual forces they contained. The afflicting creatures failed to respect anatomical boundaries of organs, skin, and bone. Charles Chesnutt made this point in his apt observation: "The lizard and snakes in these stories, by the way, are not confined to the usual ducts and cavities of the human body, but seem to have freedom of movement throughout the whole structure."[47] Descriptions of affliction render a picture of the conjured body as open to both spirit and nature. Emphasizing both the social and the religious context for suffering, the illness narratives of afflicted men and women suggest how enslaved African Americans perceived the human body within the pharmocosm.

Gruesome as the signs of conjuration were, they were not the cause of a sufferer's illness. Rather than symptoms of a disease, the snakes and spiders moving beneath the victim's skin more accurately signified the presence and power of a conjure spell. Creeping reptiles served as agents of ill will, embodied in the trick placed for the victim and enacted inside the victim.

Pain and disability therefore could not be relieved without addressing the afflictor's harming intentions. As a result, conjure sufferers sought healers who could address not only the decay of their bodies but the social conflict where affliction had begun.

Conjure Doctors and the Search for Healing

Without a conjure doctor's aid, the conjure trick could destroy both life and sanity. A Durham, North Carolina, conjure man explained that unless the victim sought a cure, he or she "either goes crazy or dies."[48] By necessity the third stage of a conjure victim's illness narrative turned temporarily from the experience of suffering to focus on the individual described by W. E. B. Du Bois as the healer, interpreter, comforter, and avenger of the plantation slave quarters.[49] Sufferers expected conjure doctors to answer several critical questions: Who had placed the hoodoo spell? Would the conjure doctor be powerful enough to overcome the trick and cure the victim before it was too late? Would the doctor turn the affliction back against the person who sent it? Each of these questions revolved around the conjurer's power to intervene in the pharmocosm by initiating processes of healing and harming.

The fact that many conjure doctors could be hired to either "cure or kill" served only to increase their stature as healers.[50] Just as Kongo sufferers enlisted *minkisi* for cures because of their healing and harming properties, so, too, enslaved African Americans consulted conjure doctors who dealt in life and death. James Washington, a Georgia root doctor and diviner interviewed in the 1930s, acknowledged the dual nature of conjuring power. "I hab a deep knowledge uh magic," he explained. "Deah's magic wut gahd yuh frum hahm an deah's ebil magic wut kin put yuh down sick aw eben kill yuh."[51] Although this twentieth-century doctor distinguished between the "good" and "evil" sides of power, antebellum African Americans were more likely to embrace a dualistic view of the conjurer's healing and harming services.[52] Many conjure doctors whose work included both affliction and healing spoke of having a "special revelation from God" and described themselves as "heaven sent" and "twice blessed."[53]

Unfamiliar with a moral world in which healing and harming were dual aspects of a practitioner's power, white medical doctors offered little hope to conjure victims. James Washington summed up the predicament: "Wen yuh bin fix, yuh [can't] git well wid regluh medicine."[54] Hardy Jones of Augusta, Georgia, agreed. "Whenever somebody fixes you, doctors never know what's wrong," he told his interviewers in 1936. "Dey think you have a new disease and call in other doctors, but none of 'em can't do you no good. De only way you kin git better is to have somebody who is already in deir good mind and know dese things can be done, to go and see 'bout you."[55] Medical doctors, asserted Hardy Jones, could not conceive of an affliction based on social conflict and spiritual power; they were incapable of knowing "dese things can be done" and therefore were ineffective as healers. Jones spoke from experience. His own affliction, like the afflictions of several other twentieth-century victims of conjuration, had ultimately resulted in incarceration in the state mental asylum.[56]

Slave society posed even greater obstacles for antebellum African Americans in search of a conjure doctor. Many planters made efforts to quash all evidence of hoodoo on their grounds. According to Virginia midwife Marrinda Jane Singleton, planters violently opposed the use of charms to ward off illness and misfortune. She recalled that conjuration "caused so much confusion among the slaves, along wid fear dat the Marsters took steps to drive it out by severe punishment to those that took part in any way."[57] The impasse between conjure practices and the beliefs of white medical doctors further suppressed the open practice of conjuration on plantations.[58] For individuals who attempted to gain help beyond the plantation's boundaries, patrollers and pass laws made travel difficult and dangerous. These hostile conditions compounded the sufferer's affliction, for the longer one languished under a conjure spell, the more difficult full recovery became.[59]

Such was the predicament of Peter, enslaved on Thomas Chaplin's modestly sized Sea Island plantation. After Peter had been sick for several months, Chaplin confessed in his journal, "God knows what is the matter with him, I do not." The white doctor, whose medicinal powders failed to cure Peter's fever, reported that Peter's "mind is worried by Negroes putting notions in his head that he is tricked." Angered by this news, Chaplin employed the language of hoodoo itself to express his own prerogative of violence: "I will trick some of them if I hear any more of it."[60] Although at least two older "negro doctors" lived in the immediate vicinity, Chaplin's hostility would have forced Peter to consult them in secret — a difficult task for the invalid patient whose affliction ultimately proved fatal.

Despite tremendous opposition, enslaved communities continued to seek protection and healing in conjuring practices. Men and women hid small charms under their clothes because, as Marrinda Jane Singleton explained, "Many of us slaves feared de charm of witchcraft more than de whippin' dat de Marster gave."[61] Archaeological excavations of "hidey holes" — underground storage areas in slave houses — provide material evidence of the sacred practices of enslaved communities. Brass amulets, pierced silver coins used to detect the presence of hoodoo work, and glass beads all signaled a hidden material culture of conjuration and the persistence of a relational view of health and illness.[62] Conjure "kits" containing the tools of the conjurer's trade have also been recovered within slave housing, suggesting the activities of ritual specialists and the reliance of enslaved communities upon them.[63]

Like the hidden artifacts of hoodoo, a conjure doctor's identity was no secret to enslaved families on nearby farms and plantations. The religious, juridical, and political leadership of conjure men and women placed them, as John Blassingame has suggested, at the "top of the slave social ladder" and secured them a measure of notoriety.[64] "It was known everywhere dat she wuz a conjurer," said Anna Grant of an older woman called "Aunt Gracie."[65] One Georgia woman recalled a conjure doctor known as "Aunt Sally the conjure woman" throughout her neighborhood, while Virginia folklorists reported that black Virginians simply preferred the respectful title "doctor."[66] Conjurers were said to be either "tall and dark" or extremely short and to have red eyes, blue gums, a piercing gaze, or some unusual feature such as a shriveled arm.[67] These striking physical attributes signified the unseen power of conjure doctors and confirmed their local prominence among enslaved communities.[68]

In contrast to the exclusivity of white professional medicine, the conjurer's power was not a male preserve. Much of the evidence above clearly suggests that conjure victims consulted both male and female practitioners. Although conjure doctors sometimes specialized in gender-specific concerns, such as childbearing or impotence, both men and women gained considerable respect as hoodoo practitioners.[69] A white doctor from Maryland wrote in 1861 that nearly every neighborhood harbored "an old negro woman who is regarded by the other negroes with profound awe and fear, on account of her supposed possession of occult powers, by which she can, at will, bring pain and death upon her enemies."[70] Despite his antagonism the Maryland doctor bore inadvertent testimony to the importance of elderly enslaved women who, alongside male conjure doctors, rendered both spiritual and healing services to their neighbors. In contrast to the white medical profession, age, spiritual revelation, and previous experiences of affliction and apprenticeship figured much more heavily in building a conjurer's reputation than did the oppositional dichotomies of manhood and womanhood.[71]

Enslaved men and women frequently traversed plantation boundaries in their search for reputed healers who shared their vision of health. Emmaline Kilpatrick of Georgia described how enslaved women crossed the nearby creek to visit an old Indian woman who made charms related to childbirth. During the spate of poisonings on the Butler family's plantation, overseer Roswell King accused the driver Elijah of making secret nighttime visits on horseback to a conjure doctor on a neighboring plantation. Similarly, when the absentee Robert Williams wanted to return home without retaliation from the plantation owner, he "wandered over to Dr. Ned Rood's quarters," where he knew he could find "a slave an' a hoo-doo doctor" to help.[72] Despite the restrictions that slave society placed on the mobility of African Americans, these discreet visits illuminated the boundaries of neighborhood slave communities that reached beyond individual plantations and incorporated free blacks and Native Americans as well. Sharing these community boundaries, conjure doctors drew on their knowledge to address the social basis of their clients' afflictions.

Conjure doctors also shared the material world of their clients and became important points of exchange within internal slave economies. While studies of the domestic slave economy tend to focus on livestock, crops, and garden produce, healing transactions also contributed to building local economies among slaves.[73] Payment for services was required and perhaps even ritually necessary. Old Bab Russ, a South Carolina conjure doctor, assembled his hoodoo "hands" (spiritually powerful packets of materials) for gaining a lover according to the following recipe:

Little pinch o' pepper,
Little bunch o' wool.

Mumbledy — mumbledy

Two, three Pammy Christy beans,
Little piece o' rusty iron.

Mumbledy — mumbledy

Wrop it in a rag and tie it with hair,
Two from a hoss and one from a mare.

Mumbledy — mumbledy

Wet it in whiskey
Boughten with silver;

That make you wash so hard your sweat pop out

And he come to pass, sure![74]

Clients of Old Bab paid both for the hand and for whiskey to feed it; the purchase with silver described in these verses appears necessary to activate Old Bab's charm.

As was the case with most economic transactions among slaves, fees charged by conjure doctors were modest. Limited evidence on the economy of healing suggests that enslaved conjurers' fees changed over time from largely in-kind payments to include cash payments as money became more available in the southern economy and in the slaves' internal economy. In 1791, for example, Virginia court testimony indicated that Ben, who "pretend[ed] to be a Cungerer & forting teller," received from his clients "a dram or some other trifle" for his services.[75] Another conjurer who appeared in Virginia court testimony in 1806 demanded a bottle of spirits and a linen shirt in exchange for sharing his art with an enslaved man.[76] As valued property useful in trading among slave communities, liquor and fine clothing may have elevated the status of these early conjurers.[77]

In the antebellum years and continuing into the postemancipation period, conjure doctors tended to collect their fees in coin. Henry Bibb reported paying small sums of money to two different conjure men in exchange for courtship charms.[78] In the 1840s William Wells Brown paid twenty-five cents for divination by an elderly enslaved man in St. Louis.[79] Likewise, Emmaline Kilpatrick reported that the men and women who crossed the creek to buy charms from the Indian woman paid her money in return.[80] When the fugitive Robert Williams asked a conjure man to help him return safely to his plantation, the doctor asked for a quarter but agreed to collect the payment later, as Williams was penniless.[81] These transactions echoed the warning of the conjure doctor in Fred Jones's longer narrative above: "I caahn do yuh no good less yuh staht off wid some silbuh."[82]

The expectation of payment revealed a distinct moral economy surrounding the conjurer's healing and harming work. Payment was necessary not only to a conjurer's livelihood but to the sufferer's cure. As a cautionary tale from Lowcountry South Carolina suggests, clients who neglected to pay risked further affliction. Zackie Knox recounted the story of a woman who neglected to pay the conjurer for a trick put on the woman's husband. In retaliation the conjurer turned the spell back on her and gave her the "wandering sickness."[83] It is not surprising that some African Americans, particularly after emancipation, condemned the hold of conjurers on the pocketbooks of impoverished individuals. Elderly Squire Irvin, a Texas man born into slavery in Tennessee, dismissed hoodoo doctors as "just highway robbers."[84] Though opinions on conjurers' fees varied, most clients assumed that conjure doctors, like white medical doctors, required remuneration.

This distinct moral economy did not necessarily extend to other African American practitioners. Herbalists and midwives, who explained their powers as a gift from God for relieving suffering, sometimes took donations or in-kind payments but worried that charging a fee would somehow taint their work. Harriet Tubman, for example, declined any compensation for her herbal remedies administered to Union troops.[85] Emma McDowell, a Virginia healer who specialized in healing bleeding and burns, explained, "I never makes no charge, if I did I would lose the magic but, of course if they gives me something I can take it."[86] Midwives who attended birthing mothers and looked after the households of enslaved and free families collected a few dollars from families who could afford it but also accepted in-kind payments of whatever poorer families could give.[87] Conjure doctors, however, required payment, and their clients expected to pay.

The search for a doctor represented the turning point in most conjuring narratives, for it was the conjure doctor who could expose the origins of affliction in social conflict and thereby initiate a cure. Under the conditions of slavery, simply securing the services of a conjure doctor required considerable and often secretive effort. Yet for many sufferers the search was critical, for only conjurers possessed the power to manipulate the web of social and spiritual forces underlying affliction. Conjure doctors offered an opportunity for enslaved men and women to address affliction in a spiritual realm outside the control of slaveholders. Furthermore, conjurers were tied to their enslaved clients not only by common belief but also by geography, shared community, and local economy. The prominent place of the conjure doctor in narratives of affliction reflected the sufferer's concern with addressing the relational dimensions of illness.

Divination and the Dynamics of Curing

Conjuring narratives culminated in the healer's attempt to cure the afflicted person. Alex Johnson of Georgia summed up this final stage as a conclusion to his own story of conjuring: "I am going to see a new root-doctor, and find out who *worked* on me, have the spell tuk off of me, and put on the person who *spelled* me."[88] Narrators retold in dramatic terms just how the conjurer detected the guilty party, ferreted out the hand that had been "put down" by the victim's adversary, and removed the fix. Most important to this analysis of the social basis of healing was the conjurer's approach to curing. Rather than focusing exclusively on the affliction within the body of the conjured person, the healer was expected to determine who "worked on" or "spelled" the sufferer. The conjure doctor and the sufferer both proceeded from the assumption that relief would come only through attention to the underlying social conflict and the spiritual origins of affliction.

The process of working backward from the illness to its origins in social conflict began with divination, the ritualized practice of obtaining hidden knowledge through supernatural assistance. Methods of divination were numerous and widespread in southern slave communities. By reading the movements or alignments of coffee grounds, cards, bones, and other materials the diviner discerned information to help an afflicted person pursue a cure. Europeans and Native Americans had their own fortune-tellers and seers whose traditions may have influenced the practices of captive Africans arriving in North America.[89] The use of English titles such as "fortune-teller," however, should not obscure the African origins of slave divination practices. In many African cultures, divination served (and continues to serve) as a primary mode of decision making and a central way of learning about and relating to the world. This interpretation of divination as a "way of knowing" provides a useful heuristic device for understanding the conjurer's work in the antebellum South.[90] Through divination the practitioner offered the afflicted person a way of knowing his or her illness that could lead to a cure.

The knowledge most clients sought from divination concerned the social origins of affliction. A sufferer most frequently wanted to know whether he or she had been tricked and, if so, by whom. In postemancipation Virginia, interviewers collected an account of a woman who had been given up for dead by a physician. As a last resort the sick woman consulted "old Lady Calloway," a diviner and conjurer. Old Lady Calloway "read her cards" to determine that the woman was "not naturally sick but 'fixed.'" The healer next pinpointed the origins of her client's sickness in a complicated dispute over coveted housing on the plantation where the woman worked. The afflicted woman and her family, in turn, judged the healer's effectiveness by her insight into social relationships. The narrator concluded, "They had faith in what old lady Calloway told them because she gave an accurate description of the persons involved and also of the condition upon which they had to move [from their house]."[91]

Varying methods of divination suggested the spiritual empowerment of all objects within a sacred world. Alex Walton, a conjure doctor residing in one of Durham's black neighborhoods, worked with cards.[92] Another Virginia conjure man combined card reading with a bug crawling in a bottle to reveal the identity of the afflicting party.[93] Bones and coffee grounds also served as common tools of divination. Ann Parker described her mother, Junny, as an African "queen" and "also a witch" who used coffee grounds to see the future.[94] Similarly, two North Carolina sisters known locally as "witches" poured coffee into a long-necked gourd for divination.[95] Though their methods varied, diviners used objects to gather knowledge previously unavailable to the client. Bodily healing was not the only purpose of divination; enslaved and free blacks used divination to anticipate slaveholder violence, to make economic decisions, and to ensure success in courtship. In each case divination provided knowledge about potential misfortune and disorder in the client's life. Conjurers and diviners offered their power to restore that order.

In the course of ferreting out the origins of affliction, conjure doctors often identified the contents and location of the conjure packet that was causing the sufferer's affliction. Virginia midwife Marrinda Jane Singleton described "charms" as sacred objects "composed of herbs, roots and scraps of cloth with certain fowl feathers" whose uses were passed on from Africa via West Indian slaves.[96] Animal parts, such as rabbit paws, chicken gizzards, or reptile skin, frequently accompanied the hair, fingernails, or footprint dust of the targeted person.[97] Alex Walton, the Durham conjure man, explained that whiskey; stale rainwater; the dried powdered skin of a toad, snake, scorpion, or lizard; and a little "secret mixture" caused reptiles to creep unbearably in the victim's stomach.[98] The woman who consulted old Lady Calloway learned that she would find a "little sack of something" in her spring.[99] Likewise, Alex Johnson pulled from under his doorstep a bag with graveyard dirt, nightshade roots, and devil's snuff.[100] Although invisibly active since the onset of the sufferer's affliction, the hoodoo bag surfaced as an enlivened agent of harm in the late stages of the conjuring narrative.

In their description of conjure hands, afflicted narrators revealed a striking resemblance between African American conjure and Kongo *minkisi*.[101] Anthropologist Wyatt MacGaffey groups *minkisi* ingredients into three categories, at least two of which are also applicable to the materials of African American conjuration.[102] First came minerals from the land of the dead, chosen because all the powers of *minkisi* derived ultimately from the dead. Graveyard dust in African American usage certainly fell into this category. So potent was graveyard dust, according to Jacob Stroyer's postbellum narrative, that slave communities used it in a poison ordeal to detect thieves. The "fathers and mothers of the slaves," wrote Stroyer, said "whatever dealing those alive had with anything pertaining to the dead, [they] must be true, or they would immediately die and go to hell to burn in fire and brimstone." When presented with a mixture of graveyard dust and water, thieves would confess rather than risk death and damnation.[103] Sometimes called "goofer dust," graveyard dust comprised a common ingredient in conjure hands aimed at making an enemy leave or even causing death.[104]

The second category of *minkisi* ingredients involved materials with important metaphorical connotations. MacGaffey writes, "Such things suggested the *nkisi*'s power to attack its victims and to produce sickness and death."[105] The frequent use of a person's hair in hoodoo hands may illustrate this principle in African American conjuration. Hair and other bodily materials from the targeted individual personalized the conjure packet, directing spiritual forces toward the intended recipient. The entangling characteristics of hair also threatened mortal danger and suggested an ability to cling around and choke the victim's heart.[106] Similarly, the popularity of devil's shoestring (*Coronilla varia*) in conjuring may have been due to its metaphorical connotations. The plant's "long, wiry-looking root resembling the smallest roots of a sweet potato vine" lent the devil's shoestring its name, which may have been associated with its powers to bind desired objects to the person using the root.[107] Metaphorical connotations can also be seen in the use of the whiskers of a cat and a dog put into a conjure packet to break up a couple.[108]

Third and finally, *minkisi* incorporated materials chosen for linguistic reasons. The names of certain West Central African plants served as puns on attributes or effects that the *nganga* wished to impart to the *nkisi*. For example, Kongo practitioners might include "*luyala* [a fruit], that it may rule [*yaala*]," or "*kisimani* [a climbing plant with red pods], that it may hold tight [*simana*]."[109] Translated into the North American English-speaking context, the linguistic implications of African American conjure materials are much more difficult to decipher or detect. The artful composition of North American conjure packets nonetheless paralleled the complexity of Kongo *minkisi*.

Taken as a whole, the conjure packet was more than the sum of its parts. A conjure packet was a "bricolage," a stunning array of mutually referential materials combined to embody and direct spiritual force.[110] The ritual process of making a conjure hand housed spiritual power within the object. Kongo ritual specialists, according to anthropologist Wyatt MacGaffey, made *minkisi* by enclosing sacred medicines in tightly wrapped packages elaborately tied for a complex visual presentation. The knots conveyed a sense of the containment of powerful forces, while the "sheer intricacy of texture and detail" suggested something remarkable and "astonishing."[111]

MacGaffey's argument that a visually striking appearance was part of the power of the *nkisi* itself resonates with lyrics in a Kentucky hoodoo song describing the conjure hand:

Take it out before der eyes,
An' you mus' be awful s'prised
And dey well think dat you is wise,
Hoo-doo[112]

As the song implied, African American conjure packets could also be elaborate and "surprising" in their construction. Many African American packets reflected an emphasis on containment, tying, and the mixture of roots, minerals, and human artifacts wrapped within cloth that echoed the ritual construction of Kongo *minkisi*. Consider, for example, the detailed description of a Mississippi conjure man's hand containing a small sandburr, a piece of Samson's snakeroot, and a piece of devil's shoestring, all wrapped in black cloth folded toward the maker, secured with white thread, and put into a red flannel bag. The colors used to make the hand further link this conjure doctor's art to certain classes of Kongo *minkisi* that signal their formidable power in red cloth and black thread.[113]

Making conjure packets in the antebellum years was a complicated process often requiring the cover of nighttime. Emmaline Heard, the source of the story about the conjurer Ned and the unfortunate young woman who caught his eye, provided valuable insight into the conjurer's work during slavery. Heard's father had been sold from Virginia to Georgia as a boy under the prevailing patterns of the antebellum domestic slave trade. Arriving at his Georgia destination, her father was boarded with "old uncle Ned," the plantation's only "bachelor" and a conjure man. Ned, like many enslaved African Americans, used the late night hours for his own purposes. Feigning sleep, Emmaline Heard's father watched each night with fascination as "old Ned" painstakingly assembled his conjuring bags:

"After a while uncle Ned would take a broom and sweep the fireplace clean, then he would get a basket and take out of it a whole lot of little bundles wrapped in white cloth. As he lay out a package he would say 'grass hoppers,' 'spiders,' 'scorpion,' 'snake heads,' etc., then he would take the tongs and turn 'em around before the blaze so that they would parch. Night after night he would do this same thing until they had parched enough, then he would beat all of it together and make a powder; then put it up in little bags."[114] This rare description of an antebellum conjurer preparing materials conveys his concern for secrecy and caution. The careful storage of the materials and Ned's recitation of their contents suggests that the process of assembling these materials possessed ritual significance.

Once the cause of affliction had been divined and exposed, the conjured person had somehow to undo or reverse the power of the hoodoo trick. Some sufferers took defensive steps, such as sprinkling red pepper and sulfur in and around the house to purify it.[115] A Georgia woman shook black pepper and potash around the spot where she had discovered a conjure bottle. She then followed up her precautions by enlisting some friends to wash her body daily with whiskey.[116] When self-help measures failed and the trick was deemed too powerful for lay efforts, the sufferer enlisted a conjure doctor's aid. Some conjure doctors sent their clients home with medicine to ingest or to apply on dangerous surfaces in the house. Durham doctor Alex Walton administered a secret mixture with nauseous effects not unlike those of the strong emetics of antebellum white physicians.[117] If a client was bedridden, the conjurer performed curing rituals at the bedside, using cupping horns, songs, and massage to withdraw the offending snakes, lizards, or other reptiles from the sick person's body.[118] Under slavery these sessions had to be conducted in secret or carried on with the grudging tolerance of white planters.

In search of a cure, both the sick person and the conjurer faced a potential ethical dilemma. Many hoodoo practitioners with healing and harming powers gave the sick person the opportunity to turn the hoodoo back against the individual who originated it. Old Lady Calloway, for example, informed her client that she would do anything but kill the person who had conjured her. In deciding whether or not to turn the trick back, the sufferer confronted the original conflict and decided if reciprocal harm would bring a cure. Speaking to interviewers in the 1930s, one Georgia woman declared that she "always treats people right" but that it had not done her any good. "Now I'se made it up in my mind to treat folks just like dey treats me. If dey do somethin' to me, I'll have it turned back on 'em," she

resolved.[119] The final stage of many conjuring narratives portrayed healing as a series of moral decisions with consequences reaching beyond the
afflicted individual to a broader community.

Some afflicted persons blended a Christian ethic of turning the other
cheek with a right to self-defense. Hector Godbold of South Carolina gave
the following advice: "It just like dis, I say fight all right, but don' never
turn no mean trick back. Turn it to God, dat what do."[120] Another Georgia
woman declined the chance to turn the trick back and make her antagonist
go mad because she felt sorry for the woman's children.[121] Matilda Henrietta Perry, afflicted with large bumps under her arms, took a similar stance.
The conjure doctor to whom Perry turned for help urged her to take the
quickest course of healing. He sang, "Give it back to her what gived it to
you an' I kin cure you." Perry refused, arguing that turning back such a
spell would jeopardize her place in heaven.[122] For some Christian believers
like Perry, seeking a conjure doctor for healing was entirely consistent with
one's faith; seeking revenge was not.

As Perry recounted, the conjure doctor eventually gave her a dose of
medicine that compelled her enemy to confess in song throughout the
neighborhood:

Oh yes! Oh yes!
I been conjurin'
Oh yes! Oh yes! Oh yes!
I been killin',
No cause, no cause, no cause,
In de worl'

Oh yes! Oh yes!
I conjured you,
I conjured you,
No cause in de worl',
No cause in de worl',
Give me yo' han',
Give me yo' han'

Upon taking her afflictor's hand, Perry began to heal. The conjure doctor's
medicine thus worked not only on Perry but also on her relationship with
her neighbor. In Perry's story the cycle of disease and restoration within
her body mirrored the fracture and resolution of community relationships.
The concluding scene of forgiveness and healing was unusual; many other

narratives recounted the adjustment of social conflicts by harming, intimidating, or sending away one's adversary. Some stories involved revenge and retaliation; others ended in gruesome death for the sufferer. Consistent among these conjure narratives, however, was the relational context of affliction and curing. From the initial scenarios of conflict to the concluding question of turning back the trick, individual health and healing was embedded in a local community and imbued with supernatural significance.

Moving from affliction to healing, the narrators of conjure stories did indeed represent their illness as "present in a life." Told from the perspective of the sufferer rather than the practitioner, conjure narratives placed illness and the search for healing within a dense web of human and spiritual relationships. In contrast to ethnographic descriptions focused on a particular system of medicine, conjuring narratives provided highly personalized accounts of affliction.[123] Sufferers suggested that the illness they experienced in their bodies was incomprehensible outside relationships of community conflict and support. So essential was the collective basis of conjured illness that the cure itself required a diviner to examine the client's past interactions with neighbors and adversaries. Detailed accounts of "unnatural illness" revealed historical tensions arising in slave communities concerning family, sexuality, and material resources.

Equally important, conjuration narratives also vividly demonstrated the spiritual importance of black doctoring in enslaved communities. Although located outside the institutional structures of the Christian church, conjuration was an important black "metaphysical tradition" at the center of the religion of enslaved communities.[124] Portrayed as a disruptive and barbaric practice by antebellum whites and as a quaint relic of a colorful folk culture by many twentieth-century folklore collectors, hoodoo has been the most consistently denigrated of all the African American doctoring arts. The complex structure of conjure packets, the delicate dualities of healing and harming, and the ethics of turning back a trick, however, all suggest a rich cosmology that gave meaning to experiences of bodily suffering. Permeable to the healing and harming forces of the pharmocosm, the human body underwent a process of physical and mental decay that failed to respond to white medical treatments. Conjuring narratives thus repeatedly affirmed the power of the pharmocosm and suggested the incomplete control that whites had over black bodies.

Herein lay the political importance of African American doctoring, for its active practice on southern plantations was a constant reminder that slaveholder power was only partial. Like the residents of Roslin Plantation who rejected the overseer's diagnosis of Calia's illness, enslaved African Americans continued to adhere to a view of health that was consistent with their cosmology and collective experience. Bondsmen and bondswomen brought this relational view of health to their work as healers and their actions as patients. In the process, plantation health matters became occasions for struggle and negotiation over broader issues of power.

II Arenas of Conflict

I just always seemed to know how to work cures and make medicines.
Folks was always coming to me and asking me to cure some illness.
When I was young and went out washing I didn't have much time to
cure folks. Then when I get too old to work steady I stay home and mix
up all kind of charms and magic remedies.
— *"Ma Stevens," ca. 1937, Georgia*

Women
Black women
Looking at white women
Never had illusions about being that
There was never any possibility
It was just not in the offering
Too far away from keeping Black folks alive
So when you look at what Black women do
You are looking at people who have to fashion a something else
A way out of no way
— *Bernice Johnson Reagon,*
    "My Black Mothers and Sisters," Feminist Studies, *1982*

CHAPTER 5
Doctoring Women

In 1832 planter Alexander Telfair instructed his overseer that, except in rare cases, an enslaved woman named Elsey should serve as the Thorn Island Plantation's doctor. "Elsey is the Doctress of the Plantation," he wrote. "In case of extraordinary illness, when she thinks she can do no more for the sick you will employ a Physician." Well into her seventies, Elsey had a reputation as a healer that reached beyond the boundaries of the plantation and earned her daunting responsibilities. She doctored all but the most severe ailments among more than thirty-five men, women, and children on the South Carolina Lowcountry plantation described by a despairing overseer as a place of "sickness and death." Elsey also served as midwife "to black & white in the neighborhood." So popular were her services that the Telfair family became anxious about collecting the large outstanding debt owed by nearby families in return for Elsey's midwifery work. Nor did her work end there, for Elsey also cared for the enslaved children, fed the poultry, and rendered tallow to make plantation supplies.[1]

As the prominence of Elsey's name in the Telfair instructions suggests, the older women whom planters called "nurses," "doctresses," and "midwives" provided crucial labor to southern plantations.[2] Their work did not necessarily exclude knowledge of conjuration, but daily sickcare bore a different relationship to plantation production and structures of power than did the clandestine practice of antebellum hoodoo. Whereas conjure doctors practiced outside the realm of plantation production and drew hostility from planters, slave nurses and midwives engaged in labor requisitioned by planters. While slaves hid conjure practices from slaveholders, bondswomen cared for the plantation's sick under occasional, if not intensive, white scrutiny. Finally, while slaveholders reluctantly conceded the fact that conjurers wielded power, they tended to view enslaved women who tended the sick not as powerful figures but as menial workers.[3] Planters frequently mentioned slave women as health workers but rarely elaborated on the content of their work. Plantation sickcare thus engendered tensions between slave women's skills and their position as subordinate health workers that were not present in the social relations of African American conjuring.

Contradictory elements of skill and servitude suffused the daily work of doctoring and, by extension, raise general questions about historical understandings of skill in slave women's labor. Nursing the sick in plantation households required experience and expertise as well as close observation and innovation. In fact, midwifery and sickcare, along with cooking and sewing, were among the few specialized labor roles reserved for enslaved women. Yet doctoring work, while indeed skillful, was at the same time fatiguing, repetitive, and dirty. Both planters and slave communities depended heavily on slave women for the bulk of daily health work. Within the gendered divisions of labor operative on southern plantations, slave women added health work to their agricultural labor, childbearing, childcare, and subsistence production activities. Daily sickcare thus represented both skilled labor and an arena of "superexploitation" for enslaved women in the Americas.[4]

Contradictions between skill and servitude in slave women's sickcare reveal similarities across time and space among societies that relegate hands-on care of the sick to subordinate groups of women. As sociologist Tim Diamond contended for late-twentieth-century care in nursing homes, classifying hands-on care of the sick or elderly as "menial" tends to obscure the complex nature of the work performed.[5] In the homes and plantations of wealthier antebellum whites, women of the enslaved and working classes supplied a large amount of the intimate and exhausting labor of domestic medicine. Household nursing tasks shared much with other domestic work generally performed by enslaved and servant women in their own homes and in the homes of the dominant classes. Furthermore, the vulnerability and dependency associated with sickcare, along with other domestic work, raised fears among slaveholders and employers of contagion, poisoning, and betrayal.[6] Enslaved women, like subordinate female health workers in other historical contexts, found that the social relations of domestic sickcare resulted in a devaluation of their skills and rendered their autonomy suspect in the eyes of the planter class.

The location of slave households within the larger plantation household meant that bondswomen nursed the sick not only because slaveholders required it but also because they were mothers, grandmothers, and next-door neighbors of the sick. Despite their legal status as property and the threat of sale and separation, enslaved African Americans nevertheless constituted themselves as families and doctored one another within their households and communities. Enslaved African Americans differed considerably from slaveholders in their recognition of the skills of doctoring women. Defining skill in relation to collective need, spiritual revelation, and teaching from older generations, enslaved African Americans left much richer descriptions of the content and meaning of slave women's health work. A general recognition and respect for slave women's doctoring skills prevailed among enslaved communities, while at the same time the gendered division of labor on plantations shifted most of the work of sickcare to black women. For every woman like Elsey who entered the written historical record, a multitude of unrecorded enslaved women worked to preserve the health of their families and neighbors.

Waiting on Them All: The Domestic Work of Plantation Doctoring

As plantation health workers, enslaved women practiced a form of domestic medicine with little relation to the metaphorical "private sphere" of women, hearth, and home.[7] Plantations contained both white and black households; they were also agricultural enterprises connected to an international market.[8] Few slave women doctors, even midwives, worked in spaces defined strictly as private, female domains. Nursing the sick took place within family dwellings—the primary connotation of "domestic" medicine—but extended into plantation hospitals and yards as well. Furthermore, enslaved healers rarely worked in settings completely free of the slaveholder's vested interests in slave health. Enslaved women did indeed provide much of the household health care of southern plantations, but their work traversed the frayed boundaries between public and private, home and market, and skill and expected subservience.

The contested social relations of plantation medicine hinged on the uneven division of health work. Slave women provided the foundation of health care for African Americans during slavery, but they were not the only plantation practitioners. Slaveholding men and women, as well as overseers, frequently intervened in matters of slave health. Yet as Alabama freedwoman Sarah Fitzpatrick recalled, enslaved women carried on the bulk of day-to-day plantation healing work. When slaves became sick, she explained, those who worked in the "Big House" received medicine from the mistress. On the plantation the overseer "is'ued out all de medicine." Above all, however, older slave women "waited on all o'em."[9] Fitzpatrick's words suggest that in addition to its spatial division between Big House and quarters, healing work was also distributed unevenly among plantation residents. Her description of enslaved women as waiting on everyone conveyed the perpetual demands of caring directly for the bodies of the sick and injured.

To the extent that they were able, slaveholding men sought to limit their involvement in the sickcare of the enslaved to examining and prescribing medicine and directing the labor of other plantation health workers. At some time most slaveowners examined and dosed sick slaves. As mentioned in Chapter 3, John Walker of Virginia ordered a commercial medicine chest and began treating enslaved men and women with the steam baths and cayenne pepper remedies of the Thomsonians.[10] Rice planter Louis Manigault carefully recorded his treatment of slaves who had fallen ill during a cholera epidemic in 1852.[11] Agricultural journals touted plantation health practices as evidence of benevolent mastery and scientific management. Few customary health practices, however, required male planters to perform the daily labor of sickcare. The involvement of white men in domestic medicine, while extensive at times, generally mirrored their position within the patriarchal society.

On larger plantations, overseers generally had more daily contact with ailing slaves. Overseer John Murphy, who supervised one of the Telfairs' Georgia plantations, wrote to his employer of the constant demands of "attending to the sick."[12] In addition to prescribing medicines, overseers vaccinated against smallpox, monitored the cleanliness of slave quarters, moved enslaved occupants to presumably healthier land during epidemics, and even regulated the activities of breastfeeding mothers.[13] They also restocked plantation medical supplies and made decisions about when to summon a white doctor. The 1837 Telfair instruction book for Thorn Island Plantation directed the overseer not to call a physician until he had tried a dose of castor oil, a dose of calomel, and a blister.[14] References to Elsey as doctress in these same instructions beg the question of who actually administered these medicines. Yet the involvement of overseers, as well as male planters, in certain aspects of plantation health work contradicts the conventional images of domestic medicine as an exclusively female sphere of labor.

White slaveholding women, on the other hand, have played an elevated role in white historical memory as the literal embodiment of plantation domestic caregiving. Many white mistresses spent considerable time in work related to the health of slaves. Will Sheets, an elderly freedman, recalled that when illness struck during slavery, "miss Carrie done de doctorin' herself."[15] Slaveholding women who lived on or near plantations visited sick children and adults in slave dwellings and sickhouses and even intervened in the health decisions of overseers. Drawing from both family tradition and standard orthodox medicines, they often made remedies or supervised their production by enslaved women. Natalie Delage Sumter, for example, recorded in her diary in 1840, "rose at 7—went in the store room below & remained there to fix all the medicines till 12."[16] Responding to minor ailments and fatal illnesses, women like Sumter treated colds with herbal teas, medicated cuts and burns, lanced infections and the gums of teething babies, and ordered special food for invalids.[17]

The remarks made by slaveholding women about their plantation health work revealed the entanglement of home and market in plantation "domestic" medicine. For white women who complained of being the "slave of slaves," nursing work figured heavily in the list of burdensome tasks. One South Carolina mistress lamented, "Morning, noon, and night, I'm obliged to look after them, to doctor them, and attend to them in every way."[18] Many women in the planter class apparently combined feelings of moral responsibility with awareness of property considerations. Solomon Northup, for example, described one white woman's reaction when her drunken husband stabbed an elderly enslaved man. While sewing up the man's wound, she upbraided her husband for his cruelty and for his carelessness with their property.[19] Others, such as Lydia Riddick of North Carolina, regarded the supervision of slave health as an irritation born of financial necessity. In a letter to her son, Riddick reported the death of a slave child: "Eugenia's baby has been dead about five weeks, I cannot say I am sorry as it would have been a deal of trouble for me, without any promise of benefit."[20] Such statements call into question the emotional context of maternal and familial motivations upon which domestic medicine is conventionally presumed to depend.

As domestic healers, white mistresses occupied a position of privileged subordination reflecting their place within the southern social order. As subordinates of planter-class men, slaveholding women sometimes incurred risks when their interventions in matters of slave health affronted patriarchal authority. Dave Lawson, formerly enslaved by a North Carolina man with a volatile temper, told a story of domestic violence erupting from plantation medical care. When the mistress smoothed salve onto the cuts of a slave woman her husband had lashed, he began to whip her too, swearing all the while that "when he want his niggers doctored he gwine doctor dem hese'f."[21] This incident of domestic violence, observed and recorded in African American oral history, suggested one white woman's intervention in slave health and the limits of her authority as a female domestic healer.

At the same time, women of the planter class derived considerable privileges from the health work of enslaved African Americans. In an 1859 journal entry Carolina planter David Gavin complained that he had removed his "best hand," Mike, from the field to attend Mr. Griffin, the overseer who suffered from a whitlow, or boil on his hand. The disgruntled Gavin reserved most of his ire for the overseer's wife as he remarked that the task of nursing Mr. Griffin should have fallen to Mrs. Griffin instead. Mrs. Griffin's failure as domestic healer of her household was only one among many offenses that caused Gavin to comment that she "seems to want as much waiting on as the mistress of the plantation."[22] From Gavin's perspective, the use of slave labor for nursing, like other domestic services, was a privilege properly reserved for planter-class women, not common whites like the overseer's wife.

Plantation mistresses assumed a managerial role in plantation health work that, although demanding enough in itself, released them from the most distasteful and laborious tasks associated with nursing. As James Bolton recalled, "When we got sick, Mistress allus had us tended to."[23] Natalie Delage Sumter, a planter in South Carolina's piedmont region, left detailed records indicating what was involved in tending the sick on her plantation. As a recent widow Sumter assumed more of the responsibilities of running her family's plantation than did most married slaveholding women. She kept track of illness within the slave quarters, sent medicines and food, and visited the sick to determine whether to summon a white doctor. Yet even Sumter, who recorded her daily work meticulously in her diary, noted visits to the sick in the slave quarters only nineteen times during the year 1840–41. Since she herself mentioned slave illness at least thirty times and physician visits only five times, it is clear that other hands participated in sickcare. Sumter's journal indicates her reliance on enslaved women to attend the sick. Once, for example, Sumter discovered that a sick woman, Milly, had not been properly attended. She promptly directed another woman, Diana, to administer the medication prescribed by a visiting physician.[24] On another September night she recorded, "after dark went to plantation to see two sick negroes & put old Anna to stay tonight with Cesar to take care of him & carried them soup."[25] Sumter's detailed records reflect a typical division of plantation healing work between enslaved and slaveholding women.[26]

On one level the sheer volume of work to be done motivated slaveholders to recruit health workers from all sectors of the enslaved population. Plantations with sizable slave quarters required daily healing work far exceeding the capacities of white residents. David Gavin's decision to assign Mike to the overseer's care indicates that enslaved men were at times enlisted in plantation health work. When epidemics erupted, even drivers helped treat the sick. A physician visiting Sea Island plantations during the 1849 cholera outbreak directed a black driver to administer calomel, opium, and cold sheet wraps to enslaved sufferers.[27] Richard James Arnold instructed his Lowcountry overseers to look to Dick, an elderly man, as a "good nurse" for cases of cholera.[28] Enslaved children of both sexes also worked at menial tasks of nursing. In keeping with the general lack of gender distinctions between slave boys and girls before puberty, one man born in the 1850s spent his boyhood waiting on the sick, cleaning the privy, and emptying chamber pots.[29]

Despite the participation of men and women, old and young, in plantation healing work, the allocation of productive and reproductive labor meant that older women bore the brunt of plantation health work. The crux of the matter was that when mistresses saw to healing work or had the sick tended to, enslaved women often did the actual labor. Enslaved African Americans sang a song that cut to the core of these disparities between the labor of bondswomen and that of plantation mistresses.

Missus in the big house
Mammy in the yard,
Missus holdin' her white hands,
Mammy workin' hard
Missus holdin' her white hands,
Mammy workin' hard.[30]

The hard work slave women did when white mistresses tended the sick has not received full recognition. In a 1930s interview with Sara Crocker, for instance, the interviewer reported, "Whenever a slave was sick, the mistress always saw to it that he was well cared for." Only as an afterthought did the interviewer add, "If any of Sara's family were sick, her mother would help care for them."[31] As Sarah Fitzpatrick recalled in the quote above, black women waited on everyone. Within the slave quarters it was they who administered food and medicines, eased pain, caught the babies, soothed and wrapped injuries, and prepared the bodies of the dead for burial.

Three factors contributed to the gendering of sickcare as slave women's work: the close relationship between sickcare and other tasks gendered as female labor, the taxing and unpleasant nature of administering antebellum medication, and the location of sickcare work. First, sickcare in nineteenth-century households, including southern plantations, was based in the world of "women's work." More precisely, sickcare involved the kind of labor usually consigned by wealthier white households to female domestic workers.[32] Enslaved healers did not merely keep watch over the sick. Antebellum nursing involved a wide range of domestic tasks. Most medicines, even pills, did not come prepackaged, and slave women often measured, mixed, and cooked medicines prior to their use. Furthermore, diet formed an important part of antebellum sickcare. Enslaved women routinely prepared special gruel and other bland foods for invalid patients. They also cleaned instruments and containers, bathed soiled bodies, and washed the fetid bedclothes of the sick. Healing work thus overlapped with the women's work of cooking, cleaning, and laundering. On southern plantations, however, this domestic nursing might be more appropriately called subsistence labor, since it was not necessarily done within individual family dwellings and was essential to the ongoing maintenance of every plantation.

Second, nineteenth-century medical therapeutics compounded the labor of nursing the sick and helped to determine who actually performed the bulk of the work. The domestic pharmacopoeia of the planter class drew heavily on the heroic measures of orthodox medical practice. Employing their medicines aggressively, antebellum professional and domestic practitioners assaulted the disease, aiming to restore the body's internal balance.[33] Standard plantation medical supplies throughout the antebellum period included powerful laxatives such as castor oil, calomel, rhubarb, and jalap as well as ipecac and tartar emetic commonly used to induce vomiting.[34] Virginia planter William Fleming Gains's plan of attack on a dysentery epidemic in 1808 conveyed the aggressive impulse of heroic therapies: "I Ipecac it, Calomel it Rhubarb & cream of tarter it blister it sal ammoniac or ammoniac it—but never lancet it nor Jallop it."[35]

Gains did not specify who would carry out his directions, but planters generally relied on enslaved women to administer prescribed treatments. Treating the sick might involve coaxing a weakened person to swallow medicine or special foods, as well as applying external poultices or ointments and giving enemas. Ellen Betts, whose healing work stretched from slavery through emancipation, recalled, "Sometime I dose with blue mass pills, and sometime Dr. Fawcett leave rhubarb and ipecac and calomel and castor oil and such."[36] Natalie Sumter, as related above, relied on Diana to administer doses prescribed by a white doctor and depended on the elderly Anna to sit up nights with the sick. Reflecting the value of these skills to planters, a South Carolina bill of sale touted the "first-rate" ability of Clarissa, a fifty-year-old midwife and nurse, who could be "trusted to mix and administer medicine."[37]

The work of caring for the sick did not end after they had swallowed their medicines, however. Bluntly put, antebellum therapies produced vomit, excrement, or blood that had to be cleaned away before the next course of medicines. Whether prescribed by a doctor or brewed at home, many common remedies produced dramatic results and required repeated doses over a span of hours or days. Medical instructions left by a South Carolina planter make plain the labor-intensive nature of sickcare: "If any of the Negroes should be attacked with the pain in the head & become seriously sick during my absence; in the first place give an Emetic of Hippo with a portion of Calomel—If danger is threatened have them cupped on the Temples—apply Blister to the Head and back of the Neck—keep the bowels moderately open with Salts dissolved in Snake Root Tea—If stupor comes on apply mustard Plaster to the legs and arms."[38] Intended to induce dysentery patients to vomit, blister, bleed, and purge, this rigorous regime of treatment raises the question of who tended the bodies, not to mention the miserable spirits, of sufferers subjected to such treatment. While slaveholders might be willing to administer medicine, enslaved women and probably the sufferers themselves, if able, were left to clean up after the medicines had produced the desired effects. Close involvement with bodily waste while caring for the sick reinforced the link between nursing and other kinds of menial domestic work.

Third, the spatial location of most doctoring work further placed the brunt of sickcare on slave women. In the rural South, as in much of the United States, most sick people recuperated or died in their own homes.[39] Proslavery sketches might depict sick bondsmen lying on clean linens in the spacious rooms of southern mansions, but most ailing slaves remained in their usual dwellings, sometimes on a blanket in front of the fireplace. Henry Baker, enslaved in Alabama until he was a teenager, described how families sought to create space for the sick in crowded rooms where three or more people often slept in one bed. He recalled, "When a 'body got sick, 'stead uv all sleepin' wid de sick pusson dey made a pallet on de floor fuh de sick pusson."[40] In addition to being crowded, slave dwellings were also dimly lit and smoky from fires. So difficult was it to see clearly, one white observer complained, that not even a pine torch at broad noon provided adequate lighting for medical examinations.[41]

On large plantations, such as those of the Georgia and South Carolina Lowcountry, planters often required enslaved sufferers to report to a hospital or sickhouse. Planters strategically located their sickhouses close to the slave quarters and near enough to the overseer's house to allow convenient monitoring, but not too close to be considered a source of contagion to slaveholders.[42] Like the quality of health care provided for slaves, the state of plantation hospitals served as ammunition in rhetorical skirmishes over slavery. Abolitionist mistress Frances Kemble decried the lack of warmth, cleanliness, and light in the Butler Island "infirmary," a two-story, four-room wooden structure that housed men and women in separate quarters and included new mothers and babies as well. The St. Simons Island hospital, with its damp earthen floor and dark, drafty interior, elicited even more passionate condemnation from Kemble.[43] Not surprisingly, proslavery advocates described plantation hospitals in more positive terms. One agricultural journal referred to the hospital on James Hamilton Couper's plantation as an "airy and warm building," a veritable monument to modern slave management.[44]

Neither side, however, disputed the fact that enslaved women remained the most consistent presence among practitioners in plantation hospitals. On Butler Island a white doctor made occasional visits, but the midwife Rose attended the sick daily.[45] Sarah Gudger, enslaved in North Carolina,

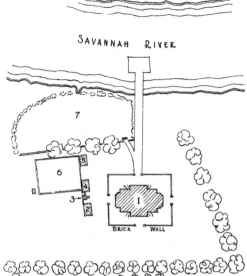

SAVANNAH RIVER

BRICK WALL

PLOT PLAN
SCALE 1"= 100'

LEGEND
1. MANSION
2. KITCHEN
3. SMOKE HOUSE
4. STABLES
5. COACH HOUSE
6. LOT
7. SUNKEN GARDEN
8. OVERSEER'S HOUSE
9. HOSPITAL
10. SLAVE HUTS
11. BRICK KILN
12. SAW-MILL
13. MILL POND
14. BURIAL GROUND

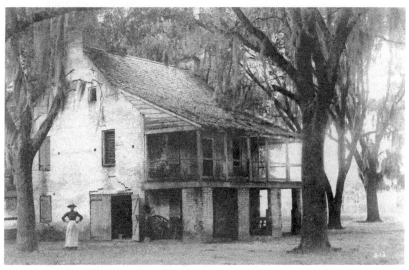

Slave hospital at the Hermitage, with unidentified woman, ca. 1883–92. The largest plantations often featured a slave hospital, or sickhouse, such as the one designed by Henry McAlpin in the 1830s to house patients from the plantation's population of nearly four hundred enslaved laborers. Plantation hospitals centralized and extended planter control over the care of enslaved patients. White doctors sometimes visited and prescribed medicines, but enslaved women provided most of the daily sickcare. (William E. Wilson Collection; courtesy of the GHS)

recalled the sickhouse as a "lil' ole house close t'de big house" where a slave nurse attended those inside.[46] Whites entered both slave houses and plantation hospitals to examine the sick but rarely remained long, except during difficult births or dangerous illnesses.[47] William Fleming Gains, one of the planters who pursued heroic remedies against dysentery, made clear his dependence on the doctoring work of enslaved women. "I have two hospitals neatly kept & fumigated every day & two excellent nurses of my own," he wrote. "I rely upon these more than any thing else, except the mercy of my God."[48] The labor-intensive, unpleasant character of plantation healing work, along with its placement within the slave quarters and plantation outbuildings, led slaveholders to designate the daily sickcare to enslaved women.

No level of skill exempted slave women from the "mudsill" tasks of nursing the plantation's sick.[49] Planters demonstrated a sense of entitlement to slave women's labor in nursing their white family members as well as individuals in the slave quarters. Harriet Newby of Virginia had firsthand

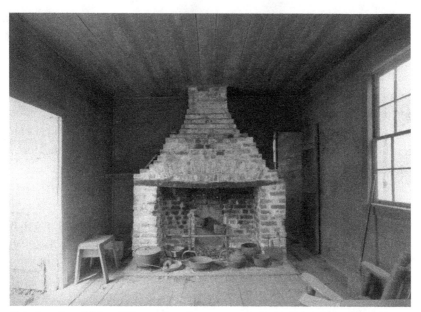

Interior view, McLeod Plantation slave quarters, James Island, South Carolina. The majority of plantations did not have hospitals built specifically for slaves. For most enslaved sufferers, sickcare took place on a pallet near the fireplace inside living quarters such as this restored slave house. The hearth provided warmth for the sick as well as a place for enslaved women to prepare medicinal teas and poultices. (Historic American Buildings Survey, Library of Congress, Washington, D.C.; photograph by John McWilliams, 1990)

experience with the fatigue and sleep deprivation inherent in sickbed attendance. In a rare letter Newby apologized to her free husband for the delay in her correspondence. Her mistress had a breast infection, she explained, "and I have had to stay with her day and night; so you know I had no time to write."[50] Likewise, Laura Smalley described the demands made on the nurse for a Texas slaveholder's child. She exclaimed, "That baby's any kind of sick that nurse had to sit up there at night and tend to it."[51] Planter families expected slave women to perform the lowest jobs in caring for white children's health. In one case Anna Garretson, a white mother in Virginia, recommended that her cousin have one of her "female servants" remove pinworms from her daughter's anus.[52] Access to this labor was the very privilege that the overseer Mr. Griffin coveted, thus leading his employer to suspect Mrs. Griffin of playing the lady.

Round-the-clock demands exacted a heavy toll from enslaved women working in the slave quarters as well as for white families. On the large plantations of the Georgia and South Carolina Lowcountry, absentee planters acknowledged their dependence on older slave women to perform most of the plantation health work. "The old Nurse Bina is a woman of the highest character[.] every body has the highest opinion of her," wrote Charles Manigault to his overseers in the 1840s. Owner of several rice plantations on the Savannah River, Manigault emphasized Nurse Binah's considerable responsibilities: "Should a Negro come to you & say he is sick you should question him as to what ails him & then tell him to go to the Nurse Bina — when you will have time to decide what is best to be given him or her."[53] The overseer was to have at least the appearance of making final decisions about medical prescriptions. Nevertheless, it was Nurse Binah who actually maintained the health of more than one hundred men and women. During the summer of 1846 many slaves, especially children, fell seriously ill from "Diarroahs & Dysentery," yet the overseer felt no need to call a physician. "Mom Banah has really managed the disease remarkably well," he reported to Charles Manigault.[54] So crucial was Binah's labor to the health of the plantation that even four years after her death in 1853, Charles Manigault continued to instruct his son Louis to follow children's health care practices adhered to by "Old Mom Bina."[55]

Overseer J. T. Cooper learned a hard lesson about the magnitude of Binah's labor when he was forced temporarily to assume her workload in 1848. That summer an epidemic of "Measles superseded by Dysentery" hit the Gowrie rice plantation. Over thirty men and women fell ill, the sickhouse overflowed, and five adults and two children died. The devastation of the slave community took a physical toll on Binah and drained her emotionally as well. According to Cooper, the "old and only nurse from constant worrying was attacked with apoplexy." To replace her, Cooper reassigned two workers from the fields to the sickhouse and other slave houses. Despite this renewed support, Cooper still found his situation "an arduous and unpleasant one." Perhaps seeking ultimately to impress his employer with his handling of the crisis, Cooper made his efforts clear: "I am up & down at all hours of the night & day & I begin to feel the effects of it."[56]

The daily work of sickcare that so drained the Gowrie overseer fell largely to enslaved women. The association of sickcare with domestic labor; the unpleasantness of preparing, administering, and cleaning up after dispensing medications; and the location of the work all defined nursing as a task of servitude. While slaveholding women in particular might expend themselves for a member of their own family, they generally avoided this type of labor in the slave quarters. The slaveholders who nursed an enslaved child or favored older person in their own house, out of a sense of benevolence, obligation, or particular affection for an individual, were the exceptions.[57] For the most part, slaveholders who became involved in the illness of their slaves attempted to separate the evaluative and prescribing aspects of doctoring from the more arduous bedside work of nursing, leaving the latter, along with related types of domestic labor, to enslaved women workers. In so doing, plantation whites revealed their own dependency on the doctoring skills of enslaved women.

Measuring Skill in Slave Communities and Plantation Books

Skill is a gendered and socially contingent attribute. The extensive historical literature on skilled slave "occupations" focuses largely on male artisans, such as blacksmiths, tanners, and coopers.[58] From North American to Caribbean plantation societies, European patriarchal notions produced a gendered division of plantation slave labor that delegated a much narrower range of specialized labor roles to enslaved women.[59] Health work occupied a prominent place among these specialized roles, which included midwives, nurses and hospital attendants, and cooks and seamstresses. Slave women's doctoring work differed considerably from the artisanal labor reserved for enslaved men, however. Older enslaved women who doctored entire slave communities practiced skilled work in the sense that they possessed accumulated experience, specialized knowledge, and some leeway for individual judgment in the implementation of that knowledge. Yet women's specialized labor did not necessarily carry with it distance from menial labor or the access to additional resources frequently identified by historians relying on a male model of skilled slave labor.[60]

The unique character of the doctoring skills of enslaved women emerged from the ways that female slave labor changed over the course of a woman's lifetime. Many specialized female healing roles involved some older women doing, in concentrated form, the work most enslaved women did on a daily basis for their families. Among enslaved families the gendered division of labor reserved a cluster of tasks related to childbearing, childcare, and sickcare largely to women.[61] Plantation doctoring certainly fell into this category; older health workers developed many of their skills first as caregivers for their own families. This lifetime of work, along with its relational context, was what lay hidden under the titles of "nurse" and "doctress" designated in planters' records.

Some enslaved women began their work as healers during their childhood while caring for younger children.[62] Ellen Betts obtained her first knowledge of sickcare as a girl in charge of the white and black children of a large sugar plantation in Louisiana. Although the title of "nurse" often designated someone who cared for children, it inevitably implied nursing children's ailments and frequently led to additional healing responsibilities. As Betts grew older, she began to nurse sick adults and even administered medicines prescribed by a visiting white doctor.[63] Sarah MacDonald, a North Carolina woman, followed a similar path as a child nurse and then a wet nurse. After emancipation she earned a living nursing the sick in white households and preparing their bodies for burial when they died. As time passed, she developed her own herbal practice and by the end of her life had established a reputation as a specialist in the cure of rheumatism.[64] Betts and MacDonald shared similar experiences as black women who accumulated healing skills over the course of their lives doing the closely related work of caring for children and attending the sick.

Despite the positive value placed on healing work within slave communities, some enslaved women actively rejected nursing work for a variety of reasons. A Georgia planter found he was unable to make "Sister Jane" work in the plantation sickhouse. "I had a little trouble here about a week ago with Sister Jane," wrote Louis Manigault to his father; "she did not attend to the sick at all, so Caramba! I put her in the field, & I tell you what it is one of the best changes ever made."[65] Louis Manigault apparently viewed the change as a demotion, but Jane may have been relieved to escape the confinement and constant demands of sickcare. Settings closely supervised by overseers and slaveholders produced particularly perilous conditions for enslaved nurses. Such was the case with "Aunt Sallie," remembered by an ex-slave from Virginia. Like Jane, Sallie was also ordered back to field work for allegedly making the white family's baby sick, possibly through the administration of medicine. Perhaps fearing further punishment, Sallie confronted the planter with a scythe, cut her way into the woods, and escaped the plantation.[66] For some slave women the work of healing remained clearly distasteful and dangerous.

Although some girls learned about sickcare as child nurses, motherhood played a much more important role in the development of enslaved women's healing skills. High infant mortality and frightening childhood diseases such as whooping cough and infant tetanus schooled enslaved mothers all too quickly in the care of sick children.[67] Elderly African Americans recalled their mothers' attention with a particularity that suggested both the emotional and physical value placed on their work. "I used to get sick a lot," recalled one elderly woman; "Mama would doctor on me with tea and grease made from weeds and marrow from bones."[68] In a similar fashion, Ransom Sidney Taylor recalled, "my mother looked after most of us when we were sick. She used roots, herbs, and grease, and medicine the overseer got in town. When my mother got through rubbin' you, you would soon be well."[69]

The wealth of curative and preventative remedies used by enslaved mothers testified to their knowledge of medicinal plants. Solomon Caldwell described his mother's precautions against childhood illness on a South Carolina plantation. "I 'member my ma would take fever grass and boil it to tea and have us drink it to keep de fever away. She used branch elder twigs and dogwood berries for chills."[70] Charlie King's mother started each day by giving her children "burnt whiskey" for "long life."[71] Enslaved women stored herb teas and "bitters" (whiskey mixed with medicinal bark) in earthenware pitchers and jugs and dispensed them daily to their children as preventative drafts. Many elderly men and women recalled their mothers tying a pungent asafetida bag around their necks to ward off sickness.[72]

Along with administering bitters and asafetida, enslaved women attempted to preserve family well-being by teaching children the meaning of signs. Signs in nature and human behavior conveyed the threat of death, the meaning of dreams, and portents of future interactions with neighbors and enemies. Within a sacred vision of health, signs served as remedies against misfortune alongside herbal medicines. For example, Harriet Collins's mother taught her a host of "doctorin' things," including the use of white sassafras tea for rheumatism and horseradish poultices for headaches. She also instructed her in reading signs for good fortune and self-protection.[73] The knowledge of signs joined the use of herbs and roots as "doctoring things" deployed against the brutality and unpredictability of enslavement.

At times the desire of mothers to preserve the lives of their children indirectly converged with slaveholders' own proprietary interests in slave health. Slaveholders somewhat reluctantly tolerated the loss of slave women's field labor when illness spread in the slave quarters. A South Carolina planter noted diminished numbers of laborers in his fields by commenting, "Much sickness among the children . . . the Mothers of Infants obliged to stay with them all day."[74] Physician and slaveholder John A. Warren worried about Sarah, the newly purchased child who had contracted typhoid fever. Illustrating the slaveholder's role in permitting or denying enslaved mothers access to their sick children, Warren noted that he had assigned Sarah's mother to attend her.[75]

Most women enslaved on plantations spent long days working on plantation crops, however, and many slaveowners, to quote historian Stephanie Shaw, simply "did not allow slave women to mother their children."[76] Plantation work schedules frequently kept mothers from providing their own families with the bedside presence they valued. In their stead, "other-mothers" in the quarters stepped in.[77] Fannie Moore, born into slavery in South Carolina, recalled that it was her grandmother who was able to steal time away for sickcare. An experienced herbalist, the grandmother came to the aid of Fannie Moore's mother, whose task of plowing the cotton fields kept her from caring for her fevered son. Moore recalled, "Granny she doctah him as bes' she could, evah time she git way from de white folks kitchen. My mammy nevah git chance to see him, 'cept when she git home in de evenin'."[78]

Secondary to the demands of field work, planters' health-driven decisions about the location of slave children further impeded slave women's ability to mother their own children. During epidemics, for example, Low-country planters removed children and sick adults from their families to inland camps considered healthier because of their higher elevation and drier ground.[79] Jacob Stroyer spent extended periods of his childhood at the "summer seat," where his wealthy owner relocated small children during the summer fever season. Separated from his father and mother, Stroyer was looked after by several women elders whose advanced age decreased their usefulness in the fields.[80]

Slave women who survived into their forties extended their work from the more immediate care of their families to attend to entire slave communities.[81] Enslaved parents often looked to these older women to doctor their children. "The [white] doctor looked after us when we were sick, sometimes," recalled Joe High from North Carolina, "but it wuz mostly done by old women."[82] If an illness lingered, according to Martha Everette, "they'd put a woman in thar ter tend ter 'em. We wuz well looked after."[83] Another woman, Polly Shine, described "the best of care." She recalled, "Maser would get us a Negro mama, and she doctored us from herbs she got out of the woods."[84]

Enslaved women also applied their healing skills to injuries sustained by the whip. Despite frequent remarks on slave health, slaveholders said little about the aftermath of the violence they called "correction."[85] For the most part, slave women doctored the welts, gashes, and bruises resulting from slaveholder coercion. "I have greased my daddy's back after he had been whipped until his back was cut to pieces," recalled Louisa Adams about the harsh conditions on a North Carolina plantation.[86] Roberta Manson, also from North Carolina, described how her mother had to grease her father's back just to remove the shirt stuck to his bloody flesh.[87] Another man described the creative care he received from several women after he was whipped by his mistress: "I was awful sore on my back and legs. The women took feathers and kept me greased in castor oil to keep my shirt from sticking to the cuts."[88] An equally resourceful use of local medicines in North Carolina called for a nightly wash of boiled Jerusalem oak applied to flogging wounds infested with maggots.[89] Significantly, much of this healing work took place at night, after the day's work in the fields. Often invisible to slaveholders, these acts of doctoring built relations of interdependence within enslaved families and increased esteem for the skills of elder women.

Older black women gained the trust of their charges in part because they lived among the men, women, and children whom they doctored. Evidence from plantation records suggests that the majority of older healers, such as Elsey, lived their entire lives in the slave quarters. Many were former field hands themselves. On a very large Georgia plantation with an enslaved population of 250 people, for example, the "Old Nurse" Sylvia lived with three children and her husband, all field workers.[90] Sale lists, with their itemized "qualifications" intended to entice buyers, also provided indirect evidence of the connections doctoring women had to communities of field workers. One such sale broadside listed fifty-year-old Nelly, advertised with her husband and four children, as field hand and midwife.[91] Evidence gleaned from the records of slaveholders suggests that when Sarah Fitzpatrick described the black "Mammies who waited on all o'em," she did not refer to the Mammy of plantation mythology who labored faithfully in the slaveholder's house but to older black women whose lives were closely interwoven with those of other field workers.

Whereas planters might enter older women in their records simply as "nurses," these same older women actually served a broader range of slave community health needs. Gus Feaster, born into slavery in South Carolina, remembered that women "too old to do any work" would "take and study what to do fer de ailments of grown folks and lil' chilluns." Although Feaster himself described the women elders as "too old to do any work," he also documented their labors for the health of their communities. These women knew how to wean, feed, bathe, and protect the health of the babies, according to Feaster; they also used pine rosin to make pills for the older men and women whose backs ached from bending and digging in the fields.[92] The highly valued services of midwives and herbalists won them positions of high status within the internal hierarchy of enslaved communities.[93]

Some doctoring women also increased their standing within enslaved communities through their ability to travel openly outside plantation boundaries. Midwifery, in particular, afforded some degree of open mobility unavailable to most slaves, especially women. Elsey's midwifery, for example, required her to travel to black and white households in the area. While we know little about the purposes to which Elsey put her mobility, her frequent travels contrasted starkly with Alexander Telfair's restrictions on most slaves "visiting" between his two plantations.[94] Another enslaved woman doctor had rare access to a horse for her sick calls. "My mother was a kind of doctor too," recalled Bob Mobley. "She'd ride horseback all over the place an' see how they was gettin' along."[95] Such mobility allowed enslaved women to see friends and kin on other plantations, carry news for those who could not travel without penalty, and perhaps even contribute to plans of escape or insurrection.

Within slave communities, older women healers also gained respect as teachers. Enslaved women figured prominently in the fireside training that schooled younger women and men in herbal lore and spiritual empowerment. The close relationship of various African American doctoring arts, such as conjuration, midwifery, and herbalism, can be seen in networks of instruction among enslaved families. A South Carolina conjure doctor acquired his knowledge of medicinal plants from his mother, a former slave and healer in her plantation community.[96] Not all fireside training was hidden from slaveholders, for planters often had a vested interest in slave women's apprenticeship in sickcare. James Henry Hammond noted in his plantation rulebook that when midwives attended the women in childbirth, "some other woman learning the art usually assists her."[97]

Doctoring knowledge often passed between mothers and daughters, and particular families became identified with plantation health work. Whenever the doctress Elsey left Thorn Island Plantation to attend a birth, her daughter assumed Elsey's place as nurse for the slave children.[98] On another Georgia plantation the "hospital nurse" Susan was the daughter of Sarah, an older woman designated as "Old Nurse" on a slave list.[99] Such evidence suggests that enslaved mothers were able to teach their daughters healing skills and that plantation owners may have even expected these duties to pass from mothers to daughters as a way of ensuring the continuity of sickcare. Enslaved women, however, had their own reasons for valuing female apprenticeships. As older enslaved women taught their remedies, they also passed along their underlying views of illness and health as relational and spiritual phenomena. A woman in the South Carolina Sea Islands expressed her commitment to her mother's knowledge with the following assertion: "My moder taught me day way, started me dat way, [I] keep up de way she started me."[100]

Slaveowner records confirm enslaved women's work as plantation healers yet do not reflect the same level of appreciation of black women's doctoring skills. Assigning one or more women to plantation health work was a standard practice. Inventories from a Virginia plantation in 1863, for example, named a sixty-three-year-old woman, Malvina, as "Doctress."[101] Similarly, in 1837 rice planter Richard J. Arnold instructed his overseer to look to fifty-four-year-old Daphney as the best nurse in case of a cholera epidemic. Daphney also spent a good part of her time at other household tasks, remaining with new mothers to assist them for a fortnight after they gave birth.[102]

By and large, however, slaveholders preferred to reserve sickcare responsibilities for women too old for agricultural work. Neither age nor disability exempted older women from a slaveholder's efforts to make efficient use of his enslaved labor force. Mary, a fifty-year-old woman listed on a sale broadside as "Plantation nurse," worked with a lame hand.[103] Sixty-year-old Binah tended the sick on the Manigault's Gowrie Plantation, despite the overseer's open acknowledgment that she was chronically disposed to "apoplexy."[104] Indeed, healing work did not necessarily even spare older women from field work, especially when harvest or planting seasons demanded all available labor. One planter's inventory, while exempting another elderly woman, rated the fifty-year-old nurse Amy as a half-hand, indicating her potential for completing at least half the normally assigned tasks in the plantation fields.[105] From the perspective of plantation labor demands, the assignment of older women to sickcare reflected planters' concessions to old age and a maximum exploitation of women's labor.

The valuation of age and wisdom in slave communities contrasted sharply with the depreciation of the bodies of older women in slaveholders' ledgers. For example, slave lists from one Virginia plantation in 1854 esti-

No.	Names	Age	Occupation	Value	No.	Names	Age	Occupation	Value
1	Erasmus	29	Foreman			*Children*			
2	Jim	28	Plowman		35	Nelly			
3	Alfred	30	"		36	Yple Buckner			
4	Henry H.	32	"		37	Cornelius			
5	Henry Jun	58							
6	John	42	Ox driver						
7	William S.	34	Field						
8	Hartwell	48	"						
9	Richard	20	"						
10	Abel	15	"						
11	Matthew	15	"						
12	Andrew	16	"						
13	Venus	27	"						
14	Sally	22	"						
15	Maria	18	"						
16	Martha	25	"						
17	Margaret	13	"						
18	Becky	13	"						
19	Hanna	13							
20	Betsy	47	Cook						
21	Angelina	57	Milk maid						
22	Julianna	35	Cook for ngrs.						
23	Malvina	63	Doctress						
24	Minerva	46	Seamstress						
25	Dawson	11							
26	Angelina	8							

Slave list, Beldale Plantation, Powhatan County, Virginia, 1863. Women who provided sickcare to entire plantation communities typically came from the ranks of enslaved elders. In this list of thirty-seven individuals, recorded during the Civil War, Malvina, the oldest woman, is designated as plantation "doctress." The same volume indicates that a white doctor, Dr. Bryant, visited the plantation only eleven times that year, with no visits from March to July. (Philip St. George Cocke Papers; reproduced by permission of VHS)

mated the market value of fifty-three-year-old "Nurse" Maria at $200. The same plantation book listed Nancy (no age recorded), a "Nurse for Sick," at $250 while valuing "prime" women field hands at $400.[106] Another plantation book sorted men and women into categories of prime laborers, half-laborers, and "useless." Among the eleven useless adults were three woman who worked at plantation subsistence tasks, including Cotto, who nursed; Mary, who cooked; and the blind Sarey, who tended the poultry.[107] Registering value in relation to crop production and market price, planters' books literally made invisible the important social reproduction and subsistence labor of older women.

Older slave women were expected not only to produce health but also to move between many kinds of work related to plantation subsistence. Slave women charged with making medicines and caring for the sick, as we have seen, frequently were responsible for childcare. On the Manigault's Gowrie Plantation, Binah's doctoring work extended to care of children. Others entered the records as weavers, dairy women, and cooks.[108] Rather than doing one particular kind of work, older women moved among a cluster of subsistence labor responsibilities. Isabel, age sixty-eight, appeared in a Virginia plantation book in 1854 as a spinner and seven years later as a nurse.[109] The doctor Elsey at Thorn Island Plantation combined domestic production and poultry work with her midwifery and childcare duties.[110] The woman described by her son Bob Mobley as a "kind of doctor" on a Georgia plantation also worked as the slave quarters cook.[111] On St. Helena Island the midwife Judy also laboriously ground and processed the arrowroot crop into gruel for babies and invalids.[112] Older slave women thus spent their later years as healers engaged in multiple subsistence tasks.

Understanding the connections between doctoring work and the subsistence activities of older women highlights the space — both literal and metaphorical — in which the work took place. For male artisans, skilled work occurred in workshops representing a middle ground between "fields" and "quarters."[113] The middle ground for older slave women was not the workshop, however, but the yard. Doctoring women often worked in the plantation yard adjacent to the slaveholder's residence and relatively close to slave dwellings, the sickhouse, and the overseer's residence. In the plantation yard stood the smokehouse, the kitchen, and the dairy and laundry areas — all places where doctoring women might have additional work to do.[114] Laboring in and around these plantation outbuildings, enslaved women drew on an expertise in childcare, botanical knowledge, and productive processes acquired throughout their lives as bondswomen. The yard was thus occupied by women who did not fit neatly into the "field" versus "big house" divisions of labor that appear frequently in the historiography. Neither did their skilled labor necessarily gain them the resources often associated with male artisanal skilled labor.

Enslaved African Americans and white slaveholders measured the healing skills of slave women in starkly different terms. Enslaved communities not only recognized skill but also attributed authority to older black doctors. This acknowledgment of older women's authority was based on criteria not generally recognized by whites: spiritual empowerment, respect for elders, and recognition of herbal expertise. White planters, however, viewed enslaved women's doctoring skills with ambivalence. Within plantation work regimes, enslaved women's doctoring was associated with other menial subsistence tasks and assigned to older women not considered fit for regular field work. While some slaveholders acknowledged their dependence on slave women's health work, few were prepared to grant slave women the kinds of medical authority attributed to white practitioners, male or female.

Race, Gender, and Medical Authority

Middling to wealthy white Americans in the antebellum period generally recognized two parallel sources of medical authority. The first, rooted in colonial domestic medicine practices and strengthened by newer antebellum ideals of motherhood, was the moral authority of white women as domestic medical practitioners guided by maternal interest. White doctors made a second claim to medical authority vested in learned knowledge, class standing, professional training, and male entitlement. While both categories of authority were subjects of contention throughout the nineteenth century, white mothers and white medical men could nevertheless draw on established conventions in the dominant society to sanction their work.[115] Black women's authority to heal, however, consistently fell outside both of these categories, for white southerners denied medical authority to enslaved women healers both in terms of maternal moral authority and in terms of professional expertise. Hence, white hostility to enslaved women's healing activities drew on two pairs of oppositional images: between white mistresses and slave mothers, and between white doctors and older slave nurses.

Planter images of the slave mother emerged from a broader ideology of southern womanhood that defined black and elite white women in direct opposition to one another. Hazel Carby has argued that "two very different but interdependent codes of sexuality operated in the antebellum South, producing opposing definitions of motherhood and womanhood for white and black women which coalesce in the figures of the slave and the mistress."[116] Of critical importance was — to borrow a phrase from Elsa Barkley Brown — "the relational nature of those differences," one image depending upon the other.[117] Images of the devoted and compassionate mistress caregiver and the servile but callous slave mother strongly influenced planter-class notions of black and white womanhood.

In their racialized ideologies of womanhood, antebellum slaveholders denied to enslaved women the moral authority that they extended to white mistresses as motherly domestic healers within their families. On one hand, planter ideology portrayed the white mistress as a civilizing force whose sexuality was tamed but whose sense of motherhood was so strongly developed that it extended beyond her own offspring to childlike and dependent slaves. At the opposite pole of planter ideology, the enslaved woman appeared as a primitive figure possessing a rampant sexuality but a sense of motherhood so flawed that it could endanger the health of her own children. In stark contrast to images of the all-caring mistress, dominant ideology portrayed enslaved women's healing work as subservient labor rendered incompetently and without maternal feeling.

Romanticized notions of white women's nursing work became one of the main supports for the idealized image of the bounteous southern lady, obscuring the extent of the labors of enslaved women. An extreme voice in racial-medical ideology, physician Samuel Cartwright argued that white women's care of slave children was the primary cause of antebellum slave population growth. Plantation mistresses, according to Cartwright, were the "presiding genius over civilization, morality and population."[118] Sir Charles Lyell, a British traveler in the 1840s, described plantation mistresses sitting up "all night" with sick slave children.[119] White historians took up this theme in twentieth-century writings, embellishing images of the planter's wife who did "more than her share," who responded "at an instant's call," and who inspired such gratitude that "slaves usually refused medicine from any hands other than those of their own mistress."[120] It was not merely coincidence that such praise for the plantation mistress also disparaged enslaved mothers' abilities to care for their own sick children.

The elevation of the white mistress as superdomestic healer for the entire plantation contrasted sharply in white southern thought with assumptions about the incompetence of enslaved mothers. Many slaveholders simply assumed that slave women were unable to care independently or compassionately for sick family members. South Carolina planter Henry A. Middleton Jr. incorporated suppositions about slave women's deficiencies into his elaborate scheme of incentives for the Weehaw Plantation population. Middleton awarded enslaved mothers cash bonuses when their children lived beyond infancy, implying that cash would provide the incentive otherwise lacking to ensure their children's survival. Middleton's journal entries in the late 1850s note Christmas payments of one dollar each to enslaved mothers with infants of one month and one year, in addition to bonuses paid to child nurses for "infants that live."[121] The Weehaw Plantation's monetary incentives welded newer public health and plantation management ideas to older and more common white assumptions about slave women's capacity to mother.

Far more common were direct attacks on slave women's lack of care. Slaveholders and overseers frequently charged enslaved women — and particularly mothers — with callousness, incompetence, and ignorance. An overseer on the Manigault plantations, possibly looking to exonerate himself in the eyes of his employer, pinned the death of two small babies on their mother. He complained, "I think it more the mother fault than anything else buy night leting them get uncovered in those coold nights of last week."[122] Planter William Massie responded to the death of a young boy on his Virginia plantation by entering the notation, "[Romulus] died by waste caused by the unnatural neglect of his infamous mother."[123] On the occasion of other infant deaths, Massie charged the mothers with "neglect" and "Barbaras cruelty." In another incident he accused a mother of having "mashed" her five-month-old boy — a common charge levied against slave mothers suspected of rolling over and suffocating their infants in bed.[124]

Charges of incompetent mothering dwelled on neglect, ignorance, and lack of mother love as broad racialized gender traits rather than as behaviors of individual women. Stephanie Shaw aptly notes in her study of mothering under slavery that "neither the biological fact of motherhood, nor the traditional gendered construction of mothering applied to them as far as slaveholders were concerned."[125] J. Hume Simons, a Charleston physician and author of a southern domestic medicine manual, warned white readers to guard against slave women who, when allowed to leave the fields to nurse their children, would use their time for sleep instead.[126] Samuel Cartwright wove the theme of maternal deficit into his litany of the failings of African Americans as a race. He charged that slave mothers with sick children deviated from the natural maternal impulses of white women. "They let their children suffer and die, or unmercifully abuse them," he wrote. Linking the depravity of slave mothers to the racialized maternal bounty of white mistresses, he credited the survival of black children to the intervention of southern mistresses with their nursery rules.[127] Charles Lyell, too, sketched "negro mothers" as a group "often so ignorant or indolent, that they can not be trusted to keep awake and administer medicine to their own children," hence creating the need for the vigilance of their mistresses.[128]

Julian Chisolm, ruminating just after the Civil War on changes brought by emancipation, went so far as to characterize slaveholders before the war as providing "foster parental care" to enslaved children whose parents, according to Chisolm, took no part in nursing their sick children.[129]

Many planters and physicians presumed that slave women were too incompetent and insensitive to care for adult kin as well. South Carolina planter Thomas Chaplin expressed exasperation over what he perceived as carelessness in an enslaved woman with a sick husband. "Isaac had not the fever in the morning," he wrote, "but his precious wife [Amy] went off to church instead of coming to me for quinine for him as she was directed, & consequently the fever came on again in the evening." As a devout Christian, Amy's concern for her husband's illness may very well have increased her desire to attend Sunday morning worship in search of spiritual support. Furthermore, her skepticism about Chaplin's medicines may have motivated her lapse in treatment. Yet Chaplin, focused as he was on his intended course of quinine treatments, could see Amy's actions only in terms of her disobedience toward him and as heedless disregard for Isaac's health.[130] In this light Amy's failure to follow Chaplin's orders could only be construed by Chaplin as both a failure of familial care and a disregard for Chaplin's authority.

The chorus of condemnation of black women as family healers did little, however, to prevent slaveholders from regularly using enslaved women as health workers in white households and plantation slave quarters. Yet stereotypes in planter ideology eclipsed the social relations of plantation healing work.[131] On one hand, images of the mistress as a devoted supermaternal figure obscured the broad extent of slave women's healing work and rendered invisible the bonds of affection and care within slave families. Images of the callous slave mother worked in tandem with those of romanticized mistresses, clouding enslaved women's emotional investment in their healing work and denigrating their knowledge while sanctioning the heavy exploitation of their skills. In stark contrast to images of the Mammy who directed her competence and emotional attachments toward the white family, the image of the neglectful slave mother obscured both skill and mother love.[132]

The discourse that placed solicitous mistresses in opposition to callous slave mothers also posed the knowledgeable professional white doctor opposite the dependent black servant nurse. Rather than denying slave women moral authority and capacity for mother love, this opposition between white doctors and slave nurses denied older slave women the capacity for autonomous action and medical expertise. Unlike idealized descriptions of plantation mistresses that denied the maternal abilities of black mothers, medical advice literature to planters openly acknowledged that enslaved older women were indispensable to plantation health care — indispensable, yes, but necessarily subservient as well. The ideal nurse for children and sick slaves, advice writers noted, should be a "good tempered notable old woman," an "experienced old woman," "intelligent and otherwise suitable" and "trusty."[133] The classic image of the old nurse depicted a female slave who worked "faithfully" under the authority of overseer, slaveholder, or physician.

Here again, social relations of healing diverged starkly from stereotypical images. While slaves were often required to report illness first to the master or overseer, in most cases it was an enslaved woman who talked to the sick about their complaints and administered medicines. As the practitioners most intimately connected with the members of their plantation community, older enslaved women had knowledge and experience that was often useful to white visiting doctors. For example, one South Carolina physician, W. F. McKain, reported that he had prescribed vermifuge (antiworm) medicines for an enslaved girl at the suggestion of the plantation nurse, who must have observed the symptoms of worms in the small child.[134] Given the variable training of antebellum white doctors and their status as visitors to the plantation, it would not have been unusual for enslaved women to provide useful advice to white practitioners. Yet the antebellum social order left little room for either planters or white doctors to acknowledge the independent judgment of elderly, enslaved doctoring women.

As a result, plantation advice literature strained to accommodate contradictions between a labor scheme that made planters dependent on the health work of enslaved women and a social order that assumed slave women's subordination. Medical advice literature, on one hand, revealed the reliance of planters on the health work of slave women by stressing their competence as health workers. Slave nurses and midwives were "sensible," "prudent," even "strong in principle," and with their life experience they could competently deliver babies and care for sick children.[135] South Carolina physician and planter Phillip Tidyman wrote of enslaved men and women who possessed "a knowledge of the virtues of medicinal plants" and could "judiciously" and "with much efficacy" apply their remedies.[136] Such laudable descriptions supported the widely recognized role that enslaved women played in the health work of plantations.

Yet the same genre of advice literature issued warnings about the dangers of slave nurses, directly contradicting themes of competence. The same advice literature that touted the "faithful" and "experienced" older slave nurse also characterized the enslaved healer as frequently "ignorant" and "inattentive to her charge." The enslaved nurse, the authors argued, required constant oversight and particular instructions lest she endanger sick slaves by her "extreme ignorance and temerity."[137] While Phillip Tidyman praised blacks' herbal knowledge, he went on to lament the tendency of enslaved men and women to hide their symptoms from whites and confide instead "in quacks of their own colour," whose claims to possess a cure led to the ruin of their patients' health. Considerations of age lay at the heart of these charges made by medical writers who portrayed elderly women healers as weak, inept, and ignorant. An 1848 planter medical guide published in South Carolina, for example, warned readers to choose a strong and "able" woman, "not as is commonly the case, a decrepit old woman," to attend the sick.[138]

At the heart of the contradictions in plantation advice literature lay the issue of enslaved women's intellect and autonomous authority. By stressing both the indispensability of older women's health work and the dangers of their "ignorance," planter literature implicitly portrayed slave women as competent only in relation to white medical authority. Under proper supervision, enslaved women were essential plantation workers. Acting on their own, however, slave women posed a triple threat of ignorance, irrationality, and deceitfulness. H. W. Moore, a South Carolina medical student, presented both the virtues and the dangers of enslaved nurses in his thesis on "plantation hygiene":

> And here it might be well to state, in a few words, the propriety, and advantage of supplying plantations with suitable nurses. There are usually persons on every place who affect this title with little show of reason. With capable and willing nurses, the labors of the physician would be less burdensome and more efficacious. Among the educated, the Practitioner finds intelligence to comprehend his views, and willingness to assist him in carrying them out but among ignorant negroes, the case is far different. They are much given to malingering and deception. Reliable nurses should be at hand to see to the proper fulfillment of the directions of the physician.[139]

Moore defined both "suitable" and "ignorant" nurses according to their relationship to the authority of white doctors. Slaves who claimed the title of healer without a planter's designation, Moore implied, were inherently dangerous because they evaded appropriate supervision by physicians. His complaint of slave healers' deceitfulness suggested that a suitable nurse should be judged not so much by the degree of her skill but by her alacrity in following orders.

The contradictory characterization of enslaved nurses as capable and ignorant, reliable and deceptive, reflected planters' fears concerning their inability to control slave women's work. Midwives, in particular, came under scrutiny as essential health workers who nevertheless possessed the troubling potential for evading direct white supervision. Enslaved midwives provided the bulk of care to birthing mothers and newborn babies. Thus, physicians often derided slave midwives for failing to follow directions and blamed them for birth complications and reproductive disorders.[140] P. M. Kollock, a Savannah physician, "severely reprimanded" a slave midwife for refusing to discard her own practice of dressing the navel with a scorched rag after the umbilical cord had fallen off. Concerned about infant trismus, Kollock instructed the midwife in washing and dressing the navel with ointment. When the woman returned to her original method, she was "threatened with punishment."[141] While Kollock intended his account as a story of medical discovery, the incident also highlighted the animosity of white doctors and planters toward older slave women with established therapies of their own.[142]

Out of the documentary historical evidence, a stereoscopic view of enslaved women's healing work emerges. On one side, plantation records and medical reports such as Kollock's project images of older slave women who worked at midwifery, sickcare, and other tasks of the plantation yards because they were too old for childbearing and for the fields. Whether they identified women healers as absolutely essential or practically useless, planter records portrayed slave women as subservient health workers who served the needs of the productive plantation. The nature and location of slave women's healing work obscured the degree of skill involved in their labor. A second contrasting view of the same women comes from interviews with formerly enslaved men and women. From this perspective, slave women's doctoring work represented the culmination of a lifelong acquisition of skills as mothers and apprentices to older healers. Their work appeared as valued services to neighbors and family members, not as a direct outcome of planter orders.

Side by side, these two images merge to form a richly textured and multidimensional view of enslaved women's doctoring. In many cases it appears that women sanctioned by their communities as nurses were tolerated as well by white planters. Yet perceptions of their activities varied greatly. From the perspective of enslaved sufferers, old age entitled women healers to authority, and healing skills drew on spiritual empowerment and the instruction of older kin. In stark contrast, planters rejected the link between slave women's skills and their authority, denied their familial ties, and perceived claims of spiritual empowerment as superstition. Ultimately slaves and slaveholders not only measured skill differently but also disagreed about the ends to which enslaved women's healing knowledge should be directed.

Within the planter ideology of mastery, independent knowledge on the part of enslaved women healers was inherently threatening and posed magnified dangers. As defined by the chattel principle, slave health was either a boon or a threat to planter wealth. Suspicious planters feared that the autonomous actions of an enslaved nurse might endanger the lives of other slaves and therefore the planters' property. Worse still, from a slaveholder's perspective, a "deceitful" nurse could also assist other enslaved men and women in feigning illness or obtaining medicines not sanctioned by white authority. Any suggestion of independent care for the body signaled a potential threat to the slaveholder's control over enslaved laborers.[143] In other words, conflicts between masters and slaves over proper treatments and practitioners went to the heart of planter interests in curtailing African American self-determination. Ironically, medical encounters between slaves and slaveholders—the very relationships that paternalist rhetoric portrayed as cementing bonds of mutual duty and obligation—became fraught instead with distrust and danger.

*To be cured, the sick person in "Nginani Na" ("What Do I Have?")
is being treated by a* sangoma. *The worried patient thinks: "I must be
very sick, the diviner is loud when he talks to the ancestors about my
condition. What could I have? A headache? Some strange pains?"
We all feel helpless during a doctor's examination.*
—*Miriam Makeba,* Sangoma, *liner notes, 1988*

*In a non-colonial society, the attitude of a sick man in the presence
of a medical practitioner is one of confidence. The patient trusts the
doctor; he puts himself in his hands. He yields his body to him. He
accepts the fact that pain may be awakened or exacerbated by the
physician, for the patient realizes that the intensifying of suffering in
the course of examination may pave the way to peace in his body.*
—*Franz Fanon,* A Dying Colonialism, *1959*

*If here we attempt to answer the question, whether medicine cures
more than it kills? The nerve of the candid medical man will tremble
in pronouncing the decision.*
—*J. Dickson Smith,*
  "Abuse of Medicine," Savannah Journal of Medicine, *1859*

CHAPTER 6

Danger and Distrust

In January 1806 a Pittsylvania County jury in the state of Virginia found an enslaved man named Tom guilty of the capital offense of "having prepared and exhibited Medicine." Testimony from Pompey, a slave witness, also implicated Amy, a slave in a white Danville household. According to Pompey, Tom had supplied Amy with a substance—described in the records as "truck," "medicine," "stuff," and a "preparation"—that she allegedly gave to her owner's two children with fatal results. The court even went so far as to examine a sample of Tom's medicines, obtained by Pompey, who feigned interest in Tom's "art of conjuring or poisoning" in order to procure a specimen. Despite the fact that James Patton, a local white physician, was unable to identify the composition of the medicine except for some nonpoisonous elements, Tom was pronounced guilty. He was sentenced to be "hanged by the Neck until he be dead."

Amy, too, received a death sentence, but the testimony of James Patton caused the court to consider sparing her life. Asserting his firsthand knowledge of any severe illnesses in the neighborhood, Patton testified that the two white children "died with the croup and not of poison." Furthermore, he argued that Amy, as a domestic slave, was "not in the habit of going from home" and so could not have consulted with Tom, who lived in another household. Hearing this and other testimony for Amy's good character, the court recommended her sentence to the mercy of the governor. Details of this case entered the historical record through the appeal of Amy's sentence and by virtue of the fact that Tom's owner petitioned the governor to reduce or commute his slave's sentence. The trial and the petition for appeal drew an entire neighborhood, including judge, jury, white doctor, slaves, and masters, into an extended contemplation of the motives and potential threat of enslaved practitioners.[1]

The prosecution of Tom and Amy exposed the underlying dangers of practicing medicine in a slave society. As the work of conjuration plainly illustrated, the doctoring arts had a destructive side. Slaveholders realized with some trepidation that they could not fully contain the harming capacities of African American doctoring any more than they could completely suppress the independent authority of enslaved nurses. Despite the exchange of herbal remedies between blacks and whites, interracial healing encounters generated many anxieties about the dangerous potential of medicines. Wherever healers and sufferers encountered each other across the lines of color, class, and servitude, sufferers feared their vulnerability to the actions of healers.

Life in antebellum slave society placed peculiar constraints on several common concerns in healer-sufferer relationships. As scholar Doris Wilkinson argues, "Universally, the healing arena incorporates the relational imperatives of trust and faith in those on whom one depends for care."[2] Yet the social relations of plantation medicine just as readily reinforced distrust and suspicion. Enslaved African Americans harbored deep suspicions about white physicians, slaveholder medicines, and white medical institutions. Slaveholders, in turn, feared that enslaved healers would use their close proximity and healing knowledge to harm members of white households. In innumerable ways both subtle and dramatic, the context of chattel slavery heightened fears about the harming capacity of medicines and made distrust commonplace in plantation healing encounters.

For enslaved African Americans, slaveholders' legal ownership of their persons immeasurably complicated their encounters with white practitioners.[3] We have already seen that bondsmen and bondswomen distrusted the financial motives underlying slaveholder medical decisions. Comparing the conditions of enslavement to the circumstances of domestic animals, former slaves condemned the dehumanizing premise of white medical treatment that violated their relational vision of healing. The institutions of southern slave society also violated the idealized expectations for doctor-patient relationships held by white doctors, further undermining the possibility of patient trust.

Antebellum medical theories of disease emphasized the doctor-patient relationship as an integral part of diagnosis and treatment. White professional doctors and many of their patients viewed illness as environmentally influenced and patient-specific. According to this theory of specificity, illness manifested itself differently in each patient's case, depending on variables such as the patient's temperament, region, race, gender, and class.[4] The physician, therefore, aimed to diagnose and treat an illness as it developed uniquely in each patient. Southern doctors, like their counterparts elsewhere in the United States, embraced this principle. One southern medical journal of the 1850s, for example, contended that the "science of medicine" could only be learned "by close observation and constant attendance at the bedside of the sick." Thus, the author continued, the physician's most important lessons came not from books but from insight gained through intimate familiarity with the patient.[5] The quality of the doctor-patient relationship, in this view, contributed to the efficacy of the healer.

As the first step toward effective healing, white professional doctors placed a premium on inspiring their patients' trust (more commonly expressed in antebellum usage as "confidence"). Couched in paternalist rhetoric, professional doctors tied patient confidence to the mutual attributes of patient dependence and physician authority.[6] The 1847 "Code of Medical Ethics" of the American Medical Association, reprinted in southern medical journals, outlined the reciprocal relationship of doctors and patients. Physicians should "inspire the minds of their patients with gratitude, respect and confidence," it announced, while patients should defer to "regular" medical authority by strictly obeying the physician's directions.[7] As nineteenth-century medical doctors came under fire from health reformers, new medical sects, and license repeal movements, their search for a stable professional identity elevated the importance of patient deference and physician authority.[8]

Among professionally active southern physicians, the expectation of patient deference to medical authority often rested as much on the practitioner's social position as on medical expertise. The medical authority of well-educated southern physicians was bolstered by their social position as white, upper-class, and often slaveholding men. It was inevitable that southern medical doctors would take these social identities with them into their doctoring work. Furthermore, the confluence of male professional identity with southern codes of manly honor underscored concerns with patient respect and professional reputation among white medical practitioners. The idealized physician-patient relationship was thus reinforced by other paternalistic and unequal relationships in southern society between independent propertied men and persons legally classified as dependents.[9]

In the case of enslaved patients, the antebellum ideals of physician authority and patient deference reached their most extreme expression. The institution of slavery turned the dyad of patient and physician into a three-way relationship between patient, physician, and slaveowner. An enslaved person could not be defined as a white doctor's *patient* independent of the equally important relationship of the slaveholder as the physician's *client*. This rendered the enslaved person "medically incompetent," unable, at least in theory, to initiate or prevent treatments without a slaveowner's consent.[10]

While the medical incompetence of slaves was, of course, a legal fiction, it nevertheless eviscerated the notion of consent for enslaved patients. Even for white, middle-class patients the mid-nineteenth-century concept of informed consent contained ambiguities. Since medical theory posited the doctor-patient relationship as important to the healing process itself, physicians sometimes withheld news about diagnosis or treatment from their patients when they deemed this information might impede healing.[11] Part of the physician's duty, according to the 1847 code of ethics, was to weigh honesty against the responsibility to "avoid all things which have a tendency to discourage the patient and to depress his spirits."[12] The will of the slaveowner rendered such fine points of debate irrelevant for enslaved patients. In legal terms a slave had no independent voice in determining treatment, no recourse in resisting an undesired treatment, and no grounds for seeking restitution for neglect or inappropriate treatment.[13]

When it came to the practical work of doctoring, however, some white doctors demonstrated a concept of dual consent, which considered an enslaved patient's wishes alongside the slaveowner's decisions. A case of strangulated hernia in a young enslaved man prompted a dual consideration of consent by surgeon Charles Bell Gibson of Virginia. Writing for his medical peers, Gibson described the hernia operation and his deliberation over whether to remove the man's undescended testicle during the same surgery. He decided that "an unwillingness to risk complication of the danger of the operation, besides the feeling that *I had no right to castrate a man without his consent, or that of his master,* prevailed against the temptation to lop off this misplaced testis."[14] Another Virginia physician described the case of a black man, age thirty years, who came to the Richmond infirmary with a tumor of the jawbone. The author wrote that the operation was quickly performed by the infirmary surgeon, the "master and the patient both wishing to have the tumor removed as soon as possible, and the health of the boy being remarkably good in every other respect."[15] The fact that these case histories appeared in medical journals published for professional peers warns against their use as direct proof of exchange between enslaved patients and white physicians. There is no corroborating evidence to suggest how these enslaved men negotiated their treatment with white surgeons. Yet case histories provide, at the very least, evidence that perhaps surgeons, in particular, wished publicly to represent consent, even of enslaved persons, as a part of their practice.

Sometimes slaveholders supported enslaved patients' refusal of surgery. Juriah Harriss, a professor at Savannah Medical College, for example, favored an operation to remove two "large pendulous tumors" on an enslaved woman's ears. Perhaps because the tumors did not threaten her life or seriously threaten her value, the slaveholder agreed to the woman's refusal of surgery. "The owners would not force her to have the operation performed," reported the physician.[16] It is significant that Harris used the phrase "would not" rather than "could not," for at other times white doctors and slaveholders brutally disregarded the will of African Americans concerning the fate of their bodies.

Surgical case histories reported in southern medical journals reveal the frailty of any notion of consent by African Americans. Such was the case when an adolescent boy in South Carolina, described as a "favored servant," injured his genitals by falling from a tree. After anesthetizing the wounded patient with chloroform, the physician repaired the injury and removed the young man's testicle without his consent. The patient was told only that his wound had been sutured, and not until a week later, reported the doctor, did "he became aware of his loss."[17] More appalling still was the 1845 account of an operation on a New Orleans "negro woman" for a hardened mass in her breast and lymph nodes. According to the author's dispassionate description, "She was frightened nearly to death, and could not be prevailed on to submit with any composure. While she was writhing and screaming with all her power, Dr. S., with characteristic firmness, proceeded with his incisions, and removed the entire mamma, as also an indurated axillary gland."[18] This horrific description did not indicate whether the black woman operated on was enslaved or free. However, it was all too clear that her consent was not an issue for the physician. Surgery proceeded in the face of her unquestionable objection and terror.

Under slavery the burden of medical consent shifted from the enslaved patient to the slaveholding client. Although white professional doctors theoretically emphasized the individuality of the patient and idealized the doctor-patient relationship, enslaved African Americans frequently found that the relationship most honored was that between the doctor and the slaveowner who employed him. Enslaved men and women responded to the distorted healer-patient relationship with suspicions that white doctors did more harm than good.

African American Distrust of White Medicine

African Americans' distrust of white medical treatment stemmed from direct experience with medical abuse and neglect. Needless to say, not every medical encounter between enslaved patients and white practitioners produced a confrontation. In the southeastern coastal states, physicians' account books and the diaries of male and female slaveholders documented white doctors routinely examining and prescribing medicines for enslaved patients.[19] Yet distrust was a common thread running through most encounters between white practitioners and enslaved patients. Enslaved sufferers held misgivings about slaveholder medicine and white practitioners and often preferred the remedies of African American healers. Furthermore, enslaved men and women articulated the dangers of white medical institutions and medical science through oral traditions concerning the violation and theft of black bodies.

Across the South enslaved men and women rejected treatments administered by slaveholders and made clear their preference for African American doctoring.[20] One Mississippi planter who was unable to contain an outbreak of illness on his plantation confessed, "The negroes unfortunately for Themselves and Equally so for us had no confidence in our treatment—they said it was certain death to take our medicine and we were compelled to stand by and See them die."[21] Likewise, the husband of an enslaved patient attended by Savannah physician Richard Arnold was warned by visiting members of the woman's church that Arnold's prescribed medicines would prove fatal to his wife.[22] In South Carolina, planter Henry Ravenel reported that sick men and women on his plantation threw the white doctor's remedies out the window and substituted a black root doctor's medicines instead.[23] Some frustrated slaveholders responded with the lash. Charlie King, formerly enslaved in Georgia, told his interviewers that those who refused the slaveholder's salts or oil risked a beating with a rawhide whip.[24] Efforts to control the medicines taken by enslaved patients thus created a climate in which medical relations became, as Theodore Rosengarten has put it, "relations of force."[25]

Most objectionable to enslaved sufferers were the harsh purgatives prescribed by physicians and planters. Anyone dosed with heroic medicines such as ipecac, jalap, or tartar emetic soon felt their strong effects. Many antebellum whites, in fact, also disliked and rejected heroic therapies. For enslaved African Americans, however, purgative medicines took on the additional symbolism of planter control and bodily objectification. Jenny Proctor, an elderly Alabama woman, recalled with distaste the cathartic treatments frequently administered in her youth: "We had to take the worst stuff in the world for medicine, just so it was cheap. That old blue mass and bitter apple would keep us out all night."[26] Proctor's negative memories associated the unpleasantness of antebellum remedies with the economic incentives of the slaveholder to find "cheap" medicine. Henry Bibb's master used a noxious red pepper tea with powerful laxative action. According to Bibb, "If the slave should not be very ill, he would rather work as long as he could stand up, than to take this dreadful medicine."[27] In their rejection of heroic medicines some enslaved African Americans questioned the efficacy of purgatives, viewing them instead as poisonous substances that punished the body.[28]

In some instances slaveholders literally and intentionally employed medicine as punishment. The institution of slavery put control of African American bodies, albeit incomplete, in the hands of slaveholders through law, labor systems, and social custom. This context of physical control blurred the line between medicine and plantation discipline, between treatment and torture. Consider James Pennington's description of the "treatment" of a man who had been shot by an overseer while seeking to escape a beating. The man returned to the plantation thinking that his wounded condition would protect him from further assault. Instead, wrote Pennington, "he was locked up that night; the next morning the overseer was allowed to tie him up and flog him; his master then took his instruments and picked the shot out of his leg, and told him, it served him just right."[29] Part of the force of Pennington's description lay in its violation of the supposed bonds of mutual obligation idealized in antebellum patient-healer relationships. The image of the bleeding man subjected to violent "treatment" while hanging from the whipping post powerfully exposed the lie of the planter's paternalistic provision of care from cradle to grave.

The thin line dividing medical treatment and discipline vanished entirely in the punitive use of emetic and purgative medicines. Some enslaved laborers had to choose between the unpleasant effects of medicine and other types of corporal punishment. When Charles Grandy complained of sickness in order to mask the fact that he had not performed his required field work, a suspicious "boss" ordered him to take a dose of vomit-inducing ipecac. Grandy felt sick for several days yet managed in this difficult way to avoid being whipped.[30]

Slaveholders also used medicine in forms of torture unrelated to even the suggestion of illness. South Carolina freedman and later congressman Robert Smalls graphically described how slaveholders could turn commonly used medicines to purposes of dehumanization. At least one planter exacted punishment by placing several slaves in stocks arranged one above the other. Then, Smalls testified, "they would all be required to take a large dose of medicine and filth down upon each other."[31] Utter degradation was the aim as well of a South Carolina planter, Gooch, whose atrocities were detailed by fugitive Moses Roper. Roper's narrative includes an account of Gooch forcing a woman to drink an enormous dose of castor oil and salts and then incarcerating her under an overturned coffinlike box for the night, effectively burying her in her own waste.[32] Slave masters' technologies of power drew readily on plantation medicine chests.

Emetic medicines could also be employed as an intrusive form of slaveholder surveillance. In the 1850s Virginia planter Thomas Eugene Massie recorded his grandfather's use of medicines to guard against theft in his orchards. Massie recalled how his grandfather once made an unsuspecting young boy, "Little Peter," take a "strong dose" of tartar emetic. The dose caused Peter to vomit, thus revealing the cherries he had eaten that day while picking the fruit.[33] Thomas Massie recorded the episode as a humorous anecdote meant to amuse family members, yet it unintentionally revealed techniques of bodily control not always associated with the disciplinary arsenal of the planter class. By removing physical self-control, violating bodily integrity, and allowing slaveholders access to the interior of slave bodies, purgatives and emetics became tools of slaveholder dominance rather than measures for restoring health.

The disciplinary impulse that encouraged the use of medicine as punishment also propagated metaphors of punishment as medicine in white southern speech. When two enslaved women on the auction block persisted with comments that discouraged buyers, an outraged slave trader wrote of his inclination to retaliate with violence: "I will have to use some of Dr. Hall's medicine of North Carolina. You know what kind of medicine that is. . . . They want braking and I had as well brake them as anybody."[34] In mid-nineteenth-century Petersburg, Virginia, newspapers described the lashing of free black men and women for legal offenses as "medicine" and "nine drops of the essence of raw hide."[35] Adopting these figures of speech, white southerners placed themselves metaphorically in the position of doctors who sought to heal enslaved men and women of their lack of deference through the medicine of violence. Punitive metaphors of treatment brought the destructive side of medicine sharply into focus and revealed intimate associations between medicine and violence.

Medical science, including its practitioners and its institutions, provoked even greater distrust on the part of enslaved and free black southerners. On the whole, enslaved individuals exhibited complex and varied attitudes toward white doctors. Antebellum narratives and twentieth-century interviews reveal that some African Americans spoke matter-of-factly, even positively, about the presence of physicians on plantations. North Carolinian Emma Blalock praised a local white doctor, perhaps viewing him as an exception to the rule. He was "a feelin' man," she said, explaining that he could cure quickly because "he wus good an' 'cause he wus sorry fer you."[36] Other informants implied the desirability of a physician's presence by criticizing slaveholders for failing to call a medical doctor when emergencies arose. John Brown, the fugitive from Georgia who published his account of slavery in 1855 for a northern readership, decried inhumane treatment of enslaved men and women who were "indifferently clad" and were doctored only by "some old 'Aunt' or 'Uncle' who has 'caught' a little experience from others; and that not of the best."[37] Despite the evidence of benign interactions with white medical doctors, black southerners nevertheless held strong reservations about the ability of white physicians and medical institutions to exert healing power over their bodies.

Antebellum African Americans had sound reasons for mistrusting white men of science. Without legal possession of their persons, enslaved men and women became vulnerable to medical interventions consented to only by slaveholders. Poverty and racial subjugation created a similar vulnerability to medical experimentation for free African Americans in southern cities as well. In an era preceding an established ethical code for human experimentation, white practitioners subjected African American patients to procedures they would not have attempted on middle- and upper-class whites. From southern plantations to urban hospitals, medical doctors tried unproven medicines, perfected surgical techniques, and pursued theories of racial difference using African American men and women.[38]

The emergent fields of obstetrics and gynecology directed white medical attention in particular at African American women. Confronting public doubt about the respectability and efficacy of male interventions in female reproduction, white physicians performed procedures on enslaved and poor black women that would have been socially unacceptable on middle-class white women. The large majority of cesarean sections in the nineteenth-century South, for example, were carried out on African American women at a time when the operation remained highly experimental and usually fatal for either mother or infant, and sometimes both.[39] Similarly, aspiring surgeon J. Marion Sims conducted experimental surgery in Montgomery, Alabama, on a small group of enslaved women who suffered from vesico-vaginal fistula. The owners of the women had bound them over to Sims's custody, where they underwent a long series of trial operations between 1845 and 1849. One of the women, Anarcha, endured thirty operations in that five-year period. When Sims left his Montgomery practice, his successor, Nathan Bozeman, continued to test the performance of various sutures used to close vesico-vaginal fistula, again by operating on enslaved women.[40]

The Montgomery experiments raise many troubling questions about the operations that established Sims in the annals of gynecological surgery. First and foremost is the problematic question of medical consent in a slave society. Although Sims himself represented the women as consenting to the operations, Betsey, Lucy, Anarcha, and the others entered the crude Montgomery hospital through an agreement between Sims and their owners. Many of the women were very young, not even twenty years old when the operations began. They had been removed from their rural communities and sent to Sims's urban residence for treatment. Since Sims relied on heavy doses of opium to sedate the women after surgery, opium addiction may have also played a role in the women's long stay with Sims. Furthermore, Sims did not use anesthesia during the procedures, although articles on the early use of inhaled ether for surgical anesthesia had appeared by the late 1840s in American medical journals. Although Sims later acknowledged the extreme pain endured by his subjects from postoperative infections, he also remarked publicly that the surgery itself was "not painful enough to justify the trouble and risk" of administering anesthesia. In this latter conclusion he was no doubt influenced by antebellum theories that represented black women as less sensitive to pain than white women.[41]

The same differential theories of pain and lack of legal consent encouraged white doctors to experiment on enslaved men as well. Numerous case histories in southern medical journals indicate that white doctors routinely tried new treatments on enslaved patients. Georgia physician Crawford Long, for example, became well known as a pioneer in the use of ether as an anesthetic with the assistance of enslaved patients. One of Long's experiments to determine the efficacy of ether in surgery involved amputating the injured fingers of a young man; one operation was done with anesthesia, and the other without.[42] A particularly abusive incident of medical experimentation on a healthy enslaved man appears in the firsthand account of Georgia fugitive John Brown. As a young man Brown fell under the control of Doctor Thomas Hamilton when his master "lent" Brown to Hamilton as a token of gratitude. Over the course of several months Hamilton brought Brown to the point of collapse, subjecting him to excessive heat and painful blistering in the name of scientific investigation.[43]

Hamilton's experiments revealed tensions between southern medical theories of racial difference and southern practices of medical investigation. At times Hamilton viewed Brown as a universal medical specimen. For example, Hamilton subjected Brown to extremely high temperatures in the attempt to develop a sunstroke medication, presumably to be marketed to white and black southerners. However, in other sessions amounting equally to torture, the physician treated Brown as a racially distinct subject. Brown described how the physician peeled off layers of his skin to determine how thick "my black skin went." Sims's experiments contained a similar paradox, as black women's racialized lack of sensitivity to pain contributed to their use in experiments designed to benefit white women. Such were the contradictions of southern medicine, which in theory espoused the idea of racial distinctiveness but in practice used black bodies in experimentation and dissection to learn about the human body in general.[44]

Southern medical schools only compounded African American suspicions of white medical science. The faculty of southern medical schools relied heavily on indigent free and enslaved African Americans as specimens for teaching, observation, and exhibition. African American patients in urban hospitals became objects of display in lecture halls, hospital rounds, and surgical demonstrations.[45] Even more dreadful to antebellum African Americans, however, were dissections of cadavers that linked hospitals and white physicians not with healing but with death and mutilation.

For much of the history of Western medicine, practitioners of scientific dissection have relied on the bodies of the poor and powerless. In antebellum America, when dissection of human cadavers was illegal yet increasingly popular in the medical school curriculum, southern medical schools procured an illicit supply of corpses drawn disproportionately from populations of free and enslaved African Americans.[46] The medical college in Charleston, South Carolina, for example, advertised the availability of cadavers and the "great opportunities for the acquisition of anatomical knowledge" as a strength of its curriculum. An 1860 notice announcing a new "negro hospital" in Charleston pointed out that the hospital's location near the medical college would assist aspiring medical students in "acquainting themselves with the diseases peculiarly incident to a class from which the majority must expect to derive their largest number of patients." The notice went on to boast that the hospital would provide unparalleled "material" for "studying the personal and race peculiarities of the African."[47] Charleston physician T. Stillman may have had both experimentation and dissection in mind when he placed the following newspaper advertisement in 1838: "Wanted fifty negroes. Any person having sick negroes, considered incurable by their respective physicians, and wishing to dispose of them. . . . The highest cash price will be paid on application as above."[48] It is not surprising that medical schools and hospitals where white students acquired anatomical training gained reputations among black southerners as fearful places of dismemberment and even organ stealing.[49]

So common was the medical exploitation of black bodies that the theme of dissection crossed over from medical practice and entered white antebellum print culture. Henry Clay Lewis, a white southern doctor who published his raw, humorous tales of frontier medicine in the mid-nineteenth century, recounted one such incident in the medical training of his literary alter ego, Dr. Madison Tensas. While attending a Kentucky medical school, Tensas became enamored of the daughter of one of the city's wealthy men, from whom the relationship was kept a secret. He was also deeply interested in the subject of anatomy. One afternoon Tensas happened to pass the morgue that was conveniently located under the hospital's lecture room. On impulse Tensas seized the body of a black infant lying beside his or her mother, secreted the corpse under his cloak, and eventually headed down the street to his rooms for a private dissection session. At that moment the young lady and then her father appeared, leading to a startling climax in which the aspiring doctor accidentally dropped the baby's body into the street in full view of shocked onlookers. For Lewis the theft of the black infant served merely as an amusing pretext for the outrageous culmination of the story. The child's body functioned as a familiar prop in what was intended as a grotesquely humorous tale.[50] For southern African Americans, however, the theft of black corpses from morgues and graveyards constituted a shameful desecration of the dead.

Postmortem examinations conveyed a similar sense of violation. At times white physicians performed autopsies to settle legal questions about cause of death. A South Carolina physician, for example, billed the state ten dollars in 1858 for a "Post Mortem Examination on negro child found on A. Haddens premises."[51] North Carolina physician J. T. Craig reported assisting in a postmortem of an enslaved man who had been killed during a melee between several slaves and a slaveholder. The autopsy was apparently done to establish the cause of death, but Craig doubted that the owner would meet with any legal sanction.[52]

Apart from legal procedures, autopsies performed on African American bodies provided white physicians with opportunities for medical investigation. Influenced by developments in Parisian clinical medicine that emphasized postmortem studies, white doctors' interest in autopsies grew during the mid-nineteenth century.[53] For antebellum physicians, autopsy became an intriguing tool for understanding the effects of fatal disease on the internal organs. During an 1839 cholera epidemic, one Savannah doctor reported his futile efforts to save several enslaved victims of the disease. His only consolation, he wrote, lay in the fact that he "had exerted [himself] to the utmost, and would certainly have ample material with which to investigate the anatomical characters of the disease on the following day."[54]

White southern doctors reported routinely on the removal of organs from black bodies for the purpose of medical investigation. Georgia physician Edward Eve wished to investigate the internal effects of worms in an enslaved woman who died under his care. Just before her evening burial, Eve arrived at the gravesite, cut the woman's stomach from her body, and

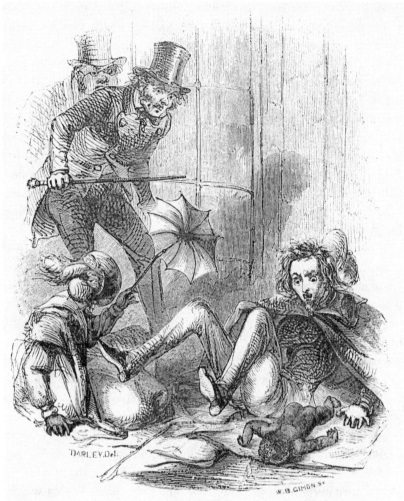

" My cloak flew open as I fell, and the force of the fall bursting its envelope, out. in all its hideous realities, rolled the infernal imp of darkness. "—*Page* 137.

Stealing a Baby. *Engraving by Darley Price. White antebellum print culture as well as medical practice reflected a callous attitude toward the dissection of black bodies. This engraving, an illustration for a tale about the theft of the body of an African American infant from a Kentucky morgue, appeared in a series of bawdy and inexpensive "humorous American works." The young author, Henry Lewis Clay, studied medicine at the Louisville Medical Institute, the likely venue for the fictional depredations of protagonist Madison Tensas. (Madison Tensas [Henry Clay Lewis],* Odd Leaves from the Life of a Louisiana "Swamp Doctor" *[1846])* "removed it to a convenient place for examination."[55] In Charleston, white physician Myddelton Michel sought to capitalize on the execution of an enslaved woman named Jane, who had been convicted of "murder by poison." While observing the official autopsy that followed her hanging, Michel saw in the procedure his own opportunity to investigate the timing and mechanics of ovulation. "I requested that the internal organs of generation of the girl Jane should be closely inspected," reported Michel. Lacking the proper instruments to examine the body closely, Michel took the "rare specimen," Jane's left ovary, away with him for further scrutiny.[56] For both men, access to the internal organs of enslaved women contributed to their professional recognition and publication in southern medical journals. For southern African Americans, however, such practices inspired indignation and dread.

From southern cities to rural plantations, African Americans viewed autopsies and dissection as an unholy theft from the dead. A white South Carolina doctor, frustrated in his attempts to perform an autopsy on a slave woman, briefly acknowledged the resistance of rural slave communities to postmortem procedures. In a medical journal article on the woman's uterine tumor he explained, "I regret extremely that I was unable to make a postmortem examination, (negroes in the country are much opposed to autopsies), and therefore cannot state the condition of the heart and veins."[57] From the perspective of enslaved communities, dissections and autopsies treated black bodies callously and retained them under white control. Postmortem examinations, furthermore, violated the correct relationship with the dead established through African American funerary rites. Members of slave communities, like many Americans of the time, placed great importance on proper mourning and burial. Within an African American sacred worldview, dismemberment and disrespectful treatment of the body risked the possibility that an offended spirit would return and cause misfortune for the living. Nineteenth-century African Americans may have also been influenced by Anglo-Christian popular beliefs that violating a corpse could prevent resurrection and entry into heaven.[58]

Moreover, the punitive desecration of black corpses by whites outside the scientific sphere had a long and painful history. During the transatlantic slave trade, white crews dismembered the bodies of Africans killed during Middle Passage insurrections. Slave traders carried out these acts of terror as a deterrent to other African captives who believed that the spirit of a mutilated person would not be able to return to Africa.[59] American slaveowners continued to employ mutilation as a tool of intimidation. A white southern doctor noted that some planters attempted to deter dirt-eating among their enslaved laborers by decapitating the bodies of those who died from this habit. Citing the effectiveness of this measure, he remarked, "The negroes have the utmost horror and dread of their bodies being treated in this manner."[60] Such punitive treatment obviously differed in intention from the dissection practices of white doctors. Yet the opening of black bodies and the parceling out of organs for medical research resonated with these historical practices of mutilation and dismemberment. Ranging from deliberate torture to banal appropriation of black bodies, the practices of slaveholder medicine, white practitioners, and medical institutions generated a healthy sense of caution and suspicion among enslaved communities.

African American oral traditions distilled truths from these historical experiences about the dangers of white practitioners, institutions, and medicines.[61] After the Civil War a genre of tales arose in the rural Southeast and cities such as Washington, D.C, describing "night doctors" who snatched black citizens off the street and took them to hospitals for mutilation and organ-stealing. As suggested by folklore scholar Gladys-Marie Fry, white authorities may have intentionally promoted urban tales of night doctors during Reconstruction to discourage African Americans from walking the streets at night. Former slave Laura Steward confirmed this argument in her description of mid-nineteenth-century hospitals. "Folks was skeared to go to hospital in dem days," she remembered. "Dey tole stories 'bout de hospital men puttin' black caps on you in the street at night, taken' you in, killin' and cuttin' you up. I guess dat was just to keep cullud folks off de streets."[62]

Night doctor tales, however, also had earlier historical origins in the experience of enslavement and antebellum racial subjugation. Given the wide proliferation of postmortem, medical display, and dissection activities focused on free and enslaved African Americans, it was not surprising that fears of malevolent white medical scientists existed in African American popular culture prior to emancipation as well. Hence the night doctor was not solely a calculating creation of white supremacists, but a terrifying incarnation of the historical relationship between African Americans and the developing field of medical science within a heavily racialized society.

Like the night doctor tales, rumors and suspicions about the violation of black corpses persisted among enslaved African Americans. Annie Burton, author of a published narrative on her childhood in slavery, reported the powerful impact of another story of postmortem violation. At the beginning of the Civil War, Burton recalled, whites in Clayton, Alabama, lynched two black men. As a child Burton refused to take castor oil prescribed by white doctors because she believed the oil had been processed from the bones of the murdered men. Later, as an adult, she saw the skeleton of one of these men assembled as a specimen in a Clayton physician's office.[63] Burton's story was hardly unique. According to an 1889 article in the *Boston Herald,* some black southerners believed that white men made castor oil from the blood of African Americans. Thus, the article continued, in "slavery times a negro would die before he would take a dose of castor oil."[64] The same theme arises in local rumors about the dissection of Nat Turner's body by white officials after his execution. At least one white newspaper at the time reported that Turner's body was delivered to white physicians for dissection, not an unusual fate for persons who died on the Virginia gallows.[65] Local oral tradition, however, holds that Turner's body was made into "grease" and his skeleton preserved as a specimen in a white doctor's collection.[66]

Constructing a lineage for elusive rumors and oral accounts is extremely difficult. On one hand, circulation of these stories in white newspapers says more about white racial ideology than it reveals about African American oral traditions. At the same time, nineteenth-century stories of white predation bear a striking resemblance to older accounts by captive Africans concerning European consumption of African bodies. Historians have long noted the persistence of African fears of "white cannibals."[67] As early as the Portuguese slave trade to the Kongo and continuing through English slaving voyages, African captives taken onto European ships feared that Europeans intended to eat them, to make oil from their bones, or to produce wine from their blood.[68] In the dislocation and terror of embarking in chains with an unknown people, African captives may have been making sense of the seeming consumption of their very lives by an alien people.[69] Though the lineage of this oral tradition is difficult to piece together, the belief that powerful whites turned black bodies into oil and other talismans persisted in nineteenth-century slave culture. In stories about castor oil, collected skeletons, night doctors, and dreaded dissections, enslaved African Americans distilled a penetrating critique of a society that consumed black men and women for their skills and labor, only to exploit their bodies once again in death.

White Fears of Black Healers

If enslaved sufferers looked with suspicion on white medical practitioners, white clients in turn viewed African American doctoring with an equal measure of distrust. The idealized physician-patient relationship allowed only white men to assume the professional authority that commanded patient deference. Yet the social relations of antebellum southern healing routinely involved white interactions with African American healers who were often women. When African Americans in subordinate social positions wielded medical knowledge as healers for white patients or white owners of slave patients, a new set of anxieties arose.

To be sure, white reliance on black healers was an everyday affair as well. As already noted, colonial planters demonstrated an interest in black herbal prescriptions and even manumitted several eighteenth-century healers in exchange for their remedies.[70] Day and night, slaveholders relied on enslaved women to prepare medicines and nurse the sick. Enslaved women elders also provided the foundation of daily health care to children and adults in plantation slave quarters. Occasionally a slaveholder hired a "negro doctor" to treat an enslaved patient with a lingering illness. Nor was it unheard of for white men and women to consult African American conjure doctors.

Yet the nagging anxiety about the independent actions of African American healers remained. Whereas slaves suspected privileged whites of employing medicine to reinforce the power they already held, slaveholders feared that enslaved healers would use their knowledge of healing to seize the power they had been denied. The authority of the enslaved healer — represented in the dependence of the white client on the slave healer's knowledge — clashed with dominant codes of deference and racial subordination. In this sense, slave healers possessed a power that generated anxiety in whites who sought their help. White antebellum society evolved a range of cultural and legal strategies intended to contain the contradictions and the implicit threat represented by authoritative black practitioners.

The fears of white southerners about the dangers of black healers surfaced primarily in the association between African American herbal knowledge and poisoning. How could they be certain, wondered many slaveholders, that slaves would not use their healing knowledge to injure or kill whites? A late-nineteenth-century newspaper article titled "Voudouism in Virginia" summed up the dilemma: "Many of them have knowledge of the properties of every tree and plant, leaf and root, found in their native fields and forests. From these they distill healing balms or deadly poisons."[71] When it came to antebellum black practitioners in general—and enslaved practitioners in particular—many slaveholding whites perceived a thin and fragile line separating medicine from poison and healing from harming.

Fears of poisoning by slaves emerged from white dependence on enslaved laborers in the intimate spaces of white households. Without changing the basic structure of southern labor relations, slaveowning households could do very little to reduce their vulnerability to personal harm. In 1836, for example, Virginia planter John Walker encountered the dangers of household poisoning in a conflict with a slave woman named Sillar. Walker had recently whipped Sillar because he was displeased with her work. Shortly after the whipping, Walker recorded in his diary, "[Sillar] said in the hearing of some of the servants . . . and one or more of the children that she would put three of us out of the way." Walker, his wife, two of his children, and two slave children soon fell ill. Walker believed the cause was some "poisonous stuff given in some way" by Sillar. Although the record does not indicate Sillar's household responsibilities, she was likely engaged in some kind of domestic work that put her in close proximity to the Walker family.[72] The overlap between healing and other types of domestic work such as cleaning, laundering, cooking, and childcare placed a range of household workers in a suspect position. Of the enslaved women and men accused of poisoning or misusing medicine, many worked in white homes as cooks and as caretakers of white children.[73]

The trials of Tom and Amy, referred to at the beginning of this chapter, provided a striking illustration of how Virginia lawmakers attempted to contain the perceived danger of medically knowledgeable slaves. It is significant that the Virginia court prosecuted Tom and Amy not on charges of poisoning but for administering medicine. Most colonial and later state statutes in the Southeast addressed poisoning under the criminal codes for persons of color.[74] Yet Virginia also passed a statute, discussed more fully below, that made the administration of medicine by both free and enslaved African Americans a capital offense. These laws exempted enslaved healers working with the consent of their masters. Thus Amy would not have transgressed the law by handling medicine in the white household where she worked as long as she did so under her master's orders. In fact, Amy probably fed and cared for the two white children daily, and her administration of remedies during their last illness would not have been unusual. Her alleged independent actions and collusion with Tom, however, brought her under suspicion. Her accusers feared and were willing to be-

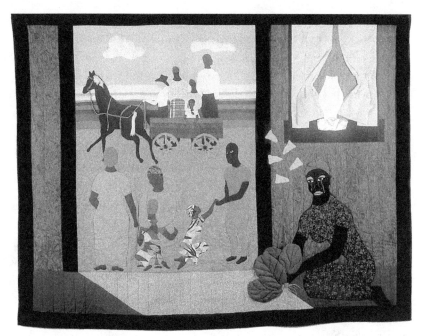

They Sold Nettie Down South. *Hand-pieced and quilted by Barbara G. Pietila, Baltimore, Maryland, 1992, 76" × 78". In this depiction Nettie's mother, an herbalist and cook for the white family who sold her daughter away, is gathering foxglove to avenge her loss. Foxglove leaves contain a potentially fatal heart stimulant used to produce the modern drug digitalis. This beautiful and arresting quilt conveys how African American arts of healing, in the hands of a skilled practitioner, also became arts of resistance. (Courtesy of the Roland L. Freeman Folkart Collection; photograph © 2001 Roland L. Freeman)*

lieve that she had used her intimate contact with the children to turn the duties of healing into an opportunity for murder. Following Amy's conviction and death sentence, her supporters sought to defend her character in terms that defined her as a subservient and obedient laborer. Calling her a "faithful servant" and depicting her as closely attached to the white household, the petition for clemency painted a portrait of Amy intended to override the image of the dangerous nurse.

As Amy's prosecution showed, white fears of poisoning produced a dangerous atmosphere for women who cared for members of white households. Former slave Nancy Williams described the whipping of a young Virginia girl who was hired out to a poorer white family who subsequently blamed their baby's illness on her.[75] Likewise Lila Nichols, enslaved as a young person in North Carolina, recounted a story of brutality unleashed by poisoning paranoia. Nichols had known a slave girl named Alice whose tasks included bringing water and food to an invalid plantation mistress. Recalled Nichols, "Missus got sick on her stomick, an' she sez dat Alice done try ter pizen her." "Ter show yo' how sick she wuz," Nichols pointedly remarked, "she gits out of de bed, strips dat gal ter de waist an' whups her wid a cowhid till de blood runs down her back." Alice was eventually sent to Richmond and sold for her alleged offense.[76] Whether or not intentional poisoning was truly involved in either incident, these stories reveal the vulnerability of enslaved household workers to legal prosecution, violence, and sale.

The convergence of concepts of poisoning and conjuration only deepened slaveholder distrust of African American medicine and enslaved healers. While some slaveholders dismissed conjuration as a mere "superstition," many nevertheless feared conjure doctors' accomplishments in the arts of poisoning. Particularly in the late eighteenth and early nineteenth centuries, "Negro doctors" or "conjurers" often appeared as immediate suspects or second parties in cases of suspected poisoning. An enslaved man named Sharper was jailed in 1773 pending a trial for attempting to "procure Poison" from a "Negroe Doctor or Conjurer." The Virginia officials examining Sharper's case charged that he had offered money to an elderly conjure doctor "to destroy White people."[77] In 1800, South Carolina courts tried and executed John, an enslaved man with a local reputation as a conjurer, for poisoning the brother of his owner. Significantly, John had previously been sentenced to one hundred lashes for another charge involving conjuring. Over the protest of John's master, the court convicted John on the testimony of slave witnesses who alleged that John boasted of giving the brother "Truck to run him Destracted, and then gave him Truck to kill him."[78]

Associations between conjuration and poisoning most likely caused Samuel A. Townes's alarmed reaction to an enslaved woman he had just purchased for plantation subsistence work. Writing home to South Carolina in 1835 from his new settlement in Alabama, Townes described his efforts to obtain a cook and a nurse for his plantation: "I made a trade with a driver day before yesterday for a cook & the evening she came to my house I found in her possession a bottle of whiskey, blue stone, brimstone, snake heads I took it to be [illegible] powdered up[,] & the pieces of various other reptiles. She had not of course any criminal intentions against me for she was delighted to come to me—but she had brought it with her as a stand by for a *rainy day*—the man took her back willingly."[79] Despite

Townes's insistence that the woman meant him no harm and was, in fact, "delighted" to be sold to him, his quick return to the slave trader clearly indicated his misgivings.

Townes's perfunctory description of the woman's possessions implied that his family, too, would immediately grasp the connotation of danger. What did the Towneses, a white slaveholding family, know about the ingredients Samuel listed, and why did he immediately associate the items with criminal intent? With the possible exception of the reptile pieces, antebellum whites did not classify any of the material as physically toxic. In fact, white plantation remedies commonly called for brimstone (or sulfur) along with other minerals and herbs.[80] Yet, as the Towneses must have known, African American conjuration also made frequent use of all the items the woman carried. The assemblage of reptile parts, whiskey, bluestone, and brimstone was undoubtedly a conjure packet, carefully composed for purposes of healing, harming, or protection.[81] While it is impossible to know how the enslaved woman intended to use it on her perilous path through the domestic slave trade of the Deep South, it is clear that Townes perceived the woman's possessions as a threat to the stability and safety of his household.

Slaveholders' fears of conjuring knowledge and household poisoning emerged again in the trial of Delphy, a Virginia slave woman. The Louisa County court sentenced Delphy to death on 10 June 1816 for "feloniously preparing and administering" poison with the intent to kill her mistress, Isabella Mitchell. Delphy worked as a milker and was "regarded as a conjurer" in her community. According to the testimony of enslaved men and women who declared themselves terrified of Delphy's powers, the conjure woman had publicly promised that "she would put her mistress out of the way" and that "her mistress, should be in the ground, before the summer was out." Aaron, also enslaved by the Mitchells, subsequently saw Delphy "beating up some bottle Glass, and boiling a decoction of pokeroot" and pouring both into a vial.[82] Not having access to the Mitchell kitchen herself, Delphy secured the cooperation of another woman, Aggy, who served the preparation to Isabella Mitchell in her daily coffee. Isabella testified in court that around the time when Delphy's public threat was reported to her, she had suffered "most violent & excruciating pains & spasisms about her stomach & bowells." Further illustrating the vulnerabilities of white families to poison, Isabella's young son had also complained of sickness after drinking the coffee, and some pigs to whom the offensive brew had been fed fell dead.[83] Though none of the Mitchell family died, Delphy's open threat and easy access to the white household frightened Louisa County slaveholders enough to convict and execute her.

In contrast with the number of enslaved women accused of poisoning within white households, African American conjurers charged with subversive activities extending across plantation boundaries were overwhelmingly male. Gender divisions of labor and patterns of mobility contributed to these distinctions. Enslaved women frequently involved in intimate care of white bodies had more opportunities for poisoning and greater vulnerability to poisoning charges while they worked as cooks, nurses, and domestics. Apart from midwives, who seem to have largely escaped suspicions of poisoning in white households, enslaved women did not usually have as much opportunity as enslaved men to travel outside plantation boundaries. The association of male conjurers with insurrection in slaveholder records may also have been influenced by white perceptions of military activity as a male domain. Slaveholders feared that the authority vested in the male healer's knowledge of medicines would extend to leadership among multiple slave communities, thereby serving as a potential organizing point for insurrection.

The link between conjure doctors and insurrection extended the threat of poisoning beyond individual white bodies to the southern body politic.[84] During the American Revolution a "Cungerer & forting-teller" called Ben gathered a "company of negroes to Joine the British" in Virginia but was caught and lashed severely for his activities. Reflecting their hostility to Ben's activities, white neighbors described him as a "fellow of bad character" and a "notorious villian."[85] In 1812 a North Carolina conjurer named Goomer also served as the "head man" for a Virginia slave conspiracy. Goomer's activities came to light in the trial of an enslaved man named Tom who was accused of murdering his master in the belief that Goomer would "conjure me clear" of danger. Furthermore, Tom's strike against his master was part of a larger insurrection plan involving up to forty enslaved men and women timed to coincide with American-British conflicts in 1812. Goomer figured heavily in the plan, not only by protecting the insurrectionists but also in providing poison for killing some slaveholders.[86]

Protection offered by a conjurer played an equally large part in Denmark Vesey's plans for a Charleston slave uprising in 1822. When Charleston officials intercepted Vesey's plot and brought the participants to trial, public reports focused heavily on the "conjurer and a physician, in his own country" known as Jack Pritchard, or Gullah Jack. According to testimony, Gullah Jack promised protection from harm to Vesey's followers and served as a military leader himself. White observers discredited Pritchard's authority as a "negro doctor" by deriding the "superstition" of his followers.[87] The hostility recorded in court reports on the appearance and character of Gullah Jack revealed the intense anxiety that white slaveholders felt about African American practitioners who escaped the confines of subservience and dependence sanctioned by white southern society.

Even when enslaved healers were not associated with conjuration, their activities provoked suspicions by fearful whites. An 1844 Tennessee court, for example, affirmed the danger of African American practitioners in the trial of Jack, an enslaved man whose practice of medicine "about the country" had come under legal question. Upholding a state law that forbade slaves from practicing medicine, the court explained that "the legislature was guarding against . . . insurrectionary movements on the part of slaves. . . . A slave under pretence of practicing medicine, might convey intelligence from one plantation to another, of a contemplated insurrectionary movement; and thus enable the slaves to act in concert to a considerable extent, and perpetuate the most shocking masacres [sic]." Given these risks, wrote the court, "it was thought most safe to prohibit slaves from practicing medicine altogether."[88] In white responses to African American healers, the public threat of enslaved men mirrored the private threat of enslaved women. Both were feared for the independent actions they might take under "pretence of practicing medicine."

From the eighteenth century on, southern legislatures sought to circumscribe the practice, mobility, and potential authority of African American healers. Among the southeastern coastal states, Virginia took a particularly aggressive stance in passing laws that addressed the practice of enslaved as well as free black healers. A 1748 law stipulated the death penalty for any "negroe, or other slave, [who] shall prepare, exhibit, or administer any medicine whatsoever." Such a measure was necessary, in the lawmakers' opinion, because "many negroes, under pretence of practising physic, have prepared and exhibited poisonous medicines, by which many persons have been murdered, and others have languished under long and tedious indispositions."[89] Medicine laws were most actively prosecuted in the eighteenth century but remained part of slave statutes until the Civil War.

Additional statutes regulated apothecary (drugstore) sales in order to restrict the medicines available to African Americans. Both Georgia and South Carolina passed apothecary laws in the mid-eighteenth century, perhaps in response to a high number of poisoning incidents during the late colonial years. In 1751 South Carolina restricted the sale of poisonous substances and prohibited druggists from employing slaves or free persons of color in jobs that involved making or dispensing medicines. The same law stipulated the death penalty for any black person instructing others in the knowledge of "poisonous root, plant, herb, or other poison whatever."[90] Antebellum legislation built on the colonial legal foundation. An 1856 Virginia law made it illegal for a druggist to sell "any poisonous drug" to a slave or a free black person without written consent of "owner or master." Georgia legislation continued to address the issue of poisonous substances sold by druggists. An 1860 version of an apothecary restriction in Georgia went so far as to forbid the sale of arsenic, strychnine, hydrocyanic acid, and aconite to anyone other than a druggist or physician and meted out harsh penalties to any person who furnished poisons to slaves or free persons of color.[91] Apothecary laws implicitly recognized that medicine had dangerous as well as beneficial uses; southern lawmakers thus attempted to restrict the ability of African Americans to deploy medicine's harming capacities.

Slaveholders could seek to ensure white security by restricting the practice of enslaved healers but could not do without their labor.[92] Accordingly, restrictive legislation revealed broad exemptions from prosecution and gradual moderation in both stipulated penalties and the sentences handed down in courts. Beginning with Virginia's colonial medicine laws, legal exemptions revealed slaveowners' reliance on enslaved healers. The initial 1748 law exempted from penalty any slave who administered medicine under "his, or her master's or mistress's order." In an extension of the notion of dual consent to African American practitioners as well, a slave healer might give medicines to slaves in another white household only if their owners also consented to the treatment.[93] Acknowledging the role of enslaved assistants in procuring and administering medicine, apothecary laws allowed a slave to purchase "poisonous drugs" from druggists with the slaveowner's written permission.[94]

Throughout the antebellum period, Virginia law continued to restrict the practice of black healers, but penalties for violating the law lessened over time.[95] In part, the decreasing severity of sentences for convictions under the medicine laws accompanied the overall moderation from the eighteenth to the nineteenth century in the number of capital crimes for slaves.[96] Additionally, poisoning prosecutions in Virginia decreased in the early nineteenth century, as violent murders, armed insurrections, and arson became the predominant charges in slave trials.[97] Even during the late eighteenth and early nineteenth centuries, when capital punishment applied, there is evidence that courts substituted other penalties for the death sentence. Several enslaved men and women convicted under the medicine laws between 1754 and 1771 were spared hanging but endured mutilations instead. In the trials of Quash and Isaac, the courts determined that no "evil Intent" or "bad consequences" were evident and thus ordered the men to be "burnt in the hand" and lashed. The slave woman Mill evaded the gallows only to receive thirty-nine lashes, public humiliation in the pillory, and the "cropping" of both ears to mark her permanently as a criminal.[98] By 1843 only the administration of medicine and deadly poison with intent to murder remained a capital offense in Virginia. Sale, preparation, and administration of medicine by a slave without consent of his or her owner had been reduced to a misdemeanor punishable by up to thirty-nine lashes.[99]

Adjustments and exemptions in the Virginia laws demonstrate how slaveholders attempted to defuse the perceived danger of African American healers by separating their labor from their authority. The law defined a legitimate slave healer as someone who practiced under the knowledge, direction, and orders of whites. This definition contrasted starkly with the authority and respect that white physicians hoped to attain in their own practice. Exemptions in the slave medicine laws revealed that white southerners feared the influence and unpredictable actions of enslaved healers as much as their medicines. Dependent on enslaved healers as plantation health workers, white planters used the law, among other methods, to harness the labor of slave doctors while aiming to eliminate their implicit threat. Laws aimed at doctoring, poisoning, and access to powerful medicines thus became tools for the impossible task of regulating the many daily interactions between black healers and persons who sought their assistance.

Within southern slave society the specter of sinister intentions on the part of the healer and the fear of vulnerability on the part of the sufferer cut both ways. Sociologist Wilbur Watson has argued that black folk medicine relies on strong "bonds of trust" between a healer and a sick person. Trust is enhanced, asserts Watson, by three important factors: first, the sick person's confidence in the healer's ability to discern the nature of the disorder; second, the sick person's faith in the practitioner's power to heal; and third, shared cultural understandings of illness between healer and sufferer.[100] Putting Watson's argument into historical perspective, the social context of slavery compromised all three of these principles for African Americans confronting slaveholder medicine.

On the most basic level, enslaved African Americans were not even sure that slaveholders or physicians could comprehend the nature of some of their afflictions, particularly those involving conjuration. Furthermore, even when they acknowledged that whites possessed the power to heal, many antebellum African Americans wondered whether they would use that power in beneficial ways. Slaveholders used their medicines, for example, to torture as well as to cure. Moreover, white medical institutions seemed as interested in consuming as in curing black bodies. Finally, the tensions between slaveholder priorities and the relational vision of healing held by enslaved communities often undermined any basic foundation of shared cultural understandings when it came to battling illness. The social relations of southern slave society thus infused interracial medical encounters with a politics of distrust.

The erosion of notions of trust in interracial medical encounters created an atmosphere in which suspicion extended beyond the healer-sufferer relationship to broader issues of planter control. Agricultural labor, by far the largest sector of enslaved labor, formed a critical arena for daily struggles over health and healing. In plantation production, however, the perceived threat lay not with enslaved healers but with enslaved sufferers whose ailments could impede the progress of cash crops. In cotton, rice, and tobacco fields, planters cast a wary eye on the physical complaints of laboring men and women.

*Once upon a time there was an old man in slavery. He told his
master that he was cripple and couldn't work. So the man let him
stay home to take care of his children. One day the master went away.
When he came home, he find the man play on his banjo, — "I was
fooling my master seventy-two years / And I am fooling him now." He
was singing this song away on his banjo. His master caught him, and
start to kill him by whipping him. So the old man went to the doctor
Negro. The next day he was to be kill'. When his master started to
whip him, everytime the man start to whip him, none of the licks
touch. And he had freedom.*
—Folk-Lore of the Sea Islands, *1923*

*At the time of sickness among slaves they had but very little attention.
The master was to be the judge of their sickness, but never had studied
the medical profession. He always pronounced a slave who said he was
sick, a liar and a hypocrite; said there was nothing the matter, and he
only wanted to keep from work.*
—*Henry Bibb,*
Narrative of the Life and Adventures of Henry Bibb, *1849*

CHAPTER 7

Fooling the Master

In the 1830s two enslaved women named Marmer and Grace
were transported from a settled plantation in Virginia into the Deep South.
Their new master, William Harrison, stopped in Alabama, where the air
bristled with the business of speculation in land and slaves. Hoping to
establish a successful cotton plantation, Harrison counted on the labor of
Marmer, Grace, and other slaves previously owned by Harrison's father-
in-law, Nathaniel Hooe. Perhaps Hooe had transferred ownership of these
men and women to Harrison as a wedding gift when he married Hooe's
daughter, Frances. Perhaps Marmer, Grace, and the others were part of
the father-in-law's investment in new territory. However they came to find
themselves breaking the ground of Harrison's newly purchased plantation,
Marmer and Grace brought with them a history of defiance as workers.

In a letter to his son-in-law concerning the "character" of the two women, Hooe disclosed a series of battles with Marmer and Grace over their claims to illness:

> Marmer of whom you speak she has been under an overseer. . . . I have herd him say he would have to Flog her to make her go out to work having counterfeited a great deal two [*sic*] much, but an excellent hand at the plough or hoe when at work, Grace a good hand to work, but hard to manage[.] I can trace her counterfeiting to 1819 the year she came to my management & you may remind her of her counterfeiting sickness, from that time under Harry King & of John Frank's begging me to take her from his management. He could not manage her, & she put me to much trouble to manage her, & at last she gained her point by being a spinner.[1]

Hooe detailed these past struggles in order to help his son-in-law control Grace and Marmer in their new surroundings. Reading between the lines of his letter, we glimpse a world in which claims of illness provided both opportunity and danger for enslaved laborers.

The drama of feigned illness emerged from the broader context of distrust in plantation medical encounters. In struggles over health and medicine, poisoning trials or incidents of medical torture represented only the tip of the iceberg. Slaveholding families commented with alarm on the unusual occurrence of a slave's murderous use of poison. Similarly, remarkable accounts of medical abuse and violated corpses circulated through enslaved communities. Far less sensational and more widespread were the everyday conflicts that arose over slaves' claims of illness, injury, or pregnancy. For millions like Grace and Marmer, struggles over illness were part of their larger efforts to resist the "management" of slaveowners.

As the correspondence between Hooe and his son-in-law revealed, planters frequently spoke of feigned illness as an issue of slave character. From the perspective of antebellum planters, control over slave labor and the management of slave health required careful attention to both the bodies and the dispositions of enslaved workers.[2] Hooe, for example, prefaced his remarks on Marmer and Grace with the reminder, "You wish information of character of the Negroes I last sent." Slave health problems became for slaveholders "an endless stream, inseparable from conceptions of the slave's personality."[3]

Feigning illness was not the only point at which white southerners linked slave character to issues of health. Samuel A. Cartwright, for example, pathologized the resistance of African Americans to slavery by naming defiance as disease. The efforts of enslaved men and women to escape the plantation, for example, became "drapetomania," defined by Cartwright as "the disease causing negroes to run away." "Rascality" among enslaved workers became "dysaesthesia aetheopica," a "disease peculiar to negroes, affecting both mind and body."[4] Despite the striking nature of Cartwright's ideas and their frequent citation by historians, beliefs about feigned illness had far greater impact on the actual relationship between slaveholders and slaves. In shaping the practice of white plantation practitioners, elaborate theories of racial medicine played second fiddle to banal assumptions about race and character.[5] However small the daily events comprising the struggle over feigned illness, they nevertheless profoundly shaped both the course of plantation production and the atmosphere of plantation health care.

Holding radically different meanings for slaves, on one hand, and slaveholders and white doctors, on the other, feigned illness was a many-faceted ailment of plantation labor relations. Feigned illness emerged from a broader struggle between slaveholders, who tried to control African Americans in the service of plantation production, and slaves, who attempted to maintain some say over their bodies and labor. For enslaved African Americans, manipulating illness claims was a strategy of resistance that offered reprieve from labor but brought with it the dangers of planter coercion. Slaveholders, meanwhile, viewed feigned illness as a defect in slave character and a plague on plantation work routines. From yet a third perspective, white doctors discussed feigned illness as a symptom of southern medical practice and a phenomenon that shaped their examination, diagnosis, and treatment of enslaved patients. Defined by whites as a false (yet contagious) "Negro" disorder, feigned illness crystallized the tensions underlying coerced labor in the antebellum South. Like other socially weighted diseases, such as tuberculosis, syphilis, and AIDS, feigned illness can be read as a socially constructed illness framed by the racial and gender ideology of the antebellum South.[6]

Perfecting and Protesting Plantation Discipline

Efforts to ferret out deception in the sickhouse contributed to overall attempts by planters to keep enslaved workers in check. In the 1840s and 1850s planters elaborated their designs for plantation discipline and control more fully under the rubric of "slave management." Many slaveholders, particularly those on plantations with large slave populations, evolved systems of rules, regulations, rewards, and punishments for their workforce. Physical violence, such as whipping, flogging, and incarceration, was only one aspect of plantation discipline broadly defined. During the late antebellum decades, advice literature on plantation management proliferated, with articles on overseers' duties, regulation of health, and systems for housing and punishment.[7] Through these measures planters attempted to exert control, to promote plantation productivity, and ultimately to maintain the social order of slave society.

At the heart of slaveholders' enthusiasm for systems of management lay the fear of deception. Management systems in large part addressed the futile effort of planters to extend their knowledge and control over all aspects of slave life. Nathaniel Hooe urged William Harrison to live on the premises of his plantation, warning that a "subaltern" overseer would not have the ability "to manage the Negroes, their Laziness, [and] their Disposition to be vicious & bad, in a great variety of ways."[8] Rice planter Louis Manigault similarly worried about his ability as a wealthy planter to exert control through several layers of plantation management including subordinate white men as well as enslaved drivers. Pondering whether to appoint a white "sub overseer" to Gowrie Plantation, Manigault considered the problem of traffic between adjoining slave communities when he and the overseer were absent. "I am *Certain*," he wrote, "there are *many things* going on that neither you nor I, nor Clark know off [*sic*]. — I know that when I am not here there is more visiting going on than we would allow." Furthermore Manigault, with some prompting from his overseer, worried that a sub overseer might "side with the negroes" and refuse to follow his superior's directions.[9] Through plantation management schemes slaveholders thus sought to develop a system that prevented deception and insubordination.

Proper management of slave health, according to many planters, required round-the-clock regulation of enslaved communities. Plantation management literature merged antebellum public health concepts with systems of plantation discipline to place a heavy emphasis on social life within slave quarters. In a medical journal article on typhoid fever, South Carolina physician W. Fletcher Holmes charged enslaved families with endangering their own health by their "irregular mode of life, monotony of diet, uncleanliness, exposure to sudden alternation of heat and cold, their crowding together in close, ill-ventilated apartments, and their want of healthy and sufficient sleep." After-sundown activities in the slave quarters received particular criticism. In the same article Holmes lamented the "cheerful gleams of torchlight, . . . the hum of the spinning wheel, and the melancholy cadence of the negro's song" emanating from slave houses late into the night.[10]

Both medical and slave management literature implied that activities taking place outside the supervision of whites threatened the health of the plantation as a whole. As a result enslaved African Americans found their habits of eating and drinking, nighttime movements, dress, and housing closely scrutinized by planters. One plantation manager, attempting to explain the cause of several slave deaths, decried the tendency of men and women to "come out of their houses at night regardless of the weather" even when under "strict injunctions" to stay indoors.[11] Although bondsmen and bondswomen might welcome a supply of warm clothes during a wet, cold winter, they were less likely to share the planter's enthusiasm for restrictions on visiting between cabins after dark. Archaeologist Larry McKee provides yet another illustration of the disciplinary potential of planter management in the upper South. A nineteenth-century reform in slave housing endorsed by many planters called for raising slave cabins off the ground to promote air circulation. This measure, however, also carried the implied goal of curtailing slave appropriation of goods commonly hidden in the root cellars of cabins built directly on the ground. Raised cabins would eliminate the clandestine use of these "hidey holes."[12] Such health reforms obviously served purposes beyond the control of disease, extending planter discipline into intimate areas of slave life.

Planters themselves overtly argued the connections between discipline and health, often posing slave health problems as the result of racialized character flaws. In an 1858 letter James Sparkman proposed, "There are difficulties incident, which are chargeable to the black race as a *people,* and which prevents the perfecting of any system of discipline by hospital or Infirmary institutions." Referring to the planters' system of health management, Sparkman believed even the most rigorous "medical police" of any plantation would be undermined by slave behavior.[13] Another South Carolina physician chose the military instead of the medical police as his preferred analogy for the management of slave health. In the *Planter's Guide and Family Book of Medicine,* Charleston physician J. Hume Simons recommended a regime of plantation hygiene based on cleanliness, sanitation, and proper housing. He pronounced himself convinced "that if more system and discipline (like regulations in an army), were pursued on plantations, the condition of the negroes, as well as that of the planter, would be materially improved."[14] As Sparkman himself recognized, however, the gap between these master plans and the reality of plantation health care remained large.

If planters were going to control slave health, they would by necessity have to control enslaved healers on whom they relied for news of illness. Planters' inability to achieve this goal often led them to blame enslaved women for plantation deaths. "Infernal stupids" was the epithet Thomas Chaplain reserved for two women upon the death of a teenage boy. The boy's mother and Old Judy, a midwife and nurse, had been attending him and did not inform Chaplain of ominous symptoms that, Chaplain complained, only the nurses could communicate.[15] Virginia planter William Massie likewise complained of finding out too late about serious illnesses of slave children. Of the death of an infant boy from "neglected putrid sore throat," Massie recorded, "indeed the writer knew not of his illness before his death."[16]

White doctors practicing on plantations similarly perceived enslaved women as impeding the goals of plantation health management. A Savannah physician, called to assist an enslaved mother's difficult labor that ended in a stillbirth, wrote that the mother "had been in labour the whole night, without the fact having been communicated by the nurse to the overseer until daylight the next morning."[17] A Virginia physician told absentee slaveholder Bowker Preston in 1834 that a young boy's death could have been prevented with earlier attention. The boy had been sick three weeks, wrote Preston: "Although about that time I was frequently at the quarters not one word was ever said to me on the subject." Perhaps these doctors were simply trying to deflect blame from their own performance.[18] Nonetheless, such charges revealed the anxieties of whites over their dependence on slave women for news about slave illness that, as Chaplin observed, they "had no way of knowing except through the nurses."

Discipline of enslaved patients eluded slaveholders as well. White physicians, planters, and overseers frequently criticized the behavior of African Americans under medical treatment. Some complained that sick slaves, like their attendants, failed to reveal their symptoms. Samuel Cartwright believed the reluctance of enslaved patients to inform whites of their illness posed an inherent threat to the health systems of any plantation. Especially in epidemics, wrote Cartwright, "the negroes themselves, when panic struck, cannot be depended upon to report or let their indisposition be known, until they are nearly half dead and can no longer conceal it."[19] Louis Manigault regretfully echoed this charge in writing about the death of an enslaved man, Brister, who "had had the symptoms of the Cholera for three days but kept it quiet until too late."[20]

Most popular among planters' complaints was the failure of sick persons to follow health-related instructions. On this failure slaveholders blamed relapses, prolonged illnesses, and even deaths. For instance, J. T. Cooper, the overseer of one of the Manigault estates in Georgia in the 1840s, reported the deaths of several "hands" from dysentery. Insisting that the Manigault slaves had brought death on themselves by ignoring his rules about drinking water and going out at night, Cooper concluded, "I look upon their deaths as suicidal acts."[21] Several years later, during an 1854 cholera epidemic, Louis Manigault relayed the attending physician's opinion of reckless health behavior in the slave quarters. Describing the need for caution in the aftermath of epidemic he wrote, "The Dr says negroes! they will overeat themselves & Clarinda was eating homony contrary to his order."[22] Tenah, a young woman on a South Carolina plantation, also bore the blame for her own death in slaveholder David Gavin's eyes. Tenah had recovered from her first illness after being treated by several physicians, but she contracted pneumonia, Gavin wrote, after "she went about for her own amusement and exercise."[23] Roswell King Jr., writing during the same time from St. Simons Island, concurred regretfully that "negroes will never adhere strictly to instruction given them, or they would do much better."[24]

Planter complaints against headstrong enslaved patients merged with nineteenth-century proslavery arguments that African Americans required the disciplinary structures of enslavement (and, by implication, the guidance of whites) in order to thrive, and even survive, as a people. Bowker Preston's physician, L. G. Cabell, again writing in 1834, informed the planter of symptoms that seemed fatal in a slave woman named Jenny. Cabell had been told (though he could not personally confirm the observation) that when Jenny had initially recovered from her mild symptoms, she "did not conform to hardly any directions I gave her." Furthermore, he went on to extrapolate from Jenny's condition to the general need for white oversight of slave health. Complaining of the "extreme ignorance & carelessness of negroes," he added, "They will never do right, left to themselves."[25] The doctrine of black incompetence in self-care came to justify planters' social control and even the institution of slavery itself.

Other professional white doctors, like Cabell, added their own unique refrain to the chorus of complaints against enslaved patients. Numerous case histories in antebellum professional journals described African Americans as being generally "unruly" and uncooperative with white practitioners. Noncompliance from enslaved patients seemed especially to insult white doctors' sense of professional dignity. Josiah C. Nott described a young black man with a broken leg: "He was the most unmanageable patient I ever saw and appeared to be perfectly regardless of consequences."[26] The *Southern Medical and Surgical Journal,* in which Nott published his article, ran other descriptions by physicians of enslaved patients who "didn't observe instructions," who deceived physicians about the cause of injury, and who lengthened the time of an operation by "[bearing] the knife badly" and being "extremely unruly."[27] As published case histories reveal, physicians condemned African Americans as difficult patients precisely because they breached the idealized relationship between the authoritative physician and the deferential patient.

Particularly frustrating for white doctors was their inability to exert authority over enslaved women's reproductive health. Another case history in a Virginia medical journal outlined Richmond doctor William Patteson's frustrations with Amy, a slave woman diagnosed with a prolapsed uterus and whose lack of cooperation threaded throughout the entire article. According to Patteson, Amy complained that the prescribed pessary was painful and, "being restive and intractable," frequently refused to wear it. After settling on a pessary that was more comfortable, Amy wore the device "rather better, but not patiently." Soon, however, Patteson discovered that Amy was pregnant, but Amy, for reasons unstated, "persistently denied" her condition and "obstinately" refused again to wear the pessary. Finally Amy gave birth to a "feeble child" who died after several days. Reflecting the interest of the planter class in enslaved women's reproductive labor, Patteson concluded that after his treatments Amy was "now perfectly well, and makes an excellent wet nurse."[28]

Other physicians who were not so sanguine about slave infant mortality questioned whether enslaved women deliberately terminated pregnancies and thus lowered the birthrate on southern plantations. Although African American sources establish slave use of herbal abortifacients, southern physicians debated to what extent slave women bore responsibility for birthrates lower than planters would have desired. E. M. Pendleton disparaged what he believed was a pervasive planter belief that "blacks have a secret unknown to the whites, by which they either produce an incapacity to bear children, or destroy the foetus in embryo." Instead the Georgia doctor blamed both overwork and "sexual indulgence" for a high rate of spontaneous abortions and sterility. Physician John Morgan agreed with Pendleton's analysis but nevertheless restated the widespread conviction that slave women willingly sought to "effect an abortion or to derange menstruation." Despite their differences, both authors recommended more attention to slave management in the service of better health. "Planters should pay more attention to the habits of their slaves, if they wish to obtain a more rapid increase," wrote Pendleton. The twin goals of plantation discipline and slave soundness left little room for the independent actions of enslaved women.[29]

The case histories of physicians and the complaints of planters, however, clearly demonstrated that enslaved African Americans eluded the discipline of planter health measures on a regular basis. Precisely because slaveholders depended on African American healing knowledge and conceded some latitude to slaves in matters of self-care, the arena of sickness and healing presented unique opportunities for resistance to planter control. Enslaved men and women refused medicines, acted contrary to orders, and concealed their serious illnesses from whites. Among such strategies of resistance was also the popular practice of claiming illness to wrest time away from the fields.

The Opportunities and Dangers of Strategic Illness

When enslaved African Americans claimed illness for their own purposes, they implicitly challenged systems of plantation discipline. Though they seemed to be opposite tactics, feigning illness and concealing signs of sickness bore underlying similarities to each other. Either action withheld health knowledge from planters and bought enslaved men and women time to act outside the control of slaveholders. Furthermore, inherent risks and potentially severe costs accompanied both actions. While concealing signs of sickness from white practitioners could result in worsening symptoms and deprivation of medical help, feigning illness risked discovery and subsequent retaliation.

Southern African American orature contained a shrewd analysis of feigned illness as a resistance strategy utilized by the oppressed and seemingly powerless. Animal tales from the Georgia coastal Lowcountry, for example, recounted one instance after another in which the trickster used sickness to throw an adversary off guard. A claim of sickness was a posture of weakness behind which the trickster achieved his desired ends. In one popular story, Buh Rabbit and Buh Wolf found themselves competing for the same young woman's favors. The inventive Buh Rabbit told the woman that Buh Wolf was no more than his riding horse. An angry Buh

Wolf rushed to Buh Rabbit's house to force him to retract his insult. There he found Buh Rabbit lying in his bed and protesting that he was too sick to go out. Buh Wolf finally forced Buh Rabbit to go see the woman by agreeing to let the ailing Buh Rabbit ride on his back. As they neared her house, Buh Rabbit sat up and dug his spurred heels into Buh Wolf's side, forcing Buh Wolf to run past the woman just like the horse Buh Rabbit had called him. The humiliated Buh Wolf slunk away, and Buh Rabbit gained the woman's hand. The appearance of sickness gave Buh Rabbit an advantage over the stronger but less clever Buh Wolf.[30]

The trickster was not above taking advantage of community norms of compassion for the families of the sick. In one story Buh Rabbit lied about his wife being sick to escape the work of building a winter provision house with other animals. Later, when cold weather arrived, he used additional trickery to live off their labor.[31] Similarly, another tale had Buh Rabbit concocting the story of his sister giving birth as an excuse to get out of work with Buh Wolf.[32] In yet another story Buh Rabbit was the one fooled when Buh Partridge tricked him out of his share of the meat from a cow they had killed; Buh Partridge pretended that two of his children had been fatally poisoned by the meat.[33] These animal tales demonstrated the bold stance of the trickster who dared use even the sacred arenas of sickness, birth, and death to outwit an opponent.

In the spirit of the trickster who deployed his wits against a more powerful adversary, enslaved African Americans used claims of illness to exploit their value to slaveholders.[34] Forcing slaveholders to respond to their assertions that they were sick, enslaved men and women manipulated the twin desires of slaveholders for both immediate profits and long-term wealth. While the labor of slaves was essential to yearly crop production, the preservation of slave health was critical to the sustained wealth of slaveholding families. The health of enslaved women had an added dimension of wealth, since they not only produced crops and sustained households, but their childbearing assured future laborers and increased property holdings for planters. Through plantation "management," slaveholders sought to balance these sometimes competing interests. There is evidence that many southern planters followed common health practices such as restricting outdoor labor in the rainiest weather, providing seasonal clothing, and reducing the tasks of pregnant women in their last trimester.[35] Frequently, however, such precautions gave way under the pressures of harvest or planting seasons when planters risked the fatigue, injury, and sickness of enslaved workers against the gathering or sowing of crops. Feigned illness was one means by which enslaved men and women turned the slaveholder's dilemma to their own limited advantage.

Frequent complaints of sickness and deception by planters and overseers suggest that enslaved workers regularly used strategic illness to ameliorate plantation work demands. Recording a daily tally of three slave women in the sickhouse, Virginia planter Charles Friend protested, "Monday is allway a sick day with us."[36] Similarly, planter Thomas Chaplin complained frequently of "pretense" among eight of approximately twenty-five enslaved men and women on the Tombee plantation. Chaplin's struggle with his finances may have made him particularly vulnerable to lost labor and thus especially vociferous in recording slave complaints of illness. In his journal Chaplin resolved, "I am determined to look more closely into their complaints, and not allow anyone to shirk from their work and sham sickness."[37] Slaves who claimed the need to "lay up" drove Chaplin to distraction as he sought ways to detect pretenders. In one journal entry Chaplin remarked that he had "caught" a man sitting up and weaving a palmetto hat in bed when he was supposed to have been ailing. According to another entry he saw Isaac out walking when he was supposed to have been seriously ill, an incident that provided evidence for Chaplin that Isaac was "playing possum."[38] Occasionally Chaplin seemed to resign himself to a loss of labor, as when Jim and Judge were "lying up." Chaplin forced them out of the sickhouse but commented that it was "no use, they will have their time out."[39] His journal remarks suggest the ability of Tombee slaves to carve out significant moments of reprieve from heavy labor, albeit under the determined surveillance of planter or overseer.

The vested interest of planters in slave reproduction added leverage to enslaved women's strategic claims of illness and pregnancy but added as well to the risks of retaliation.[40] Grace, described by Nathaniel Hooe as "hard to manage," was able to influence the type of work she did by complaining often of sickness. Grace apparently resisted the field work to which she had been assigned, for she finally "gained her point" by becoming a spinner instead. We do not know Grace's specific complaints or even if she bore any children. Yet many planters perceived women's claims of pain or disability in terms of "female complaints." General lack of understanding of the processes of menstruation, conception, pregnancy, and birth must have added to the inability of male overseers and slaveholders to detect slave women's false claims of illness. Describing her childhood on a large North Carolina slave plantation, Chana Littlejohn remembered the women "played off sick an' went home an' washed an' ironed an' got by wid it."[41]

Frances Kemble also relayed the story of a Georgia woman, Markie, who claimed pregnancy for many months and collected extra rations for her condition.[42]

The prominence of slave women as plantation health workers increased the likelihood that female complaints of illness would have their desired effect. Enslaved nurses often mediated women's claims of sickness or pregnancy with overseers and slaveholders. The large number of planter complaints about lack of notification that involved young children suggests slave women sought in particular to protect babies, young children, and new mothers from slaveholder remedies. Some doctoring women also used their intermediary position to assist members of their community who feigned illness. As an elderly woman, Polly Shine clearly remembered the protective role of the nurse on her plantation during slavery. "Of course us Negroes soon learned to play sick lots of times to get out of work, and Maser would let us off until we got better, because if we got worse and died he would lose some money," she recalled. "If Maser caught on to us making out like we were sick, he would sure give us a hard punishment. But we would be very careful not to let him catch us. We knew that old black mama would not tell on us, and if we thought the Maser was going to get the white doctor, we got better right away."[43] As Polly Shine's reminiscence indicated, careful calculations were required of those who chose pretending as a strategy of resistance. In the drama of feigned illness, enslaved men and women presented a posture of infirmity while carefully weighing the risks of detection.

Polly Shine's recollections of "hard punishment" testified to the dangers of strategic illness claims. The aura of distrust surrounding feigned illness encouraged planter suspicion of all slave complaints of unwellness. In his antebellum narrative Henry Bibb charged his owner with aspiring to be "judge of their sickness." This planter, wrote Bibb, "always pronounced a slave who said he was sick, a liar and a hypocrite; said there was nothing the matter, and he only wanted to keep from work."[44] Tines Kendricks of Georgia remembered an equally suspicious mistress. Kendricks told an interviewer, "Old Miss, she mighty stingy, and she never want to lose no nigger by them dying. Howsomever, it was hard sometime to get her to believe you sick when you tell her that you was, and she would think you just playing off from work. I have seen niggers what would be mighty near dead before Old Miss would believe them sick at all."[45]

Fearing the loss of valuable human property yet wary of medical expenses and pretended maladies, skeptical slaveholders at times refused to acknowledge even deathly illness. Tines Kendricks's young cousin died in slavery after the "Old Miss" dismissed the mother's plea that her son was dangerously ill. Likewise, in 1859 William Massie entered a begrudging obituary next to Patty's name in his slave records. At nearly eighty, Patty had died "of I know not what disease," wrote Massie. He went on to make the following accusation: "She has been saying she was sick for near a year & always pretended to be sick."[46] Apparently even Patty's death failed to convince Massie of the seriousness of her ailments.

In the climate of distrust surrounding slave complaints, the strategy of pretended illness was a double-edged sword. On one hand, claiming illness offered an opportunity for black men and women to rest their bodies, to relieve some of the extra stresses of pregnancy, to affect the pace of work, and perhaps even to reclaim time for visiting friends and family in the sickhouse. On the other hand, feigning usually only succeeded for a short while, and a planter's refusal to summon medical care, as Tines Kendricks pointed out, could be fatal. Furthermore, discovery of feigned illness could result in hardship and whippings. According to Nathaniel Hooe, Grace was ultimately able to influence the kind of work she did but had to battle owners and overseers for fifteen years to do so. The woman Marmer, also known for "counterfeiting," received several floggings from an overseer who forced her to work.[47] Pregnancy claims as well presented unique dangers for women when outward signs of pregnancy, not to mention the expected baby, failed to materialize. After more than nine months the woman named Markie in Frances Kemble's story was finally discovered to be faking and was whipped.[48] Chana Littlejohn's account, however, ended quite differently. When the overseer discovered the women's scheme and attempted to force them back to field work, Littlejohn informed her interviewer, she and her friends "flew at him an whupped him."[49]

Animal trickster tales reflected the opportunities of strategic illness, but other stories within the orature of enslaved communities warned of the dangers. Several tales centered on individuals who "fooled the master" through claims of illness and disability only to be caught and punished.[50] One Virginia story described how "Uncle Daniel" affected illness and old age in order to get a "retirement" from field work and secure the help of a young boy who waited on him. Daniel's cruelty to the young boy was his downfall, for the boy let the master in on Daniel's ruse. Now it was the master's turn to play trickster. On the pretense of setting Daniel out to convalesce in the sun, the master propped him against a haystack and set it afire. Daniel's nimble flight away from the flames exposed his deceit, and he was quickly forced back to the fields.[51] Another story circulating through-out a Virginia neighborhood warned of harsh retribution. During "slavery days" a man called "Uncle Ben" repeatedly and successfully feigned tooth-aches in order to evade work and seek rest from "runnin' bout at night." However, the slaveholder grew suspicious and finally took a pair of iron pliers and pulled almost all of Ben's teeth from his mouth.[52] Addressing the realistic dangers of challenging the slaveholder, these slave stories formed a precautionary complement to the animal tales that celebrated the triumphs of the trickster.

Finally, some tales echoed Chana Littlejohn's account of the women who turned the tables one final time. Folklorist Elsie Clews Parsons recorded a South Carolina story of an old man who posed as a "cripple" and was allowed to look after children instead of working in the fields. One day the planter discovered the man playing his banjo and boasting, "I was fooling my master seventy-two years." In retaliation the slave master determined to whip the old man each day until he died. But the old man consulted a "doctor Negro" for protection. On the day the man was to die under the lash, the slave master discovered that the whip could not touch his victim. "And he had freedom," concluded the storyteller.[53] With each twist and turn of plot, the story revealed a range of resistance strategies and outlined just as clearly their attendant dangers.

However successful feigning was as a strategy of resistance, it was im-measurably complicated by ideas slaveholders themselves brought to their interactions with enslaved workers. White responses to slaves' claims of illness were not simply reactions against African American resistance prac-tices. Instead, white assumptions about the deceptive character of enslaved men and women took on a life of their own. Preconceptions about slave character thus increased the dramatic tension between African Americans who claimed illness and the white men and women who attempted to judge the validity of those claims.

Feigned Illness through the Eyes of Slaveholders and Physicians

The belief that all enslaved African Americans possessed at least the potential for deceptiveness acquired in white antebellum racial thought an aura of indisputable truth. Derogatory assumptions about slave charac-ter, along with other racial propositions about physical differences, came to be viewed, as one medical journal put it, as truths "so universally acknowledged, as to require neither argument nor illustration in their support."[54] Moreover, in voicing their beliefs about black deceptiveness, white southerners frequently blurred the concept of individual character with collectively assigned racial traits. South Carolina planter Keziah Brevard repeatedly articulated in her diary the conviction that "Negroes are as deceitful and lying as any people can well be." Subsequent entries reiterated her obsession that "lying seems a part of a negros constitution" and that black men and women had "nothing but deception in them."[55] Suspicions of slaves' claims of illness emerged from this general white prejudice against the character of an entire population.

In the eyes of slaveholders and white doctors, "playing possum" was an expected manifestation of slave character. Hence when a perplexed William Harrison consulted his father-in-law on the eye complaint of an enslaved man named Lymus, Nathaniel Hooe alerted Harrison to the possibility of feigning. Harrison reported that he had bled Lymus and planned to take him to a doctor for night vision problems. Hooe, however, urged his son-in-law to take a second look at the complaint. "Lymus I am sure must be counterfeiting with you," he warned, "unless he has inflamation in his eyes."[56] Hooe's skepticism provides just one example of the pervasive suspicion with which slaveholders greeted slaves' claims of sickness. South Carolina slaveholder Harriott Pinckney even broached the issue openly with those enslaved on her plantation when she instructed her overseer to relay to "the people" that she had asked him about their behavior and "whether they worry you [the overseer] in pretending to be sick."[57]

Slaveholders routinely conferred with one another in their correspondence as to whether particular men or women were inclined to pretend illness. Conflating individual character with racialized traits, Socrates Maupin of Richmond wrote to his brother for advice about a hired slave man, Garland, who had complained of being ill: "You said something about his wanting medical attention. *He is a true negro in being always 'poorly'* but if he needs medical attention at any time I shall of course expect it to be rendered to him."[58] Virginia slaveholder Alexander Yuille was likewise willing to consult a white doctor for an enslaved man's complaints, but he commented with chagrin that the man had been "deseased for a length of time or at least thinks himself so."[59] Susan Hubbard informed her husband of her reassessment of an enslaved woman's illness. Franky, she wrote, "looks thin complains much and is quite disposed to be an invalid."[60] In each of these cases slaveholders considered medical care for enslaved patients but wondered whether treatment was actually necessary.

Distinctions between slave feigning and other kinds of "false" sickness illuminate the racial determinism of white theories about feigned illness. Although medical doctors had named hypochondria as a disease by the early nineteenth century, it was an illness largely reserved for privileged whites who did no manual labor. *The Planter's and Mariner's Medical Companion* informed readers that "hypochondriac disease" primarily afflicted males of a "sendentary or studious" disposition.[61] Slaveholders rarely perceived hypochondriachal tendencies in African Americans but, rather, interpreted pretended illness as deliberate deception.[62] In other words, the leisure to be respectably sick was a white elite prerogative exempting a person from the heavy demands of plantation labor. David Gavin complained heartily in his journal of an overseer's wife who, he believed, affected symptoms of illness in order to avail herself of the labor of enslaved women for laundry, cooking, and other household work. Mrs. Griffin, according to Gavin, seemed to be playing the lady instead of carrying out her domestic duties.[63] Gavin's accusation hinted at the intriguing possibility that white planters extended a racialized notion of feigned illness to poorer southern white women as well. For slaves and possibly for poorer whites, pretense in illness was not an affliction, like hypochondria, but a defect in character with criminal overtones.

Adhering to a common racial ideology, planters and white doctors nevertheless formulated the problem of feigned illness in two distinct ways, each of which reflected their respective anxieties about mastery and professional authority. For slaveholders, feigning was foremost a labor problem, defined by the threat of the deceptive worker. Physicians, in contrast, approached feigning as a difficult challenge to their medical skills and authority. These distinct formulations by planters and physicians led to separate remedies yet drew on similar assumptions about black racial traits. Ultimately the strategies of both planter and physician merged in enforcement of plantation discipline.

Planters simply assumed that enslaved African Americans would pretend to be ill in order to escape work. Slaveowners used words such as "shirking" and "malingering" to describe the threat that feigned illness posed to plantation labor regimes. Thomas Chaplin voiced his conviction that the complaints of a woman field worker, Helen, were probably caused by her desire to avoid a difficult task assignment.[64] South Carolina politician and slaveholder Charles Cotesworth Pinckney implied that feigned illness drained plantation output when he advocated Christian instruction for slaves on the grounds that Christianity would help diminish "the cases of feigned sickness so harassing the planter, [and] would augment their numerical force and consequent production."[65] Above all, planters perceived feigned illness as a dilemma of slave "management," an impediment to plantation production and labor discipline.

As both laborers and childbearers, enslaved women fell under double suspicion of "playing possum." Planters and overseers often complained of the loss of labor represented by slave women's pregnancies and "female complaints." An overseer on the Manigault rice plantation in Georgia wrote that the most troublesome aspect of slave health was "Pregnant women[.] there is now five which weaken the force very much."[66] The inability of planters to verify early stages of pregnancy merely fueled their resentment of enslaved women's claims. A South Carolina planter complaining of the field labor lost to pregnancy voiced his suspicions that female complaints were often deceitful: "Very much [vexed] with *sick women,* either real or pretended, the latter in most cases."[67]

Although it is difficult for historians to be certain, planter suspicions of feigned illness in enslaved women likely outweighed the actual incidence of feigning, thus proving more of a liability than a resistance practice.[68] Fanny Kemble, in her representation of Georgia Sea Islands slavery, charged that plantation overseers frequently dismissed the impaired health of childbearing slave women, believing the women were "shamming themselves in the family-way in order to obtain a diminution of their labor."[69] Indeed, beside the name of a woman named Betty in the Butler Island infirmary book, the word "shaming" appeared where the record keeper normally listed the nature of the malady.[70] Similarly, Thomas Chaplin complained of two women who "both *pretend* to the same thing—viz. falling of the 'body' [prolapsed uterus]."[71] Such frequent complaints suggest that, as with the issue of abortion, planters blamed enslaved women for health problems brought on by harsh labor conditions.

Thomas Chaplin's journal entries revealed the perilous tension between the twin demands of enslaved women's reproductive and field labor. Between 1845 and 1854 Chaplin often expressed impatience and exasperation over the weeks and even months that one woman, Peggy, spent "laying up" in the sickhouse. Each of Peggy's extended sick periods involved issues of reproductive health, including a pregnancy resulting in the birth of twins, breast infections, and a miscarriage. Clearly eager to expand the plantation slave population through the birth of children, Chaplin may have tolerated Peggy's many days of absence from plantation work because of her value to him as a childbearer. However, as a planter living at the edge of affluence with an overextended labor force, Chaplin also fretted over the field work he lost when Peggy stayed in the sickhouse. Four months after giving birth to a daughter, Peggy returned to the sickhouse with a "rising breast," and Chaplin remarked, "Peg still laying up. She never knows when to come out when once she gets in the house."[72] During a period of heavy field work several years later, Chaplin resentfully recorded another illness: "Peg sick, damn her. She is always sick when I am most pushed for work."[73] Though Chaplin obviously realized Peggy was not strong, he persisted in blaming her absence from the fields on deception and obstinacy rather than on pain or disability.

As with other plantation labor struggles, planter responses to suspected feigning ranged from resigned accommodation to enraged brutality. At the most benign level, slaveholders expressed distrust by discounting or dismissing African American claims to illness that did not seem to threaten disability or death. Planter correspondence frequently mentioned sick slaves and added that there was "nothing much the matter" with them or that the sick persons in question were simply "disposed to complain."[74] Overseer Roswell King took the path of least resistance at Butler Island Plantation. "Many lay by when I know from false tongue and other symptoms, it is slight," he explained, perhaps referring to the practice of examining the tongue to make a diagnosis. His treatment consisted of "a little mild medicine & a days rest; if that were not done, should loose thrice the time; even if at work, very little would be done, under the pretense of being sick & not allowed to lay by."[75] Other planters attempted to return sickhouse occupants to the fields through psychological manipulation. As a novice planter in Georgia, young Louis Manigault consulted his father about a slave woman named Nancy and her tendency to "hug the sick house." Shortly afterward, Manigault found a way to "turn her out" by telling Nancy that exercise (meaning work) was the best medicine for her malady. Whether or not Nancy believed his prescription for health, Manigault reported that she had gone out "willingly."[76]

Violent coercion, however, was never far in the background. Overseers and slaveholders often attempted to whip notions of illness out of those they distrusted. Regarding Grace's tendency to "counterfeit" sickness, Nathaniel Hooe wrote his son-in-law, "You will, to make her perform have to be tight with her, & my advice to you will be . . . not to spare her in the beginning."[77] Indeed, both Marmer and Grace endured many floggings during their lives for their persistent claims of illness. Thomas Chaplin also relied on the lash to empty his sickhouse, although it is not clear how often he carried out his periodic threats to "whip all round." In one cursory entry Chaplin observed, "Mary came out [of the sickhouse] today, or rather was *whipped out*."[78] Analiza Foster of North Carolina bitterly recalled her enslaved mother's account of a pregnant woman who fainted in the fields while plowing. The driver accused her of "puttin' on." Being cautioned by the slaveholder not to injure her baby, he dug a hole for her rounded belly and fiercely whipped the woman face down in the sand. For the Foster family this story vividly preserved harsh memories of a master who callously spent the lives of his enslaved workers.[79] The involvement of the driver further suggests that some enslaved headmen charged with pacing the day's labor may also have adopted an attitude of suspicion toward feigning aimed at women's reproductive health.

Finally, beyond the lash stood the specter of sale and separation from kin. Occasionally a planter employed this response in retaliation for feigning. Samuel Townes, writing from a frontier plantation in Alabama to family in South Carolina, declared his intentions to sell Daniel, who "pretended to be sick and did very little work for a week during a critical time in the crop." Townes reported that Daniel had "no claims on the affections of any of our family," and his fate should be governed entirely by "the suggestion of interest." Since it seems the Townes family had been looking to sell Daniel even before his week of absence from work, the accusation of feigned illness was most likely part of a larger struggle between Daniel and the Towneses.[80] Even if they were not always employed, the whip and the danger of being sold loomed as threats behind planter suspicions of African American claims to illness. Coercion and violence were thus woven into the very fabric of health care interactions between enslaved African Americans and white slaveholders.

Less directly concerned with the productivity of their clients' fields, white doctors viewed feigned illness among slaves primarily as a regionally distinct medical problem and a challenge to their professional authority. In an era that put American physicians on the defensive concerning their professional identity, the detection of feigned illness became for southern physicians another proving ground of their competence. To paraphrase Henry Bibb, white doctors also became judges of slave sickness with profound implications for their practice among enslaved patients.

Widespread planter assumptions about slave deceit added an unusual dimension to the professional relationship between the white southern doctor and his enslaved patients. White doctors not only diagnosed illness and prescribed medicines but were also asked from time to time to determine the validity of a patient's complaint.[81] In his case history of Peter, a middle-aged enslaved man, Richmond physician W. H. Taylor revealed his awareness of this peculiar duty of southern physicians. Taylor reported, "Remembering that *simulation was a characteristic of his race,* I made a rigid examination, the result of which convinced me that there was no deception attempted." Peter, already complaining of "low spirits and general depression," was subjected to a doctor's examination premised not on trust but suspicion.[82]

The writings of one South Carolina medical student suggest that the art of exposing counterfeit illness may have been seriously considered as an element of southern medical training. In an 1850 thesis titled "The Medical Treatment of Negroes," M. L. McLoud advised the southern physician to be "on his guard" with slave patients. "To detect the imposture," he argued, "constitutes a most difficult task; one which requires all his discrimination and acuteness."[83] According to this thesis, slave complaints were never to be taken at face value. Instead, a rigorous physical investigation must "pass under review and be carefully considered before the negro is pronounced to be actually sick."[84] According to McLoud, a cautious diagnosis could make or break a young doctor's career. He warned, "Every planter is well aware of this universal disposition to deception [in slaves], and if his physician does not appear to be aware of the same, his confidence in his judgment immediately abates." With experience and sound medical training, however, the physician "will the more readily detect impositions, and by the successive detection of imposture, he will secure valuable friends and rapidly rise to honorable distinction in his profession."[85] Hyperbole aside, McLoud's advice reflected the triangular relationship of enslaved patient, white doctor, and slaveowning client imposed by slavery. McLoud prioritized the confidence of the planter client over the trust of the enslaved patient, for the doctor's detection skills served to secure honor among his white peers. Establishing the planter's confidence thus depended on distrusting the enslaved patient's word.

The strategies used by white physicians in detecting deception in illness revolved around reading the signs of an enslaved person's body against his or her word. In 1846 Samuel Cartwright pondered the question of how a doctor should proceed with patients he viewed as unreliable. He advised close study of the external features of a patient to make a diagnosis using the science of "Prosoposcopia," or the "physiognomy of disease." Such an approach, he argued before an 1846 medical convention, would be to great advantage with "children who cannot, and females who often will not tell, what is the matter with them." A skilled physician, declared Cartwright, could discern many diseases simply by studying "the expression of the patient's countenance."[86] In this early speech Cartwright was not specifically discussing the treatment of enslaved patients; most of Cartwright's peculiar medical theories on the racial differences and diseases of African Americans were yet to come. Yet his recommendation touched precisely on the problem of how physicians could diagnose patients from dependent populations (such as women and slaves) presumed to be inclined toward dissemblance.

M. L. McLoud's thesis, written just four years later, tackled the issue of feigning among enslaved patients directly. He advised looking closely for "garrulity" and exaggerated expressions of pain, which he believed to be sure signs of deceit. Any person truly in pain, he surmised, would lie still and silent. Especially suspicious to McLoud were internal afflictions, such as indigestion, colic, concussions, and epilepsy. He believed enslaved men and women complained of these conditions because, in contrast to Cartwright's theories on the "physiognomy of disease," they could not be readily disproven from external examination.[87] Suspicions of illness thus produced a less patient-focused examination that differed from the usual antebellum emphasis on the patient's communication of his or her specific symptoms.[88]

Once a white doctor had convinced himself that a slave's claim to illness was false, he was likely to "treat" feigning as a medical problem. Whereas planters at times used the whip, physicians were more likely to turn to medicine and psychological manipulation. As a first line of action, McLoud suggested the physician attempt to outsmart the suspected pretender. Show no sign of suspicion, he advised, but instead use sympathy to draw out conversation; encourage suspicious patients to talk about their conditions until they betray themselves by describing "contradictory symptoms and complaints."[89] Although McLoud fastened on the problem of African American deceit, his recommendations implicated physicians themselves in a game of trying to "trick" enslaved patients into either believing themselves healed or revealing their own deception.

Some white doctors, particularly in the lower South, may have gone so far as to employ medicines in a punitive manner both to detect and to deter feigning. In his thesis McLoud endorsed the use of emetic, purgative, and foul-tasting medicines to prevent an enslaved patient from repeating complaints of illness. As supporting evidence McLoud offered the anecdote of a slaveholder who accidentally treated an enslaved woman's epileptic seizure with undiluted ammonium carbonate (spirits of hartshorn). The burning medicine brought the woman immediately out of the seizure, thus exposing her pretense. Although McLoud described this incident of dangerous medication as an accident, he implied that deliberate use of harsh remedies might prove effective in testing the patient's sincerity and act to discourage future feigning.[90]

Slaveholders at times encouraged white doctors in the punitive use of medicines as a tool for detecting feigned illness. Thomas Holloway, a South Carolina slaveholder who similarly suspected an enslaved woman of fabricating her symptoms to avoid difficult field work, consulted a physician on a "cure" for the woman's deceit. Pricy, Holloway charged, "complains of a slight pain in the head, and says she had a chill today *after dinner.*" Holloway suggested the doctor send him some medicine — "something that *will* make her sick enough tonight" to make her prefer work the following day.[91] We do not know whether the doctor actually prescribed according to Holloway's plan. Yet the request suggests that slaveholders sometimes looked to physicians to administer medicines in the interests of plantation production rather than the patient's health.

Maintaining the distinction between coercive and medical responses to feigned illness was often difficult for physicians who suspected that enslaved patients were pretending. Once a physician embarked on regulating the behavior of the enslaved patient, it quickly became possible to cross over from the harmful use of medicines to the supposed therapeutic uses of violence. McLoud approvingly related an incident on his neighbor's plantation in which a white doctor recommended the whip to "cure" a "stubborness of disposition" in a man suspected of feigning an injury. In another example he wrote of an enslaved woman given to epileptic fits; her owner did not administer harsh medicine but instead threatened a whipping. Arriving at a conclusion of "imposture," the physician attending the woman recommended her next seizure be "treated" with a "cowskin or hickory switch to scourge her on the spine."[92] Another physician attempted to draw attention to the dangers of disregarding slave complaints when he referred to the tendency of his colleagues to "prescribe a *light brushing,* and send the patient to the field" after claims of mild illness.[93]

The semantics of violent "treatment" revealed the murky ethics of medical relations under slavery. The trope of intentional pain as a punitive prescription for the illness of feigning undermined the physician's position as a healer and drew him into the process of plantation discipline. In this context of suspicion it became ultimately impossible for either physicians or slaveholders to adhere to a strictly medical approach to the illness claims of enslaved patients, for attempts to detect feigned illness joined physicians and planters in enforcing the social order of the plantation.

In the drama of feigned illness, enslaved African Americans and slaveholders manipulated for their own ends the roles of patient, healer, and trickster. Slave health care, from the planter perspective, was very much an issue of labor control. Planters' beliefs that enslaved laborers were unreliable in sickness as well as in work tended to fuse concepts of individual slave character with white racial thought on collective "negro" traits. Southern slaveholders' intensive counterattack on feigning stemmed from their desire to establish a dependable measure of slave soundness. Slaveholders employed limited accommodation, psychological manipulation, violent coercion, and punitive sale to gain the upper hand over slaves' claims of illness. In the process, techniques of labor discipline became deeply embedded in the health practices of southern slaveholders and physicians.

For their part, enslaved men and women used their knowledge of the chattel principle—the planter's investment in their bodies—to raise doubts about their soundness. By claiming illness for their own purposes, slave men and women forced slaveholders to weigh the pressing needs of planting and harvesting against their property interests in slave health and childbearing. Though feigning illness was less dangerous to enslaved laborers than outright refusal to work, it was not without cost. Animal stories and slavery tales told within plantation slave quarters taught listeners about both the opportunities and the risks of feigning illness.

The stakes were highest for enslaved women, who were suspected of duplicity both as sufferers and as healers. Planters and overseers, most of whom had no clear understanding of female reproductive health, grumbled frequently about their lack of control over slave women's pregnancy-related complaints. Midwives and sickbed attendants, too, received criticism from planters for withholding information about the sick and for sheltering those who pretended to be ill. Furthermore, the entire debate surrounding pretended illness in African Americans drew on notions of female dissemblance prevalent in the mid-nineteenth century. Antebellum whites defined "shamming" as not only a "negro" but also a female trait. Lower-class white women, too, fell under suspicion of playing the invalid to avoid domestic duties. When Samuel Cartwright made the related charge that women "often will not tell, what is the matter with them," he identified dissemblance as a gendered characteristic.[94] Directed at enslaved African Americans as a race, charges of feigning served to reinforce the myth of black dependency that would outlast the proslavery ideology it served.

Conclusion

"Sometimes we are blessed with being able to choose the time and the arena and the manner of our revolution, but more usually we must do battle wherever we are standing." The late poet Audre Lorde wrote these words in 1988 in an essay on the final stages of her battle against cancer. A brilliant writer and a passionate warrior for social justice, Lorde refused to separate her fight for health from her ongoing political work. "Battling racism and battling heterosexism and battling apartheid share the same urgency inside me as battling cancer," she wrote.[1] Lorde articulated a critical point in the history of African American health and healing. Enslaved men and women also did not choose the conditions of their struggle. On a daily basis they fought individually and collectively against a relentless assault on their humanity. Essential to their efforts were health practices that healed the body and countered the objectifying impulse of the chattel principle. As black health struggles joined other freedom fights, African American doctoring became an important weapon in the battle against the broader conditions of enslavement.

The gendered nature of slavery placed African American women in the forefront of many contested areas of plantation health. Under white southern law and custom, slave women embodied a dual form of wealth. Valued as both productive laborers and potential childbearers, bondswomen suffered multiple intrusions upon their bodily health and well-being. Enslaved women found their choice of partners restricted, their children stolen by sale, their pregnancies and other illnesses doubted, their bodies violated by rape and other violence, and their strength exploited for agricultural and domestic labor. Slaveholders' efforts to control the bodies of enslaved women exposed the power relations in which health issues were embedded. The context of slavery thus particularly confirmed Angela Davis's argument that "the pursuit of health in body, mind and

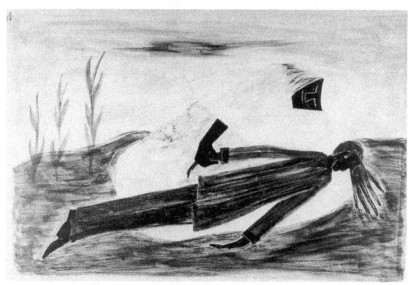

In innumerable ways slave women used healing skills to survive slavery and advance African American freedom. As portrayed in one of thirty-one panels on her life, Harriet Tubman used her herbal knowledge to serve the Union army during the Civil War. (Jacob Lawrence, The Life of Harriet Tubman, *no. 29, "She nursed the Union soldiers and knew how, when they were dying by large numbers of some malignant disease, with cunning skill to extract a healing draught from roots and herbs that grew near the source of the disease, thus allaying the fever and restoring soldiers to health"; casein tempera on hardboard, 12 × 17 ⅞ in.; collection of Hampton University Museum, Hampton, Virginia; copyright © Gwendolyn Knight Lawrence, courtesy of the Jacob and Gwendolyn Lawrence Foundation)*

spirit weaves in and out of every major struggle women have ever waged in our quest for social, economic and political emancipation."[2]

Slaveowners placed heavy constraints on enslaved women's pursuit of health and healing. Whether it was the attempts of a mother to breast-feed her baby adequately during harvest time or the efforts of older women to properly prepare a neighbor's body for burial, healing work rarely occurred in an autonomous space immune to planter interference. As the preceding chapters have shown, slaveowners had a strong and vested interest in the health practices of slaves. Enslaved sufferers seeking to define their ailments often had to consider planter and physician diagnoses. Likewise, conjure doctors and their clients by necessity conducted their business with an awareness of planter hostility to African American religious practices. Women healers had to negotiate various identities—for example "herb doctor" and "plantation nurse"—emanating from both enslaved community culture and slaveholder labor schemes. Overall the narrow confines of the doctrine of soundness posed numerous obstacles to enslaved women's pursuit of a wide spectrum of collective health needs.

Despite severe limitations on their sphere of action, enslaved women used their doctoring skills to counter slavery's degradation of the black body, family ties, and communal relations. Evidence clearly shows that enslaved women put their own stamp on work requisitioned by the master. Women elders assigned to care for young children designed remedies for enslaved adults as well. Against the grain of southern property law, enslaved mothers claimed their children by employing preventative remedies and teaching them rituals of protection. Southern bondswomen sought some measure of control on childbearing through herbal abortifacients, sparking disgruntled complaints among many planters. Older midwives, particularly on the large plantations of the Lowcountry, attempted to shelter enslaved sufferers by acting as intermediaries with white planters and overseers. In each of these situations, enslaved women exerted their authority as practitioners by using healing knowledge for their own ends.

Enslaved women's authority, like their health practices, was a subject of contention on southern plantations. Although planters depended on black women's skills and adopted their remedies, they frequently failed to recognize the basis of black healers' authority. Instead antebellum white Americans of the middle and upper classes tended to focus on two other realms of medical authority: the maternal authority of white women's domestic medicine and the professional authority of white men with medical training. Denied the prerogatives of both free motherhood and professional training, enslaved women were summarily excluded from both kinds of medical authority. Nonetheless, the status of black women as healers within slave communities suggests that enslaved African Americans recognized an important third category of healing authority, previously unexamined in the historiography of nineteenth-century medicine.[3]

The central importance of spirituality to slave health culture authorized both women and men as healers. In contrast to the dominant culture, African American concepts of healing authority did not rely on the opposing and unequal definitions of manhood and womanhood that supported both the male authority of antebellum physicians and the maternal authority of white female domestic healers. Gender hierarchies certainly existed to some degree in enslaved communities, as did gendered divisions of healing work, but healing authority itself did not rest on these differences. Instead the ability to wield spiritual power served as the measure of a healer's reputation regardless of gender. Age, experience, family ties to other healers, and mentorship by older practitioners also contributed to the collective recognition of enslaved practitioners. Spiritual empowerment, however, remained the crux of enslaved healers' authority, for it lay beyond the ownership and control of slaveholders.

Following emancipation, conflicting views of the legitimacy of slave healing authority contributed to markedly different histories of antebellum plantation medical care. In the 1930s and 1940s, African Americans with immediate memories of enslavement frequently identified respected healers within their families as the main source of medical care. According to these men and women, the health needs of enslaved communities gave rise to an ethic of self-reliance. In 1941 Mary Ross of Virginia described to an interviewer her grandmother's calm efficiency in the face of illness: "When anybody in the family had the dysentery my grandmother she won't ever bothered or skeered 'bout what to do — she knowed what to do and went ahead and done it." Collecting leaves from a nearby peach tree, Meelie Hood soaked the bruised leaves in clear water as a cure for ailing family members. What Mary Ross remembered most keenly was her grandmother's sense of confidence and her determination to use her knowledge for the well-being of her family. Ross recalled with wry humor, "You know when the old folks them days told you they was goin' to work on you, you just well be willin' to it cause that was what they was goin' to do anyhow."[4]

The value of self-reliance wove consistently through African American doctoring. One woman born into slavery remembered, "There were no doctors back there. If you got sick, you would go dig a hole and dig up roots and fix your own medicine."[5] "Dey took care o'demselves," said another elderly Virginia woman of older enslaved relatives.[6] Especially when it came to caring for sick children, slave communities looked to their own resources. Charity Austin, who worked as a children's nurse in Georgia during slavery, emphasized this point. "Then you had to depend on yourself to do for children. You had to doctor and care for them yourself. You just had to depend on yourself."[7]

Self-reliance, as Charity Austin described it, meant something different from the mythic self-sufficiency of rugged American individualism. "Doing for" one's family required a communal store of motherwit, a blend of God-given wisdom, common sense, and the instruction of older women.[8] This collective version of self-reliance drew on fireside training gained by apprenticeship with the older generation, pooled resources, and creative improvisation. It required confidence in the legitimacy of African American medical traditions and the authority of enslaved healers. As the narrator of an account of South Carolina slavery explained, "We had to find for ourselves."[9] The plural pronoun in his declaration is significant. The ethic of self-reliance, as black southerners articulated it, recognized the collective initiative that enslaved African Americans took in pursuing health under conditions often beyond their control.

During the same decades after emancipation, southern physicians, exmasters, and white historians propounded a strikingly different picture of black dependency on slaveholder health care. President of the Medical Society of South Carolina Julian J. Chisolm spoke warmly in 1867 of antebellum days when slaveowners, as the "natural guardians" of enslaved families, assumed "all responsibility" for slave sickness.[10] In the 1870s George William Bagby, Virginia's state librarian, gave popular lectures to white audiences on "the Old Virginia Negro," in which he embellished nostalgic tales of plantation life where medical relations were characterized by "mutual care and protection."[11] Sixty years later Wyndham Blanton's history of medicine in Virginia declared as simple fact, "The average negro slave was a child, anxious to shirk work and making much of his illnesses."[12] With remarkable consistency from antebellum times to the mid-twentieth century, elite whites depicted black sufferers and healers in paternalistic terms of dependency on benevolent white practitioners.

White narratives of plantation health rationalized slaveholders' supervision of black health (as well as postbellum white supremacy) by characterizing slaves as ignorant and superstitious. Julian Chisolm condemned freedmen and freedwomen as "natural children of superstition" who tended to "throw aside the advantages of medicine and accept the efficacy of charms and witchcraft."[13] George William Bagby described conjuring deaths on his aunt's plantation as "genuine manifestations of the power of occult influences upon the undeveloped brain."[14] Little had changed in this line of racial denigration by 1925, when physician S. W. Douglas dramatically informed the readers of a southern medical journal that "ignorance and superstition hang over [the Negro] with Stygian wing."[15] Confounded by the spiritual basis of healing authority, white observers delivered contorted descriptions of conjuring, divination, and other practices to depict enslaved African Americans as their own greatest health problem.

Why did these two contradictory versions of plantation health care emerge, and what accounts for their staying power in historical narratives about the Old South? How did health and healing become charged arenas within the collective memory of mastery and enslavement? The answers to these questions lie, in part, in the two opposing understandings of slave health that prevailed during the antebellum period. One view served the interests of the planter class, while the other countered the physical and ideological assault on enslaved African Americans.

Antebellum planters and the white doctors in their employ advanced a general definition of slave health as soundness that measured an enslaved person's worth according to his or her market value and potential for productive and reproductive labor. The objectification of black health extended beyond the body to include measures of character and skill as well. One does not have to regard slaveholders as crass profit-seekers to argue for the pervasive influence of soundness, for the concept accommodated notions of white honor and even humanitarianism in its definition. Hence, for example, white planters could advocate larger rations or less physical labor for pregnant slave women in the name of both the humanity and the financial interest of the slaveholder. Planters' claims to sharing mutual health interests with enslaved patients did little to lessen the impact of the chattel principle.

Self-reliant traditions of African American doctoring countered these objectifying definitions of slave health with an original and compelling view of human well-being. Unlike southern planters, enslaved men and women did not assume that they shared mutual health interests with their enslavers. On cotton, tobacco, and rice plantations of the southeastern Atlantic states, slave communities created a relational vision of health that defined well-being as more than the material worth of their individual bodies. This vision of health had roots in African notions of the self as "constituted by a web of interpersonal relationships." As scholar Albert Raboteau writes, "Our health, our fortunes, our very lives depend upon the state of our relationships with others, including those who have gone before, our ancestors, who continue to figure prominently in the progress of our lives."[16] By maintaining their vision of health in the midst of the dominant society's failure to recognize such relationships, enslaved African Americans redefined both self and community in their own terms.

The relational vision of health linked the well-being of the individual to the health of the larger community and the health of the community to its spiritual life. Sickness was not a condition to be endured alone; neither was individual healing possible without the consideration of extended social relationships. Conjuration, with its cycle of affliction and restoration, underscored the social basis of illness and healing within enslaved communities and suggested a realm of power beyond the slaveholder's control. In black herbalism, practitioners emphasized their relationship to divine guidance in a spiritually enlivened landscape. Integral to African American religion under slavery, black doctoring rested on an underlying notion of the pharmocosm, a world enlivened by both healing and harming capacities, where healers recognized a close affinity between bodily and spiritual affliction. In their adherence to the tenets of black doctoring, enslaved men and women refused, to return to Ralph Ellison's assertion, to let the masters define crucial matters for them.

For health was indeed a crucial matter. More than the absence of disease, health was an arena in which enslaved African Americans and antebellum planters struggled over religion, family, sexuality, and labor. Not every home remedy brewed became an explicitly political act. Yet persistent African American adherence to a relational view of health in the face of routine dehumanization quietly and profoundly shaped the power relations of southern plantations. With the demise of slavery the history of plantation medicine continued to bear political weight. Just as claims about slave health provided a dueling ground for abolitionists and proslavery advocates, so, too, have postbellum narratives about slavery and medicine continued to play an important role in the nation's historical memory. The history of African American health and healing is therefore by definition a political history that bears upon our larger understanding of the very institution of slavery.

Whether an arena is defined as a physical edifice or a symbolic sphere of conflict, the conditions of the arena are seldom chosen by all participants. To a certain extent the planter class determined the arena of plantation health struggles by subjecting slave health needs to the imperatives of the market. Their advantage did not win them seats as spectators, however, for slaveholders were forced to remain in the arena by their very dependence on the labor of the men and women they sought to control. Many planters attempted to use the skills and labor of enslaved healers to meet plantation health needs as defined in the interests of the slaveholder. Enslaved African Americans resisted these terms of engagement, however, by creating a sacred health culture grounded in notions of authority outside the control of the planter class and a vision of health that transcended the parameters of soundness. In doing so they transformed the struggle in the arena from a contest over the needs of the body to a wider conflict over the value of African American lives. Doing battle where they stood, enslaved men and women created an enduring art of doctoring that healed the body and preserved the soul.

Notes

ABBREVIATIONS

BMR
  Botanico-Medical Recorder, or Impartial Advocate of Botanic Medicine
CMJR
  Charleston Medical Journal and Review
Drums
  Georgia Writers' Project, Savannah Unit, ed. *Drums and Shadows: Survival Studies among the Georgia Coastal Negroes.* Athens: University of Georgia Press, 1940.
DUL
  Duke University Library, Special Collections Department, Durham, N.C.
GHS
  Georgia Historical Society, Savannah
HSP
  Historical Society of Pennsylvania, Philadelphia
JAF
  Journal of American Folklore
LC
  Library of Congress, Manuscripts Division, Washington, D.C.
LV
  Library of Virginia, Archives Research Service, Richmond
NOMSJ
  New Orleans Medical and Surgical Journal
Rawick
  George P. Rawick, ed. *The American Slave: A Composite Autobiography.* Westport, Conn.: Greenwood Press, 1972, 1977.
SCHS
  South Carolina Historical Society, Charleston
SCL
  South Caroliniana Library, University of South Carolina, Columbia
SHC
  Southern Historical Collection, University of North Carolina, Chapel Hill

Slav. Stat.
   State Slavery Statutes, 1789–1860. Virginia, North Carolina, South Carolina,
   Georgia. Frederick, Md.: University Press of America Microfiche Series, 1989.
SMSJ
   Southern Medical and Surgical Journal
UVL
   University of Virginia Library, Albert H. Small Special Collections Library,
   Charlottesville
VHS
   Virginia Historical Society, Richmond
VMJ
   Virginia Medical Journal
VMSJ
   Virginia Medical and Surgical Journal
Weevils
   Charles L. Perdue Jr., Thomas E. Barden, and Robert K. Phillips, eds. *Weevils
   in the Wheat: Interviews with Virginia Ex-Slaves.* Charlottesville: University
   Press of Virginia, 1976.
WHL
   Waring Historical Library, Medical University of South Carolina, Charleston
WPA
   Works Progress Administration

PREFACE

1. R. S. Taylor, judge of the Inferior Court, Clark Co., to Gen. Davis Tillson, assistant commissioner of the Bureau of Refugees, Freedmen, and Abandoned Land,
25 Jan. 1866, Georgia, Surgeon-in-chief, Letters Received Unentered, quoted in
Savitt, "Politics in Medicine," 57.

2. Julian J. Chisolm, "President's Address upon Retiring from the Chair," 10 Dec.
1867, typescript and manuscript, WHL, 4.

3. Richard Arnold to Miss Fannie Mims and to Miss M. W. Houston, 8 Oct. 1866,
in Shryock, *Letters of Richard D. Arnold,* 129, 131. The first letter is also quoted in
Savitt, "Politics in Medicine," 57.

4. Within the extensive literature on African American expressive arts, historical work specifically on slavery includes Stuckey, *Slave Culture,* 3–97; Levine, *Black
Culture and Black Consciousness,* 3–189; White and White, *Stylin',* 5–85.

1. Burnside, *Spirits of the Passage,* 115, 117.

2. The phrase "object of property" appears as the title of a chapter and a central concept in Patricia J. Williams, *Alchemy of Race and Rights,* 216–36.

3. Wells, *Red Record,* 75.

4. Gould, *Mismeasure of Man;* Pernick, *Calculus of Suffering;* Fredrickson, *Black Image in the White Mind;* Savitt, *Medicine and Slavery,* 281–307.

5. Byrd and Clayton, *American Health Dilemma,* 27–150.

6. Cited by permission from Kirk Johnson, "Race and Power in the Old South: Roots of African-American Medical Noncompliance" (unpublished paper, 1995 [in my possession]).

7. I use "health culture" as an umbrella phrase to indicate a range of ideas related to wellness, illness, healing, and death. I use "doctoring" and "healing" to indicate the entire spectrum of practices that enslaved communities employed to pursue bodily and spiritual well-being and protection. The repertoire of African American doctoring under slavery included herbalism, midwifery, prayer, conjure or hoodoo, divination, and sickbed attendance.

8. Savitt, *Medicine and Slavery,* 171. See also Morais, *History of the Afro-American in Medicine,* 7–20.

9. Karras, "Atlantic World as a Unit of Study"; Curtin, *Rise and Fall of the Plantation Complex;* John Thornton, *Africa and Africans in the Making of the Atlantic World,* 206–34.

10. Karen McCarthy Brown, "Afro-Caribbean Spirituality: A Haitian Case Study," in Sullivan, *Healing and Restoring,* 255–85. Brown argues that "healing is the *primary business*" of all Afro-Caribbean "religious systems" (257); see also Brandon, *Santeria from Africa to the New World;* Hurston, *Tell My Horse.*

11. For regional studies of this transformation, see Breen and Innes, *"Myne Owne Ground";* Edmund Sears Morgan, *American Slavery, American Freedom;* Gwendolyn Midlo Hall, *Africans in Colonial Louisiana,* 128. See also Barbara Jeanne Fields, "Slavery, Race, and Ideology in the United States of America." The phrases "societies with slaves" and "slave societies" come from Ira Berlin, *Many Thousands Gone,* 8. Drawing on concepts from ancient Roman historiography, Berlin defines slave societies as societies in which "slavery stood at the center of economic production, and the master-slave relationship provided the model for all social relations: husband and wife, parent and child, employer and employee, teacher and student."

12. Kathleen M. Brown, *Good Wives, Nasty Wenches, and Anxious Patriarchs,* 110.

13. Ibid., 107–36.

14. Ira Berlin, *Many Thousands Gone;* McCurry, *Masters of Small Worlds;* Bynum, *Unruly Women.*

15. I use both "physicians" and "white medical doctors" to refer to professional practitioners of antebellum medical science. Professional white doctors often em-

ployed the words "orthodox" and "regular" to distinguish their branch of medical practice from others they deemed "irregular."

16. John Harley Warner has written extensively on the significance of therapy to nineteenth-century physicians' professional identity. See Warner, *Therapeutic Perspective* and *Against the Spirit of the System*. See also Starr, *Social Transformation of American Medicine*, 47–59; Kett, *Formation of the American Medical Profession*.

17. Although the political context for these medical developments in the South was distinctive, the medical theory behind southern physicians' regionalism was not. Physicians from many regions of the United States embraced the "principle of specificity," which held that medical treatment should match the particular characteristics of individual patients and the patient's environment. See Warner, "Idea of Southern Medical Distinctiveness," 184–88.

18. Able, *Hearts of Wisdom*.

19. Murphy, *Enter the Physician*, xv.

20. McCaw, "On the Present Condition of the Medical Profession in Virginia," 45.

21. Thomsonianism was a botanical self-medication movement initiated by New Hampshire farmer Samuel Thomson in the early nineteenth century. Thomsonian diagnostics revolved around the balance of "natural heat" in the body; botanical therapies included lobelia and cayenne, in addition to steam baths, enemas, and other herbal medicines. See Kaufman, *Homeopathy in America*, 17–21; Rothstein, *American Physicians in the Nineteenth Century*, 125–51; Starr, *Social Transformation of American Medicine*, 51–54. For a history of Thomsonianism in one southern state, see Breeden, "Thomsonianism in Virginia."

Homeopathy originated in Germany with physician Samuel Hahnemann and arrived in the United States in 1825. Homeopathic medicine relied on two main assertions: first, that a substance that causes symptoms of illness in a healthy person will also cure those symptoms in a sick person and, second, that a homeopathic remedy gains strength as it is both shaken and diluted until the original plant material is present only in infinitesimal amounts. See Kaufman, *Homeopathy in America*, 23–27; Rothstein, *American Physicians in the Nineteenth Century*, 152–74.

Hydropathy, or water-cure, another self-treatment movement based on the healing properties of water along with dietary and hygienic principles, reached its height of popularity in the mid-nineteenth century. See Cayleff, *Wash and Be Healed*.

22. Ulrich, *Midwife's Tale;* Leavitt, *Brought to Bed;* McMillen, *Motherhood in the Old South*.

23. In this sense my work reflects some recent scholarship on antebellum slavery that attempts to examine how the experiences of enslavement marked enslaved individuals and communities. The best example of this scholarship is Painter, "Soul Murder and Slavery." In contrast, earlier work, such as John Blassingame's *Slave Community*, in responding to Stanley Elkins's thesis of the infantilizing impact of slavery on "slave personality," tended to stress the autonomous character of slave community life.

24. This study would have been impossible without the existing foundation of scholarship on slave community that addresses the religious, cultural, and social significance of African American healing. For seminal work, see Raboteau, *Slave Religion*, 80–86, 275–85; Genovese, *Roll, Jordan, Roll*, 215–29; Levine, *Black Culture and Black Consciousness*, 55–80; Joyner, *Down by the Riverside*, 142–49; Filomina Chioma Steady, "The Black Woman Cross Culturally: An Overview," in Steady, *Black Woman Cross-Culturally*, 21; Deborah Gray White, *Ar'n't I a Woman?*, 115–16, 124–26.

25. Raymond Williams, *Keywords*, 75.

26. Stevenson, *Life in Black and White*, 207–319; Schlotterbeck, "Internal Economy of Slavery," 172; Gomez, *Exchanging Our Country Marks*, 25.

27. Berlin and Morgan, "Slaves' Economy," 1.

28. Bay, *White Image in the Black Mind*, 113–83.

29. On the vulnerability of slaves on smaller holdings, see Stevenson, *Life in Black and White*, 173, 185; Barbara Jeanne Fields, *Slavery and Freedom on the Middle Ground*, 23–39; Rosengarten, *Tombee*, 151–52.

30. The use of the term "sufferer," rather than the clinical term "patient," as a more inclusive category for persons seeking healing comes from Good and Good, "Semantics of Medical Discourse," 187.

31. This study focuses on southern plantations, defined as cash crop agricultural enterprises with twenty or more slaves. Thus the evidence is drawn most heavily from the coastal and piedmont regions of the Southeast. Though not representative of all slave holdings, plantation slave communities had a strong cultural impact on southern African American culture; an estimated 51.6 percent of enslaved African Americans lived on plantations. It is possible that networks of slave communication, patterns of hiring, and local slave sales in these regions extended some of the dynamics of slave health discussed in this book to enslaved individuals on smaller farms and in southern towns and cities. Important questions about black doctoring and slave health in the urban South, western counties, and small farms remain for future scholars to explore. On demographic variation in the South, see Boles, *Black Southerners*, 106–39. Occasionally I have used materials from other southern states when the evidence concurred with findings for the southeastern region.

32. Gomez, *Exchanging Our Country Marks*, 149–53, 283.

33. Richard Arnold to Dr. Heber Chase, 13 Oct. 1836, in Shryock, *Letters of Richard D. Arnold;* Warner, "Southern Medical Reform," 206–25.

34. On the public health conditions of slave quarters, see Savitt, *Medicine and Slavery*, 49–148.

35. Ibid., 149–84 passim, esp. 150, 184.

36. Ibid., 149, 150.

37. Savitt and Young, *Disease and Distinctiveness in the American South.*

38. The literature on the health of African Americans in slavery is extensive and highly interdisciplinary. Major works in the biological history of Africans in the Americas include Kiple and King, *Another Dimension of the Black Diaspora;* Kiple,

African Exchange. Studies of mortality and nutrition include Steckel, "Dreadful Childhood"; Campbell, "Work, Pregnancy, and Infant Mortality"; Cody, "Note on Changing Patterns of Slave Fertility"; Kelley and Angel, "Life Stresses of Slavery"; Michael P. Johnson, "Smothered Slave Infants."

39. Good and Good, "Semantics of Medical Discourse"; Kleinman, "What Is Specific to Western Medicine?"; Kleinman, "Meaning Context of Illness and Care," 161–62; Good, *Medicine, Rationality, and Experience,* 28, 54–62. Good advocates an approach he calls "critical phenomenology," which combines the meaning-centered approach with critical anthropology's focus on theories of illness as ideological mystification.

40. Gomez, *Exchanging Our Country Marks,* 194.

41. Ibid., 50, 112, 128, 146–48.

42. Fanon, *Dying Colonialism,* 121, 125. Fanon also argued in the same chapter that when Western medicine came to the Algerian populace as an extension of the revolution rather than an oppressive regime, the people dropped "old superstitions" and embraced the rationalism of scientific public health. In this conclusion Fanon, a trained psychiatrist, surely underestimated the character and persistence of popular health traditions.

43. James C. Scott, *Domination and the Arts of Resistance,* 1–16. This open definition of medical conflict draws on Nancy Hunt's work on the asymmetry and mutability of colonial medical encounters. See Hunt, *Colonial Lexicon,* 11, 24, 323.

CHAPTER 1

1. Pennington, *Fugitive Blacksmith,* in Bontemps, *Great Slave Narratives,* 196, 198.

2. Savitt, *Medicine and Slavery,* 310.

3. Historians who have argued that slaveholders' capital investments in slaves assured relatively high-quality health care by slaveholders include Sikes, in "Medical Care for Slaves"; Marshall, in "Plantation Medicine"; Phillips, in *American Negro Slavery,* 261–65. Bennett Wall also emphasized slaveholder provision of health care to enslaved laborers but stressed the "personal relationship" of slaveholder to slaves, rather than economic interest; see Wall, "Medical Care of Ebenezer Pettigrew's Slaves." Carter G. Woodson countered the paternalistic interpretation of slave health with a description of slaveholder abuse and neglect; see Woodson, *Negro in Our History,* 107. Other dissenting arguments include Stampp, *Peculiar Institution,* 314–15; Swados, "Negro Health on the Ante Bellum Plantations"; Shryock, "Medical Practice in the Old South."

4. John A. Warren to John D. Warren, 20 Dec. 1858, Warren Papers, SCL.

5. "Charleston Work House," 22 May 1857, and John A. Warren to John D. Warren, 20 Dec. 1858, ibid.

6. Thomas Farr Capers and T. Savage Heyward to John D. Warren, 5 Jan. 1859, ibid.

7. L. W. W. Cants to Capt. John D. Warren, 8 Feb. 1859; Charles Pinckney to John D. Warren, 10 Feb. 1859; John A. Warren to John D. Warren (ca. 1859), ibid.

8. Charles Pinckney to John D. Warren, 13 Feb. 1859 (emphasis in original), ibid.

9. Charles Pinckney to John D. Warren, 10 Feb. 1859, ibid.

10. John A. Warren to John D. Warren, 19 Feb. 1859, ibid.

11. Capers and Heyward to John D. Warren, 15 Mar. 1859, ibid.

12. "Private Sale of One Negro Slave on Dock," 23 Mar. 1859, and Capers and Heyward to John D. Warren, 30 Mar. 1859, ibid.

13. Wright, *Political Economy of the Cotton South,* 24.

14. Harriss, "What Constitutes Unsoundness?," 145. Todd Savitt briefly mentions the nonhealing roles of physicians in the domestic slave trade in his paper "Medicine in the Old South" (in my possession).

15. The history of slave sales has been greatly enriched by the recent work of Ariela Gross and Walter Johnson, whose books I draw on to discuss the concept of soundness in slave markets and court disputes. See Gross, *Double Character;* Walter Johnson, *Soul by Soul.*

16. Richard D. Arnold, "On the Epidemics of Savannah, Georgia, in 1847 and 1848," *CMJR* 4 (1849): 147; Harriss, "What Constitutes Unsoundness?," 295; Cartwright, "Diseases of Negroes," 212.

17. Harriss, "What Constitutes Unsoundness?," 294; Gross, *Double Character,* 128–29.

18. Tadman, *Speculators and Slaves,* 187; Gross, "'Pandora's Box'"; Walter Johnson, *Soul by Soul,* 135–61.

19. Dolben's Act of 1788 required the presence of a trained surgeon on board every British slave ship. Ship physicians received bonuses for limiting the mortality of captive Africans. See Sheridan, *Doctors and Slaves,* 98–126; Behrendt, "British Slave Trade." In the Angolan slave trade Portuguese law required the presence of a chaplain aboard slaving vessels, but African healers were most often hired as nurses, surgeons, and translators in ships' infirmaries. Not until 1813 did Brazilian-bound ships routinely carry trained physicians. See Miller, *Way of Death,* 407, 409, 435.

20. Gross, *Double Character,* 132–35; Tadman, *Speculators and Slaves,* 186; Stevenson, *Life in Black and White,* 179.

21. Walter Johnson, *Soul by Soul,* 135–61.

22. John A. Warren to John D. Warren, 4 Feb. 1859, Warren Papers, SCL.

23. Capers and Heyward to John D. Warren, 21 Feb. 1859, ibid.

24. Samuel Browning to Archibald Boyd, 4 June 1849, Boyd Papers, DUL.

25. Harriss, "What Constitutes Unsoundness?," 148–49; Gross, *Double Character,* 72.

26. *McDaniel v. Strohecker,* 19 Georgia 432 (Jan. 1856), cited in Catterall, *Judicial*

Cases Concerning American Slavery, 3:48. For other court cases concerning sound-ness, see Catterall, *Judicial Cases Concerning American Slavery,* 2:409, 309, 316.

27. Gross, *Double Character,* 132–39.

28. Harriss, "What Constitutes Unsoundness?," 147.

29. Capers and Heyward to John D. Warren, 21 Feb. 1859, Warren Papers, SCL.

30. Samuel R. Browning to Archibald Boyd, 2 Jan. 1849, Boyd Papers, DUL.

31. Gross, *Double Character,* 136–37; Walter Johnson, *Soul by Soul,* 118–34.

32. Genovese, "Medical and Insurance Costs of Slaveholding"; Savitt, "Slave Life Insurance"; Wright, *Political Economy of the Cotton South,* 128–50.

33. Insurance Policy No. 292, 1855, Greensborough Mutual Life Insurance Com-pany, North Carolina Collection, University of North Carolina, Chapel Hill.

34. Allen, Aetna Life Insurance Company Policy, 11 Aug. 1856, SCHS.

35. Savitt, "Slave Life Insurance," 589.

36. A[rchibald] Alexander Little to Andrew G. Grinnan, 28 Mar. 1850, Grinnan Family Papers, VHS.

37. For a discussion of liability and precedent in slave hiring law, see Wahl, *Bonds-man's Burden,* 49–77.

38. Savitt, *Medicine and Slavery,* 184–95.

39. *Well v. Kennerly,* 4 McC 123, cited in "Memorandum of Law Relating to Physi-cians and Surgeons. (In South Carolina)," *CMJR* 3 (1848): 47.

40. Benjamin Evans to John D. Warren, 17 Feb. 1861, Warren Papers, SCL.

41. K. Washington Skinner to Charles Manigault, 28 Aug. 1852, Manigault Papers, DUL.

42. William Cain to Minerva Caldwell, 26 Apr. 1842, folder 2, Caldwell Papers, SHC.

43. Rosengarten, *Tombee,* 450, 488, 653. For other references to slave sickness phrased in terms of labor lost, see also Elisha Cain to Mr. Telfair, 5 Nov. 1829, Telfair Family Papers, GHS; L. Weed to Rev. Henry J. Brown, 4 Nov. 1848, Brown Papers, UVL; Friend Diary, 2 Feb. 1846, Friend Family Papers, VHS.

44. Young, "Ideology and Death on a Savannah River Rice Plantation," 705.

45. Pollard, *Complaint to the Lord,* 31–47. For examples of work done by elderly or disabled men or women, see "List of the Gordon Gang," n.d., Ravenel Plantation Papers, 1835–1866, Ford-Ravenel Papers, SCHS.

46. T. Savage Heyward to John D. Warren, 20 Dec. 1858; W. W. Johnson to John D. Warren, 24 Feb. 1859; and Capers and Heyward to John D. Warren, 21 Jan. 1860, Warren Papers, SCL.

47. Statement A, Jan. 1854, Commissioner's Report #9, Estate of Dr. James McClurg, Wickham Family Papers, VHS.

48. John Chesnutt to Col. A. F. Brisbane, 10 Jan. 1795, Chesnutt Letterbook, LC.

49. Douglass, *Narrative of the Life of Frederick Douglass,* 61–63. Leslie Pollard concludes that old age provoked the greatest collision between "capitalist and pater-nalist notions of slaveholders"; see Pollard, *Complaint to the Lord,* 32. See also Savitt,

Medicine and Slavery, 201–7; Genovese, *Roll, Jordan, Roll,* 519–23; Owens, *This Species of Property,* 47–49.

50. *Acts Passed at a General Assembly of the Commonwealth of Virginia,* sec. 3, chap. 34 (Richmond, 1824), collected in *Slav. Stat.*

51. Deborah Gray White, *Ar'n't I a Woman?,* 66–70; Jacqueline Jones, *Labor of Love, Labor of Sorrow,* 13–29; Robertson, "Africa into the Americas?," 20–28.

52. Holmes, "Typhoid Fever," 60.

53. Gross, *Double Character,* 101–2.

54. A. R. Bagshaw to Charles Manigault, 14 Aug. 1844, Manigault Papers, DUL.

55. 25 June 1861, Greenwood Plantation Journal, LC (emphasis in original).

56. Leigh Pruneau, "'I've Lost Many': Field Women's Work, Pregnancy, and Neonatal Mortality on Lowcountry Rice Plantations" (paper presented to the Fourth Southern Conference on Women's History, Charleston, S.C., 13 June 1997 [in author's possession]). See also Cody, "Cycles of Work and of Childbearing," 61–78; Shaw, "Mothering under Slavery"; Roberts, *Killing the Black Body,* 22–55.

57. Two other women on the Massie plantations also died after having "run mad" or "been crazy" for a period of time; see Massie, Slave Record Book, 27 (Betsy), 25 (Sally), 28 (Emily), LV.

58. Alfred Oliver Eggleston to John P. Mettauer, 27 Sept. 1835, Mettauer Papers, VHS.

59. James Neal to John P. Mettauer, 1 Aug. 1839, ibid.

60. R. Ruton to Rev. Henry J. Brown, 1 Feb. 1849, Brown Papers, UVL.

61. William Osborne Good to Dr. Thomas Massie, 16 June 1852, Massie Family Papers, VHS.

62. Gavin Diary, 25 Nov. 1855, SHC.

63. Ibid., 14 Nov. 1859. See also 4 Apr. 1851 and 27 May 1862, Massie, Slave Record Book, LV.

64. T. P. Baily, "Surgical Cases," *CMJR* 14 (1859): 742.

65. W. H. Robert, "Surgical Cases Occurring in the Practice of L. A. Dugas," *SMSJ* 33 (Feb. 1839): 292.

66. Pennington, *Fugitive Blacksmith,* in Bontemps, *Great Slave Narratives,* 202.

67. Albert, *House of Bondage,* 22, 49.

68. Botkin, *Lay My Burden Down,* 101. Quotations from the WPA collections appear in this study as they do in their original written form, unless otherwise noted. Depending on the interviewer and editor, the speech representations were often distorted and stereotyped. It is important, therefore, to keep in mind the possible biases represented in editors' written representations of the interviews. While attempting to take into account the potential problems of memory and editorial license inherent in the WPA collections, I continue to believe that these interviews comprise an invaluable source for studies of African American life under slavery. See also Blassingame, *Slave Testimony,* xlii–lvii; Yetman, "Background of the Slave Narrative Collection."

69. Bay, *White Image in the Black Mind,* 119, 124.

70. Molefi Kete Asante defines "orature" as "the comprehensive body of oral dis-course on every subject and in every genre of expression produced by people of African descent" (Asante, *Afrocentric Idea,* 83–84).

71. *Southern Workman* 26 (1897): 210, quoted in Levine, *Black Culture and Black Consciousness,* 131. Additional tales concerning slaves' appropriation of the master's goods can be found in Abrahams, *Afro-American Folktales,* 265, 278; Dance, *Shuckin' and Jivin',* 186, 187; Botkin, *Lay My Burden Down,* 10, 11.

72. Genovese, *Roll, Jordan, Roll,* 605–8; Lichtenstein, "'That Disposition to Theft.'" Oral sources on the theft of Africans by European slave traders are discussed in Genovese, *Roll, Jordan, Roll,* 605; Dance, *Shuckin' and Jivin',* 10; Levine, *Black Culture and Black Consciousness,* 87; Stuckey, *Slave Culture,* 7; Gomez, *Exchanging Our Country Marks,* 199–208.

73. John Brown, *Slave Life in Georgia,* 97–99. See also Tadman, *Speculators and Slaves,* 184–86, 189.

74. William Wells Brown, *Narrative of William W. Brown,* 43.

75. John Brown, *Slave Life in Georgia,* 99; Albert, *House of Bondage,* 105; Northup, *Twelve Years a Slave,* 251.

76. Walter Johnson, *Soul by Soul,* 162–88.

77. A. J. McElveen to A. B. Oakes, 21 Oct. 1856, quoted in Drago, *Broke by the War,* 133–34. For further discussions of the predicament of traders, doctors, and lawyers who depended on slaves in sale and courtroom disputes, see Gross, *Double Charac-ter,* 140–43.

78. *Slave Narratives,* 3. Botkin, *Lay My Burden Down,* 103.

79. Northup, *Twelve Years a Slave,* 321.

80. James L. Smith, *Autobiography,* 2–3.

81. Botkin, *Lay My Burden Down,* 101, 103.

82. Ibid., 83.

83. John Brown, *Slave Life in Georgia,* 7.

84. See Chapter 6.

85. Elisha Cain to Mr. Telfair, 16 Jan. 1860, Telfair Family Papers, GHS.

CHAPTER 2

1. Chireau, "Conjure and Christianity in the Nineteenth Century," 239.

2. "Invisible institution" comes from Raboteau, *Slave Religion.*

3. E. G. Crumpe, "Mount Sterling," to William Jerdone, Louisa County, 17 June [no year], Jerdone Family Papers, Swem Library, College of William and Mary, Wil-liamsburg, Va. I am grateful to Linda Sturtz who first bought the Jerdone papers to my attention.

4. Moss, *Southern Folk Medicine,* 81–86, 155–56.

5. Philip Brooks to William Jerdone, 23 July 1837, and to W[illiam] H. Barnes,

24 July 1838, Jerdone Family Papers, Swem Library, College of William and Mary, Williamsburg, Va.

6. Examples of doctors' rheumatism prescriptions can be found in the entries under "Rheumatism Acute" and "Rheumatism Chronic," Barnes Prescription Book (ca. 1860), SCL.

7. Levine, *Black Culture and Black Consciousness*, 74.

8. A classic study on the secularization of popular concepts of health in the United States is Rosenberg, *Cholera Years*.

9. Numbers and Amundsen, *Caring and Curing*, 539–62; Braude, *Radical Spirits*, 142–61; Numbers, *Prophetess of Health*, 31–76.

10. "Black sacred culture" comes from Chireau, "Uses of the Supernatural," 171.

11. Levine, *Black Culture and Black Consciousness*, 31–32; Sobel, *Trabelin' On*, 13; Mbiti, *African Religions and Philosophy*, 1–5, 75–91, 166–203; Creel, *"Peculiar People,"* 3; Webber, *Deep Like the Rivers*, 118–30.

12. Stuckey, *Slave Culture*, 10–17.

13. Levine, *Black Culture and Black Consciousness*, 30, 133.

14. Ibid., 80.

15. Stuckey, "Through the Prism of Folklore."

16. Theophus H. Smith, *Conjuring Culture*, 5.

17. Ibid., 44.

18. Ibid., 105.

19. Ibid., 143.

20. Botkin, *Lay My Burden Down*, 243. This story resonates strongly with the plagues sent against Pharaoh in the Exodus story.

21. "Negro Tales," box A688, folder: Virginia, Negro Lore, WPA Folklore Project, LC.

22. For a discussion of pharmaconic properties in antebellum African American discourse, that is, the employment of words tonic to the cause of antislavery and toxic to the cause of slaveholders, see Theophus H. Smith, *Conjuring Culture*, 90–95.

23. Raboteau, *Slave Religion*, 10.

24. Simon Kavuna, cahier 58 (1915), quoted in MacGaffey, "Eyes of Understanding," 21.

25. *Slave Narratives*, 124. The dual healing and harming power of conjurers figured significantly in the regulation of personal relationships within enslaved communities and will be discussed in Chapter 4.

26. Raboteau, *Slave Religion*, 287. The subject of cultural continuities from Africa to African America has a long and contentious history. See Herskovits, *Myth of the Negro Past*; Frazier, *Negro Church in America*. Discussions of the Herskovits-Frazier debate include Raboteau, *Slave Religion*, 48–92; Holloway, *Africanisms in American Culture*, ix–xiii.

27. Frey and Wood, *Come Shouting to Zion*, 35–62, quote on 62; Genovese, *Roll, Jordan, Roll*, 228; Raboteau, *Slave Religion*, 43–92.

28. Gomez, *Exchanging Our Country Marks*, 244–90. While recent literature tends to agree that early colonial slave populations were largely untouched by Christianity, historians disagree as to how extensive Christian conversion was in the first three decades of the nineteenth century. See, for example, Frey and Wood, *Come Shouting to Zion*, 119, compared with Gomez, *Exchanging Our Country Marks*, 256.

29. Frey and Wood, *Come Shouting to Zion*, 56–59; Kathleen M. Brown, *Good Wives, Nasty Wenches, and Anxious Patriarchs*, 354.

30. For groundbreaking work on the impact of Islam on North American slave cultures, see Gomez, *Exchanging Our Country Marks*, 59–87. By the advent of the Atlantic slave trade, West Africans had been absorbing Islamic practices into their healing systems for several centuries. For an analysis of the Islamization of Hausa medicine, for example, see Ismail H. Abdalla, "Diffusion of Islamic Medicine into Hausaland," in Feierman and Janzen, *Social Basis of Health and Healing*, 177–94.

31. Philip D. Morgan, *Slave Counterpoint*, 620–31. Morgan's richly documented study argues that in the context of slavery, sorcery (a magical means of harming) became dominant. The latter interpretation, I believe, relies too heavily on Eurocentric views of the malevolence of African spiritual practitioners. It also misses the curative dimensions of slave "sorcery," which become apparent in Theophus Smith's formulation of the pharmocosm. In stressing the duality of harming and healing traditions, I am deliberately reinterpreting Morgan's evidence to arrive at a different picture of slave spirituality.

32. Chireau, "Conjure and Christianity in the Nineteenth Century," 229.

33. Sobel, *Trabelin' On*, 245.

34. Frey and Wood, *Come Shouting to Zion*, 33.

35. The discourse among whites on superstition created and maintained an "Africanism," as Toni Morrison defines the word: a "term for the denotative and connotative blackness that African peoples have come to signify, as well as the entire range of views, assumptions, readings, and misreadings that accompany Eurocentric learning about these people" (Morrison, *Playing in the Dark*, 6–7).

36. Mary P. Randolph to Lewis C. Randolph, 6 May 1858, Hubard-Randolph Family Papers, UVL.

37. For a useful and closely related discussion of secular versus sacred medical practices in Africa, see Feierman, "Struggles for Control," 107.

38. Cosslett, *Science and Religion in the Nineteenth Century;* Conser, *God and the Natural World*.

39. Letter to editor, *BMR* 8 (16 Nov. 1839): 61.

40. Rosenberg, "Therapeutic Revolution," 487.

41. Rosenberg, *Cholera Years*, 73.

42. For example, New England writer and reformer Lydia M. Child, in her 1831 publication *The Mother's Book*, advocated the importance of self-restraint in child-rearing. See also Ryan, *Cradle of the Middle Class*, 158–61.

43. Ewell, *Planter's and Mariner's Medical Companion*, 155; Folger, *Family Physi-*

cian, 52–61; Gunn, *Gunn's Domestic Medicine,* 74; John B. Blake, "From Buchan to Fishbein: The Literature of Domestic Medicine," in Risse, Numbers, and Leavitt, *Medicine without Doctors,* 12–28.

44. "Recipies," *Southern Planter* 4 (1844): 39–40.

45. Pettigrew, *On Superstitions,* 90.

46. G. S. M., "Connection between Body and Mind," *BMR* 8 (13 July 1840): 299–300. For additional discussion of body and mind relationships, see letter to editor, *BMR* 8 (16 Nov. 1839): 60–61, and "Body and Mind," *BMR* 7 (28 Dec. 1839): 105–6.

47. Folger, *Family Physician,* 62; see also Gunn, *Gunn's Domestic Medicine,* 74.

48. Lydia A. Riddick to Charles Riddick, Nov. 1852, folder 1, Riddick Family Papers, SHC.

49. Walter Channing, "Spiritualism," *VMJ* 9 (1857): 45–50, reprinted from *Boston Medical and Surgical Journal.* Mesmerism, so named after German physician Franz Anton Mesmer, emphasized bringing individual magnetic forces into line with universal forces. See Butler, *Awash in a Sea of Faith,* 234–35.

50. See, for example, Robert Morris's record of a trip to Norfolk for an exhibit in phrenology, mesmerism, and clairvoyance, in Morris Diary, 19 May 1848, VHS. For an account of a New Orleans family seeking a mesmerist in Philadelphia to cure their deaf daughter, see Ellen Martin to Elizabeth S. Martin, 17 July 1844, Martin Papers, SHC.

51. Jon Butler argues that race and class lines in the United States exerted a strong influence, thus preventing cross-fertilization between various "occult" practices, such as hoodoo and spiritualism, in the antebellum period. See Butler, "Dark Ages of American Occultism," 59.

52. Gilman, "Black Bodies, White Bodies."

53. Folger, *Family Physician,* 230.

54. Castle, "Inaugural Dissertation on Cholera Infantum," 3–6, Toner Papers, LC.

55. McCaw, "On the Present Condition of the Medical Profession in Virginia," 45. For other metonymic uses of "old women," see "Editorial and Miscellaneous: Medical Ethics in Virginia," *VMJ* 7 (1856): 257; J. B. McCaw, "On Sick Headache," *VMJ* 8 (1857): 36; Pendleton, "On the Comparative Fecundity of the Caucasian and African Races," 355; E. C. Baker, "A Case of Vicarious Menstruation from an Ulcer on the Right Mamma," *Southern Journal of Medicine and Pharmacy* 2 (1847): 152–55. "Editorial and Miscellaneous: Medical Cossacks," *VMJ* 11 (1858): 335, refers to "old nurses" (meaning midwives) who admire the "irregular troops" like army camp followers.

56. D. F. N., "Quacks and Quackery," *Thomsonian Recorder* 2 (2 Aug. 1834), 360–61; "Medical Superstition," *Thomsonian Recorder* 1 (3 Nov. 1832): 80–81; J. F. Peebles, "The Rise and Progress of Thomsonianism," *Stethoscope and Virginia Medical Gazette* 1 (Jan. 1851): 17.

57. Antebellum medical journals were not entirely hostile to home remedies. For example, a Virginia doctor recommended urine as an effective wash used by "old

women of this neighborhood" for chapped nipples. See George William Semple, "Urine as a Local Application," *VMJ* 8 (1857): 196–97. For a positive discussion by a physician of "old women's" low-intervention approach to treatment, see "Review of *On Nature and Art in the Cure of Disease* by Sir John Forbes, 1858," *CMJR* 13 (1858): 658.

58. E. Warren, "Lactation in an Old Woman," *VMSJ* 3 (May–Dec. 1854): 384–85.

59. Castle, "Inaugural Dissertation on Cholera Infantum," 3–6, Toner Papers, LC; Pettigrew, *On Superstitions,* 89.

60. W. H. Robert, "Amputation of the Penis," *SMSJ* 3 (Jan. 1839): 209.

61. Murphy, *Enter the Physician,* 225.

62. Ewell, *Planter and Mariner's Medical Companion,* 24; see also Buchan, *Domestic Medicine,* xi; Warner, *Therapeutic Perspective,* 43–46.

63. McCaw, "On the Present Condition of the Medical Profession in Virginia," 45.

64. Ewell, *Planter and Mariner's Medical Companion,* 25.

65. McCaw, "On the Present Condition of the Medical Profession in Virginia," 42.

66. Brevard Diary, 31 July 1860, SCL.

67. Ibid., 9 Nov. 1860.

68. Gavin Diary, 2 Aug. 1856, SHC. Attitudes toward the interpretation of dreams varied among slaveholding whites. The communication of portents through dreams was an important theme in Methodism but may have been fading (at least among Methodist itinerants) by the early nineteenth century. See Butler, *Awash in a Sea of Faith,* 238–39. Some evidence indicates that even in the mid-nineteenth century, although poorer white men and women also placed great significance on dreams, they were not self-conscious of their interpretations as "superstition," as were more wealthy and formally educated white southerners. See, for example, I. P. to "My Dear Wife," 5 May 1864, folder 2, Confederate Papers, SHC.

69. Silverman, *Life and Times of Cotton Mather,* 244–50.

70. See, for example, M—, "Moon-ology: Superstitions and Humbugs," *Southern Planter* 10 (1850): 182–83; Wyatt-Brown, *Southern Honor,* 160. Ritual intercessions against natural disaster nevertheless continued among some white southerners. For an example of a written charm against fires and lightning, see "Art against fire" (ca. 1840), Daniel G. Cushwa, Cushwa Family Papers, VHS.

71. Rawick, 14:356–57.

72. H. H. Townes to Mrs. Rachael Townes, 17 Nov. 1833, Townes Family Papers, SCL.

73. Ibid., 24 Nov. 1833.

74. Merrill, "Essay on Some of the Distinctive Peculiarities of the Negro Race," 90, 35. See also Cartwright, "Remarks on Dysentery among Negroes," 155.

75. McCaa, "Observations on the Manner of Living and Diseases of the Slaves," 7–8 (emphasis in the original), WHL. Samuel Cartwright also wrote about "negro superstition" as a kind of disease. Among the many articles that addressed Cart-

wright's obsessions with African spiritual belief and biological difference were "Diseases of Negroes" and "Dr. Cartwright on the Caucasians and the Africans."

76. On the conflation of biology and culture within white Victorian notions of civilization, see Bederman, *Manliness and Civilization*, 28–29.

77. Van Deburg, *Slavery and Race in American Popular Culture*, 9–14, 29. Winthrop Jordan presents a moderated view of Van Deburg's argument, reminding us that even at the height of the popularity of images of noble savages, Africans were never seen as possessing purely noble qualities; see Jordan, *White over Black*, 27. See also Curtin, *Image of Africa*.

78. Notes from Frederick Dalcho, M.D., *Historical Account of the Protestant Episcopal Church in South Carolina*, 1820, cited in Scrapbook (ca. 1926), Bennett Papers, SCHS.

79. C. C. Jones, *The Religious Instruction of the Negroes in the United States* (1842; reprint, New York, 1969), 127–28, quoted in Levine, *Black Culture and Black Consciousness*, 61.

80. Corporation of Charleston, *Account of the Late Intended Insurrection*, 24.

81. "Voudouism in Virginia," n.d., clipping in George William Bagby Scrapbook, 1866–76, George William Bagby Papers, VHS, 110.

82. See Wyatt-Brown, *Southern Honor*, 315; *Reel v. Reel*, 2 Hawks 63, June 1822, and *State v. Martin Posey*, 4 Strobhart 103 and 142, Nov. 1849, cited in Catterall, *Judicial Cases Concerning American Slavery*, 2:43, 413. On the interracial clientele of conjurers, see Genovese, *Roll, Jordan, Roll*, 217–18. Whites continued to seek out African American root doctors into the twentieth century. See Floyd Marmaduke, "Some Negro Superstitions on the Coast," 14–15, talk before the Savannah Historical Research Association, 26 Feb. 1936, Savannah Historical Research Association Papers, GHS; Puckett, *Folk Beliefs of the Southern Negro*, 275; Chesnutt, "Superstitions and Folklore of the South," 371.

83. William Wells Brown, *Narrative of William W. Brown*, 91. James L. Smith similarly consulted a black doctor, who was also a fortune teller, just before his escape from Virginia; see his *Autobiography*, 37.

84. Morrison, *Playing in the Dark*, 11–12.

85. Jacobs, *Incidents in the Life of a Slave Girl*, 69. Superstition in enslaved communities was a sensitive subject for the authors of antebellum slave narratives. On one hand, they sought to depict slavery as a realm of ignorance from which the enslaved urgently needed to be rescued. On the other hand, authors of slave narratives were cautious about playing into the hands of critics who would define superstition as a black racial characteristic. James Pennington, a former fugitive and Presbyterian minister, for example, carefully distanced himself from belief in "superstitious proverbs"; see Pennington, *Fugitive Blacksmith*, in Bontemps, *Great Slave Narratives*, 229–30.

86. *Weevils*, 120.

87. Botkin, *Lay My Burden Down*, 46. See also Mellon, *Bullwhip Days*, 85.

88. Botkin, *Lay My Burden Down,* 46.

89. Arens and Karp, *Creativity of Power,* xv, 96, xxi.

90. Lula Russeau interview, Federal Writers' Project, 1938, SHC.

91. Rawick, supp., ser. 1, 4:584. African American women's references to spiritual domains of knowledge are abundant in nineteenth-century slave narratives and in early twentieth-century interviews with former slaves. See, for example, Egypt, Masuoka, and Johnson, *Unwritten History of Slavery,* 212, 316; Kate Drumgoold, *A Slave Girl's Story: Being an Autobiography of Kate Drumgoold* (New York, 1898), in Gates, *Six Women's Slave Narratives,* 14.

92. Botkin, *Lay My Burden Down,* 46.

93. Clifton Johnson, *God Struck Me Dead,* 60. For further discussion of spiritual revelation in herbal medicine making, see Chapter 3.

94. Clifton Johnson, *God Struck Me Dead,* 97. Among the Fisk University interviews, not only does spiritual power play an important role in healing, but conversely, healing images and metaphors also play an important role in conversion. For examples, see ibid., 150, and Egypt, Masuoka, and Johnson, *Unwritten History of Slavery,* 223.

95. Humez, *Gifts of Power,* 1–50.

96. This song was collected in the late 1930s in Augusta, Georgia. The folder in which it was deposited is not marked specifically as "Negro folklore," as some surrounding folders are. Although the song is located within a collection focused primarily on African American folklore materials, it may have been sung by whites as well. See "Folk Songs (Richmond Co.)," box A593, folder: Georgia, Songs, Ballads, and Rhymes, WPA Folklore Project, LC.

97. Charles S. Johnson, *Shadow of the Plantation,* 195.

98. *Drums,* 69. The revelation of remedies through dreams was common for many southerners. For example, Mary Bethell, a Methodist North Carolina slaveholder, wrote of the positive effects of cold morning baths, a remedy given to her in a dream. Bethell attributed the revelation "as from God," however, rather than from ancestors. See Bethell Diary, 28 June 1864, SHC. See also Friedman, *Enclosed Garden,* 40–53.

99. Marie Campbell, *Folks Do Get Born* (New York: Rinehart, 1946), 244–45, quoted in Wilkie, "Secret and Sacred," 85.

100. Elizabeth W. Pearson, ed., *Letters from Port Royal, 1862–1868,* quoted in Jacqueline Jones, *Labor of Love, Labor of Sorrow,* 40.

101. Blassingame, *Slave Testimony,* 648.

102. Joyner, *Down by the Riverside,* 64–65; Stuckey, *Slave Culture,* 31; Mbiti, *African Religions and Philosophy,* 81; Blassingame, "Status and Social Structure in the Slave Community," 149; Genovese, *Roll, Jordan, Roll,* 519–23. In addition to their spiritual power, elders also played an important role in enslaved communities through work such as childcare, instruction, and doctoring. See Pollard, *Complaint to the Lord,* 49–50.

103. The issue of gender and authority among slave women healers is discussed in greater detail in Chapter 5.

104. Regarding spirits, see Jack Waldburg interview, *Drums*, 68–69; Agnes Cullen interview and Martha Coleman interview, box 2, folder 6, items 377, 379, WPA Folklore Collections, UVL.

105. Thompson, "Kongo Influences on African American Artistic Culture," 152–57; Thompson, *Flash of the Spirit*, 103–58; Gomez, *Exchanging Our Country Marks*, 148–49.

106. Vlach, *Back of the Big House*, 18–32, 153–82.

107. Creel, "Gullah Attitudes towards Life and Death," 69–97; Creel, *"Peculiar People,"* 311; Robinson, "Faith Is the Key and Prayer Unlocks the Door."

108. Peters, *Lyrics of the Afro-American Spiritual*, 87.

109. Northup, *Twelve Years a Slave*, 288, 321, 367. In another variation on the theme of medical neglect, some authors of antebellum slave narratives emphasized the barbarity of slavery by highlighting the lack of Christian comforts, such as Bible reading, given to dying slaves. See Bibb, *Narrative of the Life and Adventures of Henry Bibb*, 122; John Brown, *Slave Life in Georgia*, 27; *Anti-Slavery Reporter* 2 (29 Dec. 1841): 273–75, reprinted in Blassingame, *Slave Testimony*, 217; Mary Prince, *The History of Mary Prince, a West Indian Slave* (London, 1831), in Gates, *Six Women's Slave Narratives*, 8, 10, 14, 18–19.

110. See Chapter 5 for a more detailed discussion of women's remedies for whipping victims.

111. Faulkner, *Days When the Animals Talked*, 34–39.

112. Smith and Holmes, *Listen to Me Good*, 26.

113. For a description of the centrality of church social ties to sickbed attendance among twentieth-century African Americans in rural Alabama, see Charles S. Johnson, *Shadow of the Plantation*, 193.

CHAPTER 3

1. Throughout this chapter I use Etienne Wenger's definition of "repertoire" as "a community's set of shared resources" to refer to the body of slave herbal knowledge. According to Wenger, *Communities of Practice*, 83, a community's repertoire includes "routines, words, tools, ways of doing things, stories, gestures, symbols, genres, actions or concepts that the community has produced or adopted in the course of its existence, and which have become part of its practice."

2. Doctor Lewis lived at Whites Mill in King William County and was legally part of the estate of the deceased John Whites. Sources do not indicate whether Doctor Lewis controlled any of his own earnings. See 1, 5, 19 July 1833, Plantation Journal, Walker Papers, SHC.

3. 7 June, 12 Aug. 1834, ibid.

4. A small number of southern botanical scientists promoted the study of local plants. Their concerns, however, centered on taxonomy, not on practical medicinal use. See Stephens, *Science, Race, and Religion in the American South.*

5. 24 May 1834, Plantation Journal, Walker Papers, SHC.

6. Stewart, *"What Nature Suffers to Groe,"* 135–36, 142, 178.

7. William Berly to Joel Berly, 18 May 1855, Berly Family Papers, SCL. Antebellum "Indian doctors" were popular practitioners who claimed to practice indigenous medicine but were not necessarily Native Americans themselves. See Crellin and Philpott, *Herbal Medicine Past and Present,* 27.

8. Peter Wood, "People's Medicine in the Early South"; Savitt, *Fevers, Agues, and Cures,* 7–14.

9. Valverde, "Aztec Herbal of 1552"; Risse, "Transcending Cultural Barriers."

10. Anne Fausto-Sterling, "Gender, Race, and Nation: The Comparative Anatomy of 'Hottentot' Women in Europe, 1815–1817," in Terry and Urla, *Deviant Bodies,* 23–26; Kincaid, "In History," 4–6.

11. Crellin and Philpott, *Herbal Medicine Past and Present,* 16.

12. Voeks, *Sacred Leaves of Candomblé,* 22.

13. McClure, "Parallel Usage of Medicinal Plants."

14. Voeks, *Sacred Leaves of Candomblé,* 26–27; Grimé, *Ethno-Botany of the Black Americans,* 19, 21, 26, 92, 107. Other Old World plants with both food and medicinal uses include winged yam, pigeon pea, sorghum, oil palm, watermelon, akee, and black-eyed pea.

15. Richard Donn White, "'We Didn Know No Clinic,'" 103, 185; Voeks, *Sacred Leaves of Candomblé,* 24, 26.

16. The impact of Native American medicine on the pharmacopoeia of Western medicine requires further research. See Crellin and Philpott, *Herbal Medicine Past and Present,* 22–25; Duffy, *Healers,* 1–8. Crellin and Duffy argue that the influence of Indian botanical knowledge on Western medicine has been romanticized. Their critiques, however, do not seriously consider the importance of spirituality in Native American herbal practices, nor do they address the impact of American Indian medicines on ordinary white domestic medicine, rather than on the therapies of orthodox physicians. See also Risse, "Transcending Cultural Barriers."

17. Peter Wood, *Black Majority,* 121–22; Gwendolyn Midlo Hall, *Africans in Colonial Louisiana,* 97–118; Grimé, *Ethno-Botany of the Black Americans,* 186, 187, 190.

18. Mellon, *Bullwhip Days,* 94.

19. Berkeley and Berkeley, *Reverend John Clayton,* 24–25; Philip D. Morgan, *Slave Counterpoint,* 619.

20. William Gooch to English authorities, 29 June 1729, reprinted in Kemper, "Documents Relating to the Boundaries of the Northern Neck," 306–7; "Virginia Council Journals," 103–4. Virginia planters sought an alternative to the mercury treatments used widely in eighteenth-century Europe for syphilis. Papan was also called James Pawpaw; see Philip D. Morgan, *Slave Counterpoint,* 625.

21. See 24 Nov. 1749 to 14 Mar. 1750, *Journal of the Commons House of Assembly, March 28, 1749–March 19, 1750,* 293, 302–3, 316, 320, 326, 461; Chappell, "'Doctor Caesar' and His Cure for Poisons."

22. 6 to 12 Mar. 1755, *Journal of the Commons House of Assembly, Nov. 12, 1754–Sept. 23, 1755,* 144–45, 179; Philip D. Morgan, *Slave Counterpoint,* 625. Indigenous societies in the Southeast may also have associated snake handling with healing. See John Brickell's eighteenth-century description of a North Carolina colonist cured by a Native American practitioner with herbs and a large defanged rattlesnake, in Brickell, *Natural History of North-Carolina,* 402–4.

23. *Weevils,* 310.

24. Rosengarten, *Tombee,* 399. See also Fielder Hampton interview, in Rawick, supp., ser. 1, 11:121.

25. Porcher, *Resources of the Southern Fields and Forests,* viii.

26. Ibid., 52, 62–63, 69, 80, 106, 230, 393, 421; Goodson, "Medical-Botanical Contributions of African Slave Women."

27. Gutman, *Black Family in Slavery and Freedom,* 80–82; Grimé, *Ethno-Botany of the Black Americans,* 122; Porcher, *Resources of the Southern Fields and Forests,* 62–63; John H. Morgan, "Essay on the Causes of the Production of Abortion."

28. McMillen, *Motherhood in the Old South,* 135–64; Weiner, *Mistresses and Slaves,* 79–80.

29. Emoline Glasgow interview, in Rawick, 2(2):135.

30. Mom Agnes James interview, in Rawick, 3(3):9; Authur Colson interview, in Rawick, supp., ser. 1, 3:220.

31. Henderson Diary, 3 Sept. 1855, Steele Papers, SHC.

32. Rawick, 2(2):89.

33. Sally McMillen asserts that occasions of nursing and childbirth served as moments of "special intimacy" for black and white plantation women, "dissolving for a moment racial barriers." She provides little evidence to support the assumption that intimacy dissolved racial barriers, however. See McMillen, *Motherhood in the Old South,* 57, 70, 130, 134, 185. The social relations of the healing work of slave women and slaveholding women are discussed at length in Chapter 5.

34. Louisa Collier interview, in Rawick, 2(1):221. See also Alice Battle interview, in Rawick, supp., ser. 1, 3:42.

35. Bethell Diary, 1 Jan. 1853, SHC.

36. Ewell, *Planter's and Mariner's Medical Companion,* 49, 137–39.

37. Murphy, *Enter the Physician,* xv, 31.

38. Rawick, 2(1):334; Bookman Family Remedy Book, 1834–1885, SCL; Prescriptions, folder "section 32," Douthat Family Papers, VHS; Commonplace Book, Elizabeth (Lumpkin) Motley Bagby Papers, VHS. On plantation remedy books, see Lacy and Harrell, "Plantation Home Remedies"; Carrigan, "Early Nineteenth Century Folk Remedies"; Moss, *Southern Folk Medicine.*

39. Recipe Book, n.d., Telfair Family Papers, GHS, 55.

40. "Recipe for dropsy," n.d., Miscellany, Brookes Papers, DUL.

41. "Home Remedies for Diseases of Man and Beast," 68:28, 43, Lenoir Family Papers, SHC. Caesar's remedy appeared also in the following: "The Negro Ceasars Cure for Poison," Recipe Book, William Gibbons Jr., Telfair Family Papers, GHS, 79; Banister Cookbook, Cocke Family Papers, VHS; "Cure for Rattlesnake Bite," *Southern Cultivator* 13 (1855): 228. See also Moss, *Southern Folk Medicine*, 93, 124–26.

42. Wall, "Medical Care of Ebenezer Pettigrew's Slaves," 454; Moss, *Southern Folk Medicine*, 33, 36, 45–56.

43. For an analysis of the impact of an expanding antebellum market economy on southern planters, see Young, *Domesticating Slavery*, 10–14, 124; Rosengarten, *Tombee*, 183, 187.

44. Yetman, *Life under the "Peculiar Institution,"* 201.

45. Stewart, *"What Nature Suffers to Groe,"* 135–36, 178.

46. Leland Ferguson, in "The Strength of these Arms: Black Labor/White Rice," North State Public Video, 1988.

47. "Granny" Cain interview, William Ballard interview, Anderson Bates interview, and Hector Godbold interview, in Rawick, 2(1):28, 42, 167, 2(2):146.

48. Gus Feaster interview, in Rawick, 2(2):50, 52.

49. Porcher, *Resources of the Southern Fields and Forests,* 421.

50. *Weevils,* 309.

51. Rawick, 14:286.

52. *Weevils,* 294.

53. Jane Arrington interview, in Rawick, 14:48; box 2, folder 6, item 379, WPA Folklore Collections, UVL; Westmacott, *African-American Gardens and Yards,* 25, 84, 96–97, 183.

54. Box 2, folder 6, item 372, WPA Folklore Collections, UVL; Egypt, Masuoka, and Johnson, *Unwritten History of Slavery,* 244. This woman made a tea out of jimsonweed for a neighbor whose period had stopped. Jimsonweed is a highly toxic plant in the nightshade family. It is possible she was using the plant as an abortifacient. See also Foster and Duke, *Field Guide to Medicinal Plants,* 86, 312; Cadwallader and Wilson, "Folklore Medicine among Georgia's Piedmont Negroes," 220–21.

55. Rosengarten, *Tombee,* 477, 491, 512, 513, 590. See also James Bolton interview, in Rawick, supp., ser. 1, 3:78; George Harris interview, in Rawick, 14:372. Slave women processed arrowroot into powder using a repetitive process of grating, soaking, straining, and drying. See "Arrowroot Powder Receipt," Misc., Telfair Family Papers, GHS.

56. Rawick, supp., ser. 1, 4:631.

57. Rawick, 14:355. Additional evidence of slaves going to the woods for medicine includes Sylvia Cannon interview, Mom Louisa Collier interview, Julia Rush interview, and Louisa Adams interview, in Rawick, 1:193, 2(1):221, 13(3):231, 14:5; *Slave Narratives,* 231.

58. Carolina Ates interview, in Rawick, supp., ser. 1, 3:27; Fannie Moore interview, in Rawick, 15:134; Mellon, *Bullwhip Days,* 97.

59. Rawick, 16:17, 9, 76, 49, quoted in McDaniel, *Hearth and Home,* 120.

60. "Plantation Remedies," box A670, folder: South Carolina, Negro Lore, Beliefs and Customs, Remedies and Cures, WPA Folklore Project, LC.

61. Porcher, *Resources of the Southern Fields and Forests,* viii; Grimé, *Ethno-Botany of the Black Americans,* 67.

62. Josephine Bacchus interview, in Rawick, 2(1):24; Egypt, Masuoka, and Johnson, *Unwritten History of Slavery,* 38, 313.

63. Deas-Moore, "Home Remedies, Herb Doctors, and Granny Midwives," 480–81; Faith Mitchell, *Hoodoo Medicine,* 27; Cadwallader and Wilson, "Folklore Medicine among Georgia's Piedmont Negroes," 222; Julia F. Morton, *Folk Remedies of the Low Country,* 109-10. Pokeweed was not used exclusively by African Americans; at least one white physician's notebook contained a remedy made from the pokeweed root and berries. See "Cure for a Cancer," McLeod Notebook, 52-53, SCL.

64. Faith Mitchell, *Hoodoo Medicine,* 27.

65. Rawick, supp., ser. 1, 3:99; Lula Russeau interview, Federal Writers' Project, 1938, SHC, 56; Egypt, Masuoka, and Johnson, *Unwritten History of Slavery,* 223.

66. Blassingame, *Slave Testimony,* 668–69.

67. Faith Mitchell, *Hoodoo Medicine,* 27.

68. Payne-Jackson and Lee, *Folk Wisdom and Mother Wit,* 21–26; Snow, *Walkin' over Medicine,* 95-113; Hill and Mathews, "Traditional Health Beliefs and Practices," 315-17; Holly F. Mathews, "Doctors and Root Doctors: Patients Who Use Both," in Kirkland, Mathews, Sullivan, and Baldwin, *Herbal and Magical Medicine,* 72-75. African American diagnostic systems based on blood, phlegm, and gall share obvious similarities with the ancient Galenic system of humors, yet it would be a mistake to assume that African American systems are simply a derivative of European humoral theory. Many diagnostic systems throughout the African diaspora are organized around the qualities and meanings of blood, which is understood to be central to the well-being and ongoing function of the body. See LaGuerre, *Afro-Caribbean Medicine,* 66.

69. Snow, *Walkin' over Medicine,* 77–80.

70. Box 2, folder 6, item 378, WPA Folklore Collections, UVL.

71. Rawick, 15:3.

72. *Drums,* 57.

73. Ira Berlin, *Many Thousands Gone,* 308.

74. *Drums,* 183.

75. Ibid., 71.

76. Ibid., 68.

77. According to Michael Gomez, an intimate connection between "land and the ancestral realm" formed a foundation for political and spiritual life among the Akan and the Igbo as well as other West Africans. The profound connection to the land, he

argued, greatly augmented the trauma of displacement under American slavery. How subsequent American-born generations drew on West African views of the land to forge their sacred orientation toward the North American landscape is an important question in need of further attention. See Gomez, *Exchanging Our Country Marks,* 112, 113, 128.

78. Brandon, "Uses of Plants in Healing," 55.

79. Voeks, *Sacred Leaves of Candomblé,* 73; Brandon, *Santeria from Africa to the New World,* 16–17. Michael Gomez's analysis of the ethnic distribution of Africans in the upper and lower South indicates that the Yoruba presence in the geographical regions of this study was relatively small. My introduction of the concept of *ashé* is not intended as an argument for exclusive Yoruba origins of African American herbalism but, instead, to demonstrate the spiritual basis of other Black Atlantic herbal practices and thereby illuminate possible underlying spiritual tenets of North American black herbalism. See Gomez, *Exchanging Our Country Marks,* 34, 54, 114.

80. Brandon, "Uses of Plants in Healing."

81. Thompson, "Icons of the Mind," 53, 59.

82. Voeks, *Sacred Leaves of Candomblé,* 24.

83. Ibid., 163–64.

84. Ibid., 69–114.

85. Mintz and Rolph Trouillot, "Social History of Haitian Vodou," 138; Thompson, "From the Isle beneath the Sea," 109.

86. The West African divinity Loko (Iroko in Brazil) appears also in Haiti, as a leaf healer and guardian of priestly authority who incorporates aspects of indigenous Arawak and Taino traditions. See Beauvoir-Dominique, "Underground Realms of Being," 158–59, 169.

87. Thompson, "From the Isle beneath the Sea," 105, 108–14. Thompson also points out that *Simbi Makaya* could also refer to an enslaved revolutionary hero, Makay.

88. These differences in Black Atlantic sacred plant traditions parallel comparative differences in the retention and transformation of African religions in North America compared to the Caribbean and Latin America. See Raboteau, *Slave Religion,* 44–92.

89. New Orleans Voodoo, although outside the geographical boundaries of this study, also offers an ideal context for an investigation of the role of plants in African American religions. See Hurston, "Hoodoo in America"; Jessie Gaston Mulira, "The Case of Voodoo in New Orleans," in Holloway, *Africanisms in American Culture,* 34–68.

90. Ferguson, *Uncommon Ground,* 110–16; Ferguson, "'Cross Is a Magic Sign.'"

91. On the importance of the Exodus story to black Christianity under slavery, see Raboteau, *Slave Religion,* 311–12; Sobel, *Trabelin' On,* 125; Theophus H. Smith, *Conjuring Culture,* 67–69.

92. Box 2, folder 6, item 372, WPA Folklore Collections, UVL. For a discussion

of southern African American beliefs about nature and gardening in the twentieth century, see Westmacott, *African-American Gardens and Yards,* 87–100.

93. *Weevils,* 310.

94. Clifton Johnson, *God Struck Me Dead,* 60.

95. Mellon, *Bullwhip Days,* 95.

96. Berlin and Morgan, "Slaves' Economy," 16–17.

97. Bass, "Mojo," 386. Plants continued to play a role in African American religious worship in the twentieth century. Bishop Mason, the founder of the Church of God in Christ, for example, posed for photographs with plants and frequently used plants, vegetables, and other natural objects in his sermons. See Patterson, Ross, and Atkins, *History and Formative Years of the Church of God in Christ,* xii, 13.

98. Anderson and Kreamer, *Wild Spirits, Strong Medicine.*

99. Jacobs, *Incidents in the Life of a Slave Girl,* 112–13.

100. Raboteau, *Slave Religion,* 213–19.

101. George Briggs interview, in Rawick, supp., ser. 1, 11:68–72; Payne-Jackson and Lee, *Folk Wisdom and Mother Wit,* 19.

102. Interview with Riley and Cameron, SHC.

CHAPTER 4

1. 17 July 1810, McKean letterbook, Business Records, Roslin Plantation Records, LV.

2. The two conflicting interpretations of Calia's affliction converge in the term "Negro Poisoning" (also "Negro consumption" or "Struma Africana"), an expression used by antebellum white doctors for a form of pulmonary tuberculosis they considered peculiar to African Americans. The name may have had its origins in the overlap between symptoms of this type of consumption (breathing difficulties, abdominal pain, and wasting away) and the signs of conjure affliction. See Savitt, *Medicine and Slavery,* 42; Haller, "Negro and the Southern Physician," 242–44; Cartwright, "Diseases of Negroes," 212–13.

3. This chapter as a whole owes a debt to the approach found in Feierman and Janzen, *Social Basis of Health and Healing.*

4. Chireau, "Uses of the Supernatural," 172.

5. African American southerners of the nineteenth and early twentieth centuries used these terms to describe the act of conjuring. Although the phrase "to witch" was used in some areas to indicate conjuration, a separate set of characteristics distinguished the witch from the conjure doctor. Witches in African American lore were living persons who left their skin at night, assumed various shapes, and "rode" their victims while they slept. Unlike conjure doctors, witches did not have paying clients and they were hardly ever associated with healing. The witch in African American tra-

ditions, almost always a woman, was a personal problem, ranging from a nuisance to a terror. Victims of witches used individual action, community rituals, incantations, and other preventative steps, but they rarely employed collective violence as seen in the New England or European witch trials. Mention of witches and conjuring activities performed by witches was much more frequent in the North Carolina WPA materials than in the Georgia, South Carolina, or Virginia accounts. See Rawick, 14:122, 128–29; *Slave Narratives*, 100; *Drums*, 4, 6, 24, 34, 35, 58–60, 95; Stroyer, *My Life in the South*, 52–53; Mamie Garvin Fields, *Lemon Swamp*, 118–19; William Grimes, *Life of William Grimes, the Runaway Slave* (New Haven: by the Author, 1855), in Bontemps, *Five Black Lives*, 79–80; Deborah Gray White, *Ar'n't I a Woman?*, 135; *Weevils*, 278.

6. Good, *Medicine, Rationality, and Experience*, 128. Good uses the concept of the illness narrative as a tool of analysis in his work with late-twentieth-century Turkish communities. One important difference between the narratives Good collected and the conjuring accounts used here is that the Turkish informants were in the midst of coping with their illness, whereas most conjuring accounts concern past encounters with conjuration.

7. Ibid., 157.

8. David H. Brown, "Conjure/Doctors," 26.

9. *Drums*, 27–28. Due to the length of this quotation, I have departed from the usual approach to Federal Writers' Project material by standardizing the spelling of the original text.

10. George McCall, "Symbiosis: The Case of Hoodoo and the Numbers Racket," in Dundes, *Mother Wit from the Laughing Barrel*, 420.

11. Kelley, "Notes on Deconstructing 'The Folk'"; Carby, "Ideologies of Black Folk," 126–28.

12. *Drums*, 29; *Slave Narratives*, 32.

13. Puckett, *Folk Beliefs of the Southern Negro*, 277–78; *Drums*, 28, 31; *Weevils*, 246.

14. Postemancipation materials collected by folklorists and WPA interviewers on conjuration during slavery instead stress the slaves' use of hoodoo against the power of slaveholders, overseers, and patrollers rather than against fellow slaves. The production of these interviews makes it difficult, however, to conclude that this accurately reflects the way conjure was used under slavery. The smaller pool of stories about conjuring within slave communities may have been due to an emphasis in the interview on slave-master relations intended by the informants and/or the collectors. Moreover, many informants may not have discussed intraracial conjuring incidents out of a concern for maintaining some privacy in the most personal areas of their lives. Among other evidence generated in the antebellum period itself, published slave narratives occasionally cited the use of roots for courtship or against slaveholders. See Douglass, *Narrative of the Life of Frederick Douglass*, 80–82; Bibb, *Narrative of the Life and Adventures of Henry Bibb*, 70–74. For perspectives on conjuring in slave narra-

tives published in the late nineteenth century, see Bruce, *New Man,* 43–59; Albert, *House of Bondage,* 94–100.

15. Gorn, "Folk Beliefs of the Slave Community," 321–22.

16. 11 Dec. 18[16?], McKean letterbook, Roslin Plantation Records, LV. On the structure of double-unit houses, see Vlach, *Back of the Big House,* 158–60. Jacob Stroyer comments on the social dynamics of families who shared a single hearth in *My Life in the South,* 42–43.

17. 11 Dec. 18[16?], McKean letterbook, Roslin Plantation Records, LV.

18. 23 Feb. 1816, ibid.

19. Gorn, "Folk Beliefs of the Slave Community," 317–18, 324.

20. Hill and Mathews, "Traditional Health Beliefs and Practices."

21. "Folklore: Cures and Magic Remedies," box A671, folder: South Carolina, Negro Lore, Beliefs and Customs, WPA Folklore Project, LC.

22. Herron and Bacon, "Conjuring and Conjure Doctors," 362, 363, 365; Puckett, *Folk Beliefs of the Southern Negro,* 237; *Drums,* 90–91.

23. Botkin, *Lay My Burden Down,* 135; Gorn, "Folk Beliefs of the Slave Community," 325–26. For a similar account told by the son of a slaveholder, see "Witchcraft," box 3, folder 1, item 48, WPA Folklore Collections, UVL.

24. James L. Smith, *Autobiography,* 4–6.

25. Berlin and Morgan, "Slaves' Economy," 17.

26. James Gunnell to Miss Telfair, 27 June, 9 Sept. 1833, 20 Mar. 1834, 2 Apr. 1836, Telfair Family Papers, GHS.

27. James Gunnell to Miss Telfair, 27 June 1833, ibid.

28. James Gunnell to Margaret C. Telfair, 2 Apr. 1836, ibid.

29. A. H. Urquhart to Miss Margaret C. Telfair, 4 Nov. 1839, ibid.

30. Steiner, "Observations on the Practice of Conjuring in Georgia," 175.

31. This section of the chapter is restricted to conflicts arising specifically under slavery, but evidence of postemancipation conflicts between men and women over sexuality, marriage, and money abound. See, for example, *Drums,* 3, 101; "A Tale of 'Spell' Moving as Told By Reverend P. L. Harvey of Lynchburg, Virginia," box 2, folder 2, item 279, WPA Folklore Collections, UVL; Julien A. Hall, "Negro Conjuring and Tricking," 241–43.

32. Chireau, "Uses of the Supernatural," 179–88.

33. "Folklore (Negro)," box A593, folder: Georgia, Negro Lore, WPA Folklore Project, LC.

34. Chesnutt, "Superstitions and Folklore of the South," 369–76.

35. Roswell King to Pierce Butler, 5 June, 10 July 1814, Butler Papers, HSP.

36. Steiner, "Observations on the Practice of Conjuring in Georgia," 177.

37. *Drums,* 25.

38. Ibid., 3.

39. Chesnutt, "Superstitions and Folklore of the South," 374.

40. Sarah Fitzpatrick interview, Alabama, 1938, reprinted in Blassingame, *Slave*

Testimony, 647. For other instances of pining away, see *Drums,* 44, 101; Julien A. Hall, "Negro Conjuring and Tricking," 241–43; Herron and Bacon, "Conjuring and Conjure Doctors," 361.

41. "Folklore (Negro)," box A592, folder: Georgia, Beliefs and Customs, Superstitions, WPA Folklore Project, LC.

42. Rawick, supp., ser. 1, 3:140. See also interview with Riley and Cameron, SHC, 2.

43. Rawick, supp., ser. 1, 4:652. References to reptiles and insects in the conjured body are ubiquitous throughout African American folklore and oral history sources. See *Drums,* 25, 41; box 1, folder 8, item 73, WPA Folklore Collections, UVL; Herron and Bacon, "Conjuring and Conjure Doctors," 361; Puckett, *Folk Beliefs of the Southern Negro,* 249.

44. Rosengarten, *Tombee,* 20 Feb. 1846, 399. Nancy apparently recovered, but Chaplin insisted that she was "not cured by old Sancho." See also Herron and Bacon, "Conjuring and Conjure Doctors," 365.

45. McCandless, *Moonlight, Magnolias, and Madness,* 15–39.

46. Coxe, *Philadelphia Medical Dictionary,* 1, 277, 298.

47. Chesnutt, "Superstitions and Folklore of the South," 373. Historical scholarship on African and African American views of the body in the Americas is difficult to locate, especially for North America. On related Afro-Caribbean ideas of the body, see LaGuerre, *Afro-Caribbean Medicine,* 64; Sobo, *One Blood.* More attention has been directed to describing and theorizing changing European and white American views of the body. See, for example, Isaac, *Transformation of Virginia,* 47–52; Duden, *Woman beneath the Skin,* 7–27.

48. "Durham's Voodoo Doctor," box A661, folder: North Carolina, Witchcraft, WPA Folklore Project, LC.

49. Du Bois, *Souls of Black Folk,* 342.

50. Zora Neale Hurston, working in the Deep South in 1929 and 1930, distinguished between root doctors, who focused exclusively on cures, and hoodoo or conjure doctors, who also used their powers to harm. Within the southeastern states and coastal islands the titles of healers varied widely, and a distinction between root and hoodoo doctors was less apparent. See Hurston, *Mules and Men,* 288. See also Sobel, *Trabelin' On,* 41–45.

51. *Drums,* 39.

52. The WPA narratives are the primary sources most used by historians surveying the range of attitudes toward conjuration held by black men and women. See, for example, Genovese, *Roll, Jordan, Roll,* 218–19; Joyner, *Down by the Riverside,* 148–50. Historical shifts involving literacy, uplift, and white supremacy, however, provide good reason to suspect that beliefs about the morality of conjuration in southern black communities changed considerably from the antebellum to the early-twentieth-century period. Class formation also contributed to the controversial

nature of conjure among African Americans. These factors make the WPA narratives a somewhat problematic source for judging antebellum attitudes about conjure. See A[lice] M[abel] Bacon, "Proposal for Folk-Lore Research at Hampton, Va.," *JAF* 6 (Oct.-Dec. 1893): 305-6; A[lice] M[abel] Bacon, "Work and Methods of the Hampton Folk-Lore Society," *JAF* 11 (Jan.-Mar. 1898): 17; Levine, *Black Culture and Black Consciousness,* 155-74.

53. "Durham's Voodoo Doctor," box A661, folder: North Carolina, Witchcraft, WPA Folklore Project, LC; Herron and Bacon, "Conjuring and Conjure Doctors," 360. See Chapter 2 for a discussion of dualism in African conceptions of power.

54. *Drums,* 39. A single exception to this rule appeared in the account of a woman who thought she was conjured and was told by a physician that she was wrong. He gave her some medicine and she reported getting better. See Harriette Benton interview, in Rawick, supp., ser. 1, 3:52.

55. "Richmond Co. Folklore Interviews—Conjuration," box A592, folder: Georgia, Beliefs and Customs, Superstitions, WPA Folklore Project, LC.

56. Ibid. See also Malissa Gilchrist interview, ibid.; "Compilation Folklore Interviews—Richmond Co.," box A593, folder: Georgia, Ghost Stories and Spiritual and Supernatural Tales, WPA Folklore Project, LC; Herron and Bacon, "Conjuring and Conjure Doctors," 361; Puckett, *Folk Beliefs of the Southern Negro,* 274.

57. *Weevils,* 267. See also Faust, "Culture, Conflict, and Community," 89.

58. In an attempt to reduce the influence of conjure doctors on enslaved sufferers during epidemics, Samuel Cartwright, for example, recommended that planters subject conjure doctors to public humiliation; see Cartwright, "Remarks on Dysentery among Negroes," 149.

59. Mellon, *Bullwhip Days,* 99.

60. Rosengarten, *Tombee,* 448, 452.

61. *Weevils,* 267.

62. McKee, "Earth Is Their Witness," 39.

63. Kenneth Brown, "Material Culture and Community Structure," in Hudson, *Working toward Freedom,* 95-118; Wilkie, "Secret and Sacred."

64. Blassingame, "Status and Social Structure in the Slave Community," 142-43.

65. Rawick, supp., ser. 1, 3:265.

66. *Drums,* 44; Herron and Bacon, "Conjuring and Conjure Doctors," 361.

67. Ibid.; Puckett, *Folk Beliefs of the Southern Negro,* 201; Bass, "Mojo," 381.

68. According to Robert Farris Thompson, the visual portrayal of the Yoruba deity associated with herbalism, Osanyin Elewe, emphasizes the "physically ruined" body. This depiction continues in Cuban herbal arts and may have some connection to the mention of physical peculiarities of conjurers in the southern United States. See Thompson, "Icons of the Mind," 52, 54.

69. For examples of the conjurer assumed to be male, see Owens, *This Species of Property,* 158; Genovese, *Roll, Jordan, Roll,* 222-23. For an example of gender-

specific services, see F. Roy Johnson, *Fabled Doctor*, 95–101, in which twentieth-century conjure doctor Jim Jordan, described as "proud of his manhood" and father of many children, is sought as a specialist in "restored manhood."

70. W. S. Forwood, letter of 13 May 1861, in Cartwright, "Serpent Worship," 98. See also Charles C. Jones, *Negro Myths from the Georgia Coast*, 153.

71. For a view confirming the importance of female conjurers in slave communities, see Chireau, "Uses of the Supernatural," 176, 184. In many narratives, conjure men and conjure women are equally feared. However, the issue of competition for power between male and female conjurers arises occasionally in folklore collections. See Hurston, *Sanctified Church*, 37–40; Hurston, "Hoodoo in America," 404–5. A WPA collector remarked that "cunjer-men" were generally considered more powerful to the "witchcraft 'ooman" among African Americans in Charleston; see "Folklore," box A677, folder: South Carolina, Negro Lore, Witchcraft & Occult, WPA Folklore Project, LC. On the argument that gender identities based in southern black slave culture did not rely, as did Victorian middle-class gender identities, on oppositional constructions of manhood and womanhood as a basis for societal power, see Elsa Barkley Brown, "Negotiating and Transforming the Public Sphere," 107–26.

72. *Slave Narratives*, 12; Roswell King to Pierce Butler, 5 June, 10 July 1814, Butler Papers, HSP; *Weevils*, 324.

73. Schlotterbeck, "Internal Economy of Slavery." Schlotterbeck refers very briefly to economic activities, including transactions with conjurers, which "strengthened slave community life." For an overview on the North American internal economy, see Berlin and Morgan, "Slaves' Economy." For a discussion of the social function of payments to conjure doctors, see Gorn, "Folk Beliefs of the Slave Community," 323.

74. Botkin, *Lay My Burden Down*, 38–39 (emphasis added). A former slave, Henry Pyles, related this rhyme in Oklahoma. Pyles was born into slavery in Tennessee. The conjure man, Old Bab, had moved to Tennessee in the late 1860s from South Carolina. "Pammy Christy" beans came from the Palma Christi, or castor bean, plant, from which castor oil is derived. Its seeds can be toxic. My thanks to Vicki Betts, personal communication, Oct. 2000, for this identification.

75. *Calendar of Virginia State Papers*, 5:333, 338.

76. Trial of Tom and Amy, 20 Jan. 1806, Pittsylvania Co., Governor's Office, William H. Cabell, box 138, Executive Papers, State Records, LV. For a detailed discussion of this trial, see Chapter 6.

77. Genovese, *Roll, Jordan, Roll*, 559–60, 641–42.

78. Bibb, *Narrative of the Life and Adventures of Henry Bibb*, 70–74.

79. William Wells Brown, *Narrative of William W. Brown*, 91–93.

80. *Slave Narratives*, 12.

81. *Weevils*, 324.

82. *Drums*, 28.

83. WPA Mss., quoted in Joyner, *Down by the Riverside*, 149.

84. Mellon, *Bullwhip Days*, 93. See also Laura Sorrell interview, in Rawick, 15:298; Bruce, *New Man*, 52.

85. *Freedmen's Record* 1 (Mar. 1865): 34-38, reprinted in Blassingame, *Slave Testimony*, 464. Some herbalists evidently believed that accepting payment could diminish their power to heal. See Payne-Jackson and Lee, *Folk Wisdom and Mother Wit*, 12-13.

86. Box 2, folder 2, item 269, WPA Folklore Collections, UVL. Both African Americans and whites with the ability to talk out fire or stop bleeding practiced in southern communities. On African American blood stoppers, burn prayers, and wart removers, see Payne-Jackson and Lee, *Folk Wisdom and Mother Wit*, 13. One white "blow-out-fire healer" in South Carolina learned her incantations from a "very old negro woman"; see "Superstitions Obtaining among White People," box A669, folder: South Carolina, Beliefs and Customs — Superstitions, WPA Folklore Project, LC.

87. The issue of payment was complicated by slaveholders' claims to the fees earned by enslaved midwives. See the case of the doctress and midwife Elsey discussed in Chapter 5. See also Logan, *Motherwit*, 103-4.

88. Steiner, "Observations on the Practice of Conjuring in Georgia," 177.

89. Butler, *Awash in a Sea of Faith*, 21-22; Chireau, "Uses of the Supernatural," 174.

90. Peek, *African Divination Systems*, 1-5.

91. "Tale of Conjuration," box 2, folder 2, item 271, WPA Folklore Collections, UVL.

92. "Durham's Voodoo Doctor," box A661, folder: North Carolina, Witchcraft, WPA Folklore Project, LC.

93. Box 1, folder 8, item 73, WPA Folklore Collections, UVL.

94. Rawick, 15:157.

95. Ibid., 375.

96. *Weevils*, 267. The view that Africa was the source of conjuring knowledge was not uncommon among elderly freedpeople; some held that knowledge in a positive light, while others spoke of it as a "superstitious" past. See Rias Body interview, in Rawick, supp., ser. 1, 3:75; *Drums*, 28, 177.

97. Julien A. Hall, "Negro Conjuring and Tricking," 241-43; *Weevils*, 267.

98. "Durham's Voodoo Doctor," box A661, folder: North Carolina, Witchcraft, WPA Folklore Project, LC.

99. "Tale of Conjuration," box 2, folder 2, item 271, WPA Folklore Collections, UVL.

100. Steiner, "Observations on the Practice of Conjuring in Georgia," 177.

101. Thompson, *Flash of the Spirit*, 128-31; Raboteau, "Afro-American Traditions," 548-51.

102. MacGaffey, "Eyes of Understanding," 62-68; MacGaffey, "Complexity, Astonishment, and Power," 192-96.

103. Stroyer, *My Life in the South,* 57–59.

104. References to graveyard dust are widespread in folkloric evidence on conjuration. See Bass, "Mojo," 382–83; Puckett, *Folk Beliefs of the Southern Negro,* 232, 235, 236, 239, 246–48; *Drums,* 36, 42, 44, 75, 84, 93, 94, 102, 125.

105. MacGaffey, "Eyes of Understanding," 68; Steiner, "Braziel Robinson Possessed of Two Spirits."

106. Herron and Bacon, "Conjuring and Conjure Doctors," 362. Another explanation for the frequent use of hair in conjuring was that hair grows near the brain and thus when placed in a conjure bag can affect the victim's brain. See *Drums,* 39.

107. Puckett, *Folk Beliefs of the Southern Negro,* 234; Herron and Bacon, "Conjuring and Conjure Doctors," 362.

108. Bass, "Mojo," 384.

109. MacGaffey, "Eyes of Understanding," 62.

110. David H. Brown, "Conjure/Doctors," 20. In this description Brown draws on Claude Levi-Strauss's concept of a *bricoleur,* Wyatt MacGaffey's analysis of metonymy and metaphor in BaKongo *minkisi,* and Robert Farris Thompson's concept of "spirit-embedding" and "spirit-directing" medicines.

111. MacGaffey, "Eyes of Understanding," 62–68.

112. "Hoo-dooism," Mamie Hanberry, WPA Slave Narrative Project, Kentucky Narratives, 7:121–22, LC.

113. Puckett, *Folk Beliefs of the Southern Negro,* 234; Thompson, "From the Isle beneath the Sea," 111.

114. Emmaline Heard interview, WPA Folklore Project, LC.

115. Steiner, "Observations on the Practice of Conjuring in Georgia," 177.

116. *Drums,* 3.

117. "Durham's Voodoo Doctor," box A661, folder: North Carolina, Witchcraft, WPA Folklore Project, LC. See also *Drums,* 25, 41; "Folklore (Negro)," box A592, folder: Georgia, Beliefs and Customs, Superstitions, WPA Folklore Project, LC.

118. *Drums,* 27, 29.

119. "Compilation Folklore Interviews—Richmond Co.," box A593, folder: Georgia, Ghost Stories and Spiritual and Supernatural Tales, WPA Folklore Project, LC.

120. Rawick, 2(2):148.

121. "Richmond Co. Folklore Interview—Conjuration," box A592, folder: Georgia, Beliefs and Customs, Superstitions, WPA Folklore Project, LC.

122. *Weevils,* 222.

123. On the contrast between practitioner-centered and sufferer-centered analyses of medical systems, see Feierman and Janzen, *Social Basis of Health and Healing,* 2–4.

124. Robinson, "Africanisms and the Study of Folklore," 218.

1. Thorn Island Rule and Direction Book, 11 June 1832; Thorn Island Rule and Direction Book, 1837; "List of Negroes at Thorn Island," 1836; Stephen Newman to Miss Telfair, 28 Feb. 1837, all in Telfair Family Papers, GHS. Thorn Island Plantation was located in Barnwell District, S.C.

2. I have grouped enslaved nurses, doctresses, and midwives together in this chapter because of the similar work they did for their charges. Plantation records use the terms "nurse" and "doctress" somewhat interchangeably. Both referred to women (occasionally men were nurses, too) who made medicines and took care of the sick. Midwives assisted birthing mothers, but many also did sickcare as well. In the planter lexicon, "nurse" also applied to someone in charge of children.

3. The differences between conjuring and nursing in their relationship to plantation production did not, however, preclude the possibility that a woman assigned to healing work by slaveholders might also be a conjure doctor. See, for example, F. Roy Johnson, *Fabled Doctor,* 48.

4. Robertson, "Africa into the Americas?," 23; Jacqueline Jones, "Race, Sex, and Self-Evident Truths," 20, 22. On gendered divisions of labor in enslaved families, see Deborah Gray White, *Ar'n't I a Woman?,* 158–59; Jacqueline Jones, *Labor of Love, Labor of Sorrow,* 38–39; Stevenson, *Life in Black and White,* 226–57.

5. Diamond, *Making Gray Gold,* 2, 130–67. Diamond's study draws on the work of feminist sociologist Dorothy E. Smith, *Everyday World as Problematic.*

6. Davidoff, "Class and Gender in Victorian England"; Hunter, *To 'Joy My Freedom,* 187–218.

7. Elizabeth Barnaby Keeney, "Unless Powerful Sick: Domestic Medicine in the Old South," in Numbers and Savitt, *Science and Medicine in the Old South,* 276–94. Keeney suggests that the "most uniquely southern aspect" of domestic medicine was the influence of slavery, which expanded the pool of patients and challenged "gender roles and authority structures" (289), although she does not elaborate on this latter claim.

8. Fox-Genovese, *Within the Plantation Household,* 37–99; Kerber, "Separate Spheres, Female Worlds, Women's Place." On the entanglement of home and marketplace, public and private, under plantation slavery, see Hortense J. Spillers, "Changing the Letter: The Yokes, the Jokes of Discourse, or, Mrs. Stowe, Mr. Reed," in McDowell and Rampersad, *Slavery and the Literary Imagination,* 25, 28.

9. Sarah Fitzpatrick interview, Alabama, 1938, reprinted in Blassingame, *Slave Testimony,* 647.

10. 12 Aug., 7 June 1834, Plantation Journal, Walker Papers, SHC.

11. Louis Manigault, Prescription Book, 1852, Manigault Papers, DUL.

12. John M. Murphy to Mr. Hodgson, 22 Jan. 1861, Telfair Family Papers, GHS. See also "Agrnt. with J. B. Gross Overseer for the year 1844," 1 Dec. 1843, folder 14, ser., 1.2, Financial and Legal Papers, Arnold and Screven Family Papers, SHC.

13. Richard J. Arnold to Mr. Sanford, [19 May 1840], Overseer Instructions, Correspondence, folder 4, ser. 1.1, Financial and Legal Papers, Arnold and Screven Family Papers, SHC; Schwartz, "'At Noon, Oh How I Ran.'"

14. Thorn Island Rule and Direction Book, 1837, Telfair Family Papers, GHS.

15. *Slave Narratives,* 212.

16. Sumter Diary, 3 Oct. 1840, SCL.

17. Fannie Cawthon Coleman interview and Cicely Cawthon interview, in Rawick, supp., ser. 1, 3:213, 189; Mollie Malone interview, in *Slave Narratives,* 106; Rosengarten, *Tombee,* 520; Lindsey Faucette interview, in Rawick, 14:303.

18. Russell, *Diary,* 141, quoted in Stampp, *Peculiar Institution,* 314; see also 298. Also see Savitt, *Medicine and Slavery,* 160–61. Occasionally, neighboring white women healers also attended sick slaves. See J. N. Bethea to Mr. Hodgson, 1 May 1859, Telfair Family Papers, GHS; "Mrs. Eversole's Cure for Pains, Rheumatism, & Weakness in Knees," in "Home Remedies for Diseases of Man and Beast," vol. 68, Lenoir Family Papers, SHC.

19. Northup, *Twelve Years a Slave,* 366.

20. Lydia A. Riddick to son, 9 Aug. 1848, folder 1, Riddick Papers, SHC.

21. Rawick, 15:45.

22. Mike also nursed an elderly slave man on his deathbed. See Gavin Diary, 27 May 1859 to 6 June 1859, 29 Aug. 1856, SHC.

23. Rawick, supp., ser. 1, 3:86.

24. Sumter Diary, 19 Nov. 1840, SCL.

25. Ibid., 7 Sept. 1840.

26. Clinton, *Plantation Mistress,* 19–29; Anne Firor Scott, *Southern Lady,* 27–37.

27. Harris, "Report on the Treatment of Some Cases of Cholera," 581–85.

28. Richard J. Arnold to I. Swanston, 22 May 1837, Correspondence, folder 2, series 1.1, Arnold and Screven Family Papers, SHC. In addition to his nursing work, Dick also toiled in the gardens and made baskets.

29. Clifton Johnson, *God Struck Me Dead,* 28; Deborah Gray White, *Ar'n't I a Woman?,* 92–93. In addition, some enslaved boys and young men developed medical skills as assistants to white physicians. See Jacobs, *Incidents in the Life of a Slave Girl,* 61; Roper, *Narrative of the Adventures and Escape,* 12.

30. Harold Courlander, *Negro Folk Music, U.S.A.* (New York: Columbia University Press, 1963), 117, quoted in Stuckey, "Through the Prism of Folklore," 425.

31. Rawick, supp., ser. 1, 3:226.

32. For the connections between antebellum nursing and domestic service generally, see Reverby, *Ordered to Care,* 11–16.

33. Rosenberg, "Therapeutic Revolution."

34. "Medicines," "Instructions to Managers," 1854, Philip St. George Cocke Papers, VHS, 1; Elisha Cain to Mr. Telfair, 10 Feb. 1829, 16 Jan. 1831; Elisha Cain to Mary Telfair (ca. Dec. 1836), #125; J. N. Bethea to Mr. Hodgson, 10 June 1860; and John M. Murphey, "List of Medicines Wanted," 2 Dec. 1860, all in Telfair Family

Papers, GHS; Charles Izard Manigault Accounts, 12 Sept. 1834, 20 June 1848, Manigault Family Papers, SCHS; 1833 list of supplies, William W. Smith Plantation Papers, Wragg Family Papers, SCHS.

35. William Fleming Gains to Thomas Chrystie, 25 June 1808, Chrystie Papers, VHS. Gains's reluctance to use the lancet, presumably because of his patients' race, was in accordance with the prevailing medical theory that African Americans could not withstand heavy bleeding as readily as whites. Strong evidence suggests that not all physicians and planters practiced these fine distinctions. See, for example, James Turner McLean interview, in Rawick, 15:88; Savitt, *Medicine and Slavery*, 12–14.

36. Botkin, *Lay My Burden Down*, 135. Blue mass pills were made by pulverizing metallic mercury with honey of rose, then adding glycerin, powdered althaea, and licorice; see Lacy and Harrell, "Plantation Home Remedies," 263.

37. Sale Broadside, 23 Jan. 1860, De Saussure Papers, SCHS.

38. N.d., Cheves Family Papers, SCL. For similar descriptions of heroic treatments applied to enslaved patients, see Farm Notebook of Fountain Humphreys, UVL; Dr. Richmond Lewis to Major Lewis Holladay, letters from 2 Jan. to 23 July 1813 and undated letter, Holladay Family Papers, VHS.

39. In the antebellum years the exception to treatment in one's own home was confinement in almshouses and charity hospitals, which were not seen as respectable places for middle-class whites and not available to most slaves. Some hospitals for black patients existed in Charleston, Richmond, and Savannah but served only a small minority of enslaved rural African Americans. Childbirth, too, was located almost exclusively in the home. See Rosenberg, *Care of Strangers;* Leavitt, *Brought to Bed*, 87–115; Able, *Hearts of Wisdom*, 37–67.

40. Henry Baker interview, 1938, Alabama, in Blassingame, *Slave Testimony*, 669.

41. R. W. N. N., "Negro Cabins," *Southern Planter* 16 (1856): 121–22.

42. Vlach, *Back of the Big House*, 142–44, 175, 214, 221. In a letter detailing his response to several diphtheria cases, Robert Hubard mentioned that he had had a sick family moved to a more remote house "as I did not like to have the sick negroes so near my dwelling house" (R[obert] T. Hubard to James L. Hubard, 15 Nov. 1860, Hubard-Randolph Family Papers, UVL).

43. Kemble, *Journal of a Residence*, 69–72, 257.

44. *Southern Agriculturist* 6 (June 1833): 573–75, quoted in Julia Floyd Smith, *Slavery and Rice Culture*, 133.

45. Kemble, *Journal of a Residence*, 71. See also 1828 list of taskable hands, Rockingham Plantation Journal, DUL. On this plantation one woman named Teneh was assigned as "the Nurse for the Sick ones" among sixty-two persons in the slave quarters.

46. Rawick, 14:355.

47. Stowe, "Obstetrics and the Work of Doctoring," 556–57.

48. William Fleming Gains to Thomas Chrystie, 25 June 1808, Chrystie Papers, VHS.

49. The reference to slaves as the mudsill of southern society and thus its most menial workers comes from James Henry Hammond's infamous proslavery speech on the Senate floor, March 1858. See Bleser, *Secret and Sacred,* 272–73.

50. Harriet Newby to Dangerfield Newby, 11, 22 Apr., 16 Aug. 1859, *Calendar of Virginia State Papers,* 11:310–11, in Blassingame, *Slave Testimony,* 116–17. Harriet Newby's husband, Dangerfield Newby, was at the time of her writing a free man who later that year died taking part in John Brown's raid. See also Petition of Eliza or Liza Purdie, 28 Jan. 1839, Legislative Petitions, Isle of Wight County, 1776–1861, box 122, folder 67, General Assembly, State Records, LV.

51. Interview with Mrs. Laura Smalley, Recordings of Slave Narratives, Archive of Folk Culture, Library of Congress, Washington, D.C.

52. Anna Garretson to her cousin, 29 Jan. 1816, Anna Garretson Papers, SHC, quoted in McMillen, *Motherhood in the Old South,* 145.

53. Charles Manigault, "Hints for Mr. Papot," Manigault Papers, DUL.

54. Z. Haynes to Charles Manigault, 1 June, 1 July 1846, ibid.

55. Louis Manigault to Charles Manigault, 9 Apr. 1853, and Charles Manigault to Louis Manigault, 20 Apr. 1857, ibid.

56. J. T. Cooper to Habersham & Son, 20, 30 June 1848, Manigault Family Papers, SCHS. Cooper does not name the Gowrie nurse. However, a December 1848 slave roster in Manigault Papers, DUL, lists Binah, "Nurse," age sixty years.

57. See, for example, Kemble, *Journal of a Residence,* 90; William Taylor Barry to daughter, 16 Aug. 1832, Barry Letters, UVL.

58. Michael P. Johnson, "Work, Culture, and the Slave Community," 331–33; Marks, "Skilled Blacks in Antebellum St. Mary's County"; Newton and Lewis, *Other Slaves;* Genovese, *Roll, Jordan, Roll,* 388–98.

59. Jacqueline Jones, *Labor of Love, Labor of Sorrow,* 18. Caribbean historians find a similar pattern, although in sugar production, enslaved men's assignment to processing cane into sugar resulted in women often comprising a significant majority of field workers, even when overall gender ratios were heavily tilted toward men. See Robertson, "Africa into the Americas?," 21–23; Beckles, "Black Female Slaves and White Households in Barbados," 113; Geggus, "Slave and Free Colored Women in Saint Domingue," 260–61; Bush, "Hard Labor," 195.

60. In many studies of slave labor, skilled work is often either shown to be or assumed to be an avenue toward higher status, whether measured by greater material goods, ability to travel, access to market, or the exercise of authority, whether within slave communities or in relation to the delegated power of slaveholders. See Dusinberre, *Them Dark Days,* 190–210.

61. Jacqueline Jones, *Labor of Love, Labor of Sorrow,* 29, 38, 42; Owens, *This Species of Property,* 195; Stevenson, *Life in Black and White,* 238.

62. King, *Stolen Childhood,* 24.

63. Botkin, *Lay My Burden Down,* 134.

64. Rawick, 14:53–54. See also Shaw, "Mothering under Slavery," 244.

65. Louis Manigault to Charles Manigault, 17 Mar. 1854, Manigault Papers, DUL.

66. *Weevils*, 288–89.

67. Savitt, *Medicine and Slavery*, 120–22, 127–28, 137–38; Steckel, "Birth Weights and Infant Mortality"; Steckel, "Dreadful Childhood"; McMillen, "'No Uncommon Disease.'"

68. Clifton Johnson, *God Struck Me Dead*, 160.

69. Rawick, 15:339. See also Weiner, *Mistresses and Slaves*, 19–20.

70. Rawick, 2(1):171; Shaw, "Mothering under Slavery," 242.

71. *Slave Narratives*, 19.

72. Ibid., 49, 134, 212; Egypt, Masuoka, and Johnson, *Unwritten History of Slavery*, 313.

73. Mellon, *Bullwhip Days*, 94. See also Rawick, supp., ser. 1, 4:649–52, 3:28.

74. 28 Oct. 1861, Greenwood Plantation Journal, LC; Shaw, "Mothering under Slavery," 237.

75. John A. Warren to John D. Warren, 4 Feb. 1859, Warren Papers, SCL.

76. Shammas, "Black Women's Work"; Shaw, "Mothering under Slavery," 242.

77. Patricia Hill Collins describes othermothers as "women who assist blood-mothers by sharing mothering responsibilities" and who have thus been central to the institution of black motherhood. The term originally comes from Rosalie Riegle Troester. See Patricia Hill Collins, "Meaning of Motherhood," 47–49; Troester, "Turbulence and Tenderness," 163. Deborah White notes older women's childcare as part of the labor of the "female slave network"; see Deborah Gray White, *Ar'n't I a Woman?*, 127–28.

78. Rawick, 15:130–31.

79. K. Washington Skinner to Charles Manigault, 3 Dec. 1852, Manigault Papers, DUL.

80. Stroyer, *My Life in the South*, 8.

81. Given the disproportionate mortality of enslaved African Americans, historians of slavery generally locate the beginning of old age around forty-five to fifty. See Pollard, *Complaint to the Lord*, 32–33.

82. Rawick, 14:413.

83. Rawick, supp., ser. 1, 3:239.

84. Mellon, *Bullwhip Days*, 97. References to older enslaved women as healers are too numerous to list exhaustively, but see Rawick, supp., ser. 1, 4:421; Egypt, Masuoka, and Johnson, *Unwritten History of Slavery*, 38; Jacobs, *Incidents in the Life of a Slave Girl*, 98.

85. On the health effects of whipping, see Savitt, *Medicine and Slavery*, 111–14; Bankole, *Slavery and Medicine*, 33–43.

86. Rawick, 14:5.

87. Ibid., 15:101.

88. Clifton Johnson, *God Struck Me Dead*, 26. See also Northup, *Twelve Years a Slave*, 288, 368; Albert, *House of Bondage*, 92.

89. Moses Grandy, *Narrative of the Life of Moses Grandy, Late a Slave in the United States of America,* in *Five Slave Narratives,* 23, 32. Grandy also reported that enslaved families shared portions of their "fat meat," intended for cooking, as salve for wounded backs.

90. "Refuge" Plantation Slave List, 1859, Clinch Papers, LC. Another "Old Nurse" on the same plantation also lived in a family of field workers.

91. Sale Broadside, n.d., DeSaussure Papers, SCHS; see also Sale Broadside, 21 Jan. 1859, ibid.

92. Rawick, 2(2):55, 68.

93. Blassingame, "Status and Social Structure in the Slave Community," 142-43.

94. Thorn Island Rule and Direction Book, 11 June 1832, Telfair Family Papers, GHS. Some of the largest plantations, such as the Butler Island plantation described by Frances Kemble, contained several slave settlements that required enslaved women doctors to travel considerable distances even within the plantation boundaries.

95. Rawick, supp., ser. 1, 4:449.

96. F. Roy Johnson, *Fabled Doctor,* 36. See Mellon, *Bullwhip Days,* 96.

97. Hammond, "Plantation Manual," Waring Research Files, WHL. See Deborah Gray White, *Ar'n't I A Woman?,* 116, 124-26, 129.

98. Thorn Island Rule and Direction Book, 11 June 1832, Telfair Family Papers, GHS.

99. "Refuge" Plantation Slave List, 1859, Clinch Papers, LC.

100. Parsons, *Folk-Lore of the Sea Islands,* 197. See also *Drums,* 68, 131.

101. Plantation and Farm Record Inventory and Account Book, vol. a3, 1863, Philip St. George Cocke Papers, VHS.

102. Richard J. Arnold to I. Swanston, 22 May 1837, folder 2, and Richard J. Arnold to Mr. Sanford, [19 May 1840], Correspondence, folder 4, ser. 1.1, Arnold and Screven Family Papers, SHC. Younger women, too, appeared occasionally as health workers in planter records. Nan, a nurse who worked with Daphney on the Arnold plantation, was only thirty-one.

103. Sale Broadsides, 21 Jan. 1859, 13 Mar. 1860, DeSaussure Papers, SCHS.

104. J. T. Cooper to Habersham & Son, 20, 30 June 1848, Manigault Family Papers, SCHS.

105. "Plantation List, Nov. 1836," Horry Estate, Accounts and Voucher Books, Frost Papers, LC.

106. "Inventory of Negroes," 1854, Philip St. George Cocke Papers, VHS. For similar patterns in value estimation, see Slave lists, 10 May 1848 and Feb. 1849, Smithfield Plantation Book, Smith Family Papers, SCHS.

107. Slave List, n.d., "Negroes 1825," Business and Plantation Correspondence, Ford-Ravenel Papers, SCHS.

108. List of Field Hands, 9 Jan. 1845, Negro Records, 1815-60, Jones Family Papers, GHS.

109. "Inventory of Negroes," vol. 1, 1854, and vol. 2, 1861, Belmead Plantation

Book, Philip St. George Cocke Papers, VHS. See also Shaw, "Mothering under Slavery," 243.

110. Thorn Island Rule and Direction Book, 11 June 1832; Thorn Island Rule and Direction Book, 1837; "List of Negroes at Thorn Island," 1836; Stephen Newman to Miss Telfair, 28 Feb. 1837, all in Telfair Family Papers, GHS.

111. Rawick, supp., ser. 1, 4:449.

112. Rosengarten, *Tombee*, 477, 491, 512, 513, 590.

113. Berlin and Morgan, "Slaves' Economy," 1.

114. Vlach, *Back of the Big House*, 33–42; Kemble, *Journal of a Residence*, 57.

115. Abel, *Hearts of Wisdom*, 68–82.

116. Carby, *Reconstructing Womanhood*, 20–39; Deborah Gray White, *Ar'n't I a Woman?*, 28–46.

117. Elsa Barkley Brown, "'What Has Happened Here,'" 298.

118. Cartwright, "Dr. Cartwright on the Caucasians and the Africans," 55.

119. Lyell, *Second Visit to the United States*, 264.

120. Postell, *Health of Slaves on Southern Plantations*, 135; "Pamphlet on the Practical Conduct of a Great Plantation," Misc. Prose, Bennett Papers, SCHS; Waring, *History of Medicine in South Carolina*, 6; Blanton, *Medicine in Virginia in the Eighteenth Century*, 168.

121. Weehaw Plantation Journal, Cheves-Middleton Papers, SCHS.

122. L. F. Ventura to Mr. Manigault, 27 Sept. 1856, Manigault Papers, DUL.

123. Massie, Slave Record Book, 21, LV. According to Massie, Romulus had a twin, Remus, who died at six months of age from thrush and "neglect."

124. Ibid., 21, 35, 33. On "mashing," or smothering, deaths, see Savitt, *Medicine and Slavery*, 122–27; Michael P. Johnson, "Smothered Slave Infants"; Kiple and Kiple, "Slave Child Mortality."

125. Shaw, "Mothering under Slavery," 238, 245.

126. Simons, *Planter's Guide and Family Book of Medicine*, 208.

127. Cartwright, "Dr. Cartwright on the Caucasians and the Africans," 55.

128. Lyell, *Second Visit to the United States*, 264.

129. Julian J. Chisolm, "President's Address upon Retiring from the Chair," 10 Dec. 1867, Chisolm Papers, WHL.

130. Rosengarten, *Tombee*, 542, 154. See also Henderson Diary, 19 Aug. 1855, Steele Papers, SHC.

131. See Carby, *Reconstructing Womanhood*, 22, on the mystifying function of stereotypes.

132. On the images and ideologies surrounding the Mammy mythology, see Deborah Gray White, *Ar'n't I A Woman?*, 46–61; Patricia Hill Collins, *Black Feminist Thought*, 70–78; Patricia Morton, *Disfigured Images*, 153–58.

133. Ewell, *Planter's and Mariner's Medical Companion*, 36; "Instruction to Managers," 1854, Phillip St. George Cocke Papers, VHS; Hammond, "Plantation Manual," Waring Research Files, WHL.

134. McKain, "Strangulation of the Jejunum," 276–79.

135. [David Collins], *Practical Rules,* 137; Tidyman, "Sketch of the most remarkable Diseases of the Negroes," 332.

136. Ibid., 333.

137. Ibid., 207; Moore, "Thesis on Plantation Hygiene," Theses, WHL; Tidyman, "Sketch of the most remarkable Diseases of the Negroes," 329.

138. Simons, *Planter's Guide and Family Book of Medicine,* 208. See also Dr. R. H. Day, *NOMSJ* 4 (1847): 227, quoted in Fisher, "Physicians and Slavery," 44. For similar comments from a West Indian medical manual, see [David Collins], *Practical Rules,* 222.

139. Moore, "Thesis on Plantation Hygiene," Theses, WHL.

140. F[ranklin] Perry Pope, "A Dissertation on the Professional Management of Negro Slaves" (1837), 13, 14, ibid.

141. P. M. Kollock, "Case of Traumatic Tetanus Cured by Strychnine," *SMSJ* 3 (Oct. 1847): 601.

142. On white midwives and doctors, see Leavitt, *Brought to Bed;* Scholten, " 'On the Importance of the Obstetrick Art' "; Wertz and Wertz, *Lying-In;* Ulrich, *Midwife's Tale.*

143. For a similar argument about eighteenth-century slave medicine as a "rival system of authority," see Kathleen M. Brown, *Good Wives, Nasty Wenches, and Anxious Patriarchs,* 354.

CHAPTER 6

1. Trial of Tom and Amy, 20 Jan. 1806, Pittsylvania Co., Governor's Office, William H. Cabell, box 138, Executive Papers, State Records, LV.

2. Doris Y. Wilkinson, foreword to Watson, *Black Folk Medicine,* vii.

3. I am grateful to Todd Savitt for sharing with me his exploration of how slavery specifically shaped the relationship between white physician and enslaved patient. See Savitt, "Medicine in the Old South."

4. Rosenberg, "Therapeutic Revolution," 487; Warner, *Therapeutic Perspective,* 72–80.

5. Joseph LeCont, "On the Science of Medicine," *SMSJ* 6 (Aug. 1850): 459. See also Stowe, "Seeing Themselves at Work."

6. Warner, *Therapeutic Perspective,* 13–17.

7. "Code of Medical Ethics." The code of ethics was printed in the *SMSJ* following a Georgia physician's report from the 1846 and 1847 proceedings of the National Medical Convention. During the 1847 proceedings the National Medical Convention changed its name to its current title, the American Medical Association.

8. Warner, *Therapeutic Perspective,* 51–54.

9. On honor and deference, see Wyatt-Brown, *Southern Honor;* Greenberg, *Honor*

and Slavery. On the slave-master relationship as model for other social relations, see Ira Berlin, *Many Thousands Gone*, 8. For discussions of how relations between household masters and dependents were replicated in southern social relations and social institutions, see McCurry, *Masters of Small Worlds;* Edwards, *Gendered Strife and Confusion*, 6–7, 25–31.

10. Savitt, "Medicine in the Old South," 6–7.

11. Pernick, "Patient's Role in Medical Decisionmaking," 4–21.

12. "Code of Medical Ethics."

13. Pernick, "Patient's Role in Medical Decisionmaking," 18–21.

14. Charles Bell Gibson, "Notes of Surgical Cases," *VMJ* 13 (1859): 17 (emphasis mine). See also A. J. Wedderburn, "Remarks on Strangulated Umbilical Hernia, with a Case," *NOMSJ* 3 (Jan. 1847): 478.

15. Frank Cunningham, "Surgical Cases at the Medical College of Virginia," *VMJ* 9 (1857): 21. Also reflecting a dual notion of consent is T. L. Ogier, "Ligature of the Femoral Artery for the Cure of Elephantiasis of the Leg and Foot," *CMJR* 15 (1860): 191.

16. Harriss, "What Constitutes Unsoundness?," 293.

17. B. F. Davis, "Chloroform: Its Effects in a Case of Castration," *CMJR* 7 (1852): 171–73. For a case history of amputation in an enslaved man in which consent was sought only from a slaveowner, see W. W. Anderson, "A Case of Tetanus Relieved by Amputation," *CMJR* 13 (1858): 43–44.

18. "Surgery in New Orleans," *NOMSJ* 2 (July 1845): 113. Since the woman endured this operation in a New Orleans public hospital, she may have been an impoverished free woman. Free black patients may have been even more vulnerable to coercive medical treatments, since physicians did not have to concern themselves with interested slaveowners.

19. Southern archival holdings contain numerous account books detailing visits made by white doctors to enslaved patients. See, for example, Thomas Medical Account Book, Nesbitt Account Book, Pugh Account Book, and Boyd Account Book, all in SCL; Ravenel Medical Daybook, SCHS; Mettauer Papers and Southall Account Book, VHS. Physicians' account books provide evidence of treatment and cost but rarely detail interactions between doctor and patient.

20. On African Americans' distrust of white medicines and healers, see Savitt, *Medicine and Slavery*, 149; Levine, *Black Culture and Black Consciousness*, 63–65; Genovese, *Roll, Jordan, Roll*, 225–26; Owens, *This Species of Property*, 34.

21. Henry to Sarah Tyler, 27 Apr. 1849, Quitman Papers, SHC, quoted in Owens, *This Species of Property*, 31.

22. Richard Arnold to Sol Cohen, Esq., Care of Dr. Hays, Phila., 29 Sept. 1854, in Shryock, *Letters of Richard D. Arnold*, 70–71. Arnold viewed the warning as "impertinence" and believed that the women mistook his medicines for a popular patent remedy sold on the Savannah streets at the time.

23. Henry Ravenal, *Yale Review* 25 (1936): 767, quoted in Levine, *Black Culture*

and Black Consciousness, 64. See also Catterall, *Judicial Cases Concerning American Slavery,* 3:204.

24. *Slave Narratives,* 17.

25. Rosengarten, *Tombee,* 187.

26. Botkin, *Lay My Burden Down,* 103.

27. Bibb, *Narrative of the Life and Adventures of Henry Bibb,* 122.

28. Archaeologist Laurie A. Wilkie, working from postemancipation-era artifacts, argues that African American assemblages of medicinal artifacts did not reflect the emphasis on purgatives found in Anglo-American assemblages. See Wilkie, "Transforming African American Ethnomedical Traditions," 468.

29. Pennington, *Fugitive Blacksmith,* 213. A West Indian planter manual explicitly linked care of the sick with physical coercion when it recommended that planters place a pair of stocks in the men's and women's rooms of plantation sickhouses. See [David Collins], *Practical Rules,* 217-29.

30. *Weevils,* 115. Eighteenth-century planters also employed medicines as punishment. See Kathleen M. Brown, *Good Wives, Nasty Wenches, and Anxious Patriarchs,* 353.

31. Robert Smalls interview, 1863, American Freedmen's Inquiry Commission, reprinted in Blassingame, *Slave Testimony,* 379.

32. Roper, *Narrative of the Adventures and Escape,* 51.

33. Massie Commonplace Book, Massie Family Papers, VHS. Margaret Walker's novel *Jubilee,* based on extensive historical research and Walker's own family history, features a mistress who used ipecac on the slave woman assigned to assist with the annual canning and jelly making. After each dose the woman became ill, and the mistress inspected her vomit to make sure she was not eating while she worked. See Walker, *Jubilee,* 108-9.

34. Toler to Ferguson, 27 Dec. 1850, Ferguson Papers, North Carolina Department of Archives, quoted in Tadman, *Speculators and Slaves,* 185.

35. *Southside Democrat,* 21 July, 9 Aug. 1855, quoted in Lebsock, *Free Women of Petersburg,* 93. The story of Patience and the threat of "Hickory oil" is another such example. See Chapter 2.

36. Rawick, 14:108.

37. John Brown, *Slave Life in Georgia,* 158.

38. William G. Smith, "Case of Caesarean Operation," *VMJ* 7 (1856): 203-8; Savitt, "Use of Blacks for Medical Experimentation"; Fisher, "Physicians and Slavery," 45-49.

39. Savitt, "Use of Blacks for Medical Experimentation," 347; Savitt, *Medicine and Slavery,* 118; McGregor, *From Midwives to Medicine,* 42.

40. Vesico-vaginal fistula was the name physicians gave to perforations in the wall of the vagina that developed after difficult childbirth. The condition caused leakage of urine or feces into the vagina. See Sims, *Story of My Life,* 236-46. See also Sims, "On

the Treatment of Vesico-Vaginal Fistula"; McGregor, *From Midwives to Medicine,* 33–68; Savitt, "Use of Blacks for Experimentation," 344–46.

41. McGregor, *From Midwives to Medicine,* 50–51; Axelsen, "Women as Victims of Medical Experimentation"; Sims, *Story of My Life,* 237, 238; Savitt, "Use of Blacks for Experimentation," 345–46. On differential theories of pain espoused by antebellum physicians and white middle-class Americans, see Pernick, *Calculus of Suffering,* 148–67.

42. James Harvey Young, "Crawford W. Long," in *Encyclopedia of Southern Culture,* ed. Charles Reagan Wilson and William Ferris (Chapel Hill: University of North Carolina Press, 1989), 1373.

43. John Brown, *Slave Life in Georgia,* 40–46. For a somewhat apologetic discussion of the experimentation of Hamilton and Sims, see Boney, "Slaves as Guinea Pigs."

44. Savitt, "Use of Blacks for Medical Experimentation," 332. Evidence of these experiments in Alabama and Georgia supports Todd Savitt's suggestion that aggressive experimentation on and medical display of slaves was probably even more pronounced in the lower South states than in Virginia. See Savitt, *Medicine and Slavery,* 307.

45. Savitt, *Medicine and Slavery,* 281–307.

46. Savitt, "Use of Blacks for Medical Experimentation," 336–39; Savitt, *Medicine and Slavery,* 307. See also Shultz, *Body Snatching;* Breeden, "Body Snatchers and Anatomy Professors"; Blakely and Harrington, *Bones in the Basement.*

47. "Negro Hospital," *CMJR* 15 (1860): 850.

48. "Dr. T. Stillman's Medical Infirmary for Diseases of the Skin," *Charleston Mercury,* 12 Oct. 1838, quoted in Norrece T. Jones Jr., *Born a Child of Freedom,* 201.

49. Savitt, *Medicine and Slavery,* 245. African Americans' dread of urban medical schools clearly carried into the postemancipation years. An 1872 letter from a white physician to the board of trustees of the Georgia Infirmary, a white-run hospital for indigent African Americans, warned of a severe reaction from African Americans if the Savannah Medical College were to build a dissection building on the grounds of the infirmary. See Dr. Myers to John Stoddard, 18 Nov. 1872, Georgia Infirmary Minute Book, vol. 1, GHS.

50. Lewis, *Odd Leaves from the Life of a Louisiana Swamp Doctor,* 131–37.

51. 27 Nov. 1858, Barnes Account Book, 9, SCL.

52. J. T. Craig to Lizzie Craig, 9 Jan., 17 Apr. 1854, Craig Papers, SCL.

53. Warner, *Therapeutic Perspective,* 185–87.

54. Harris, "Report on the Treatment of Some Cases of Cholera," 581–85. For another description of a postmortem on a five-year-old slave girl on a plantation near Camden, South Carolina, see McKain, "Strangulation of the Jejunum," 276–79.

55. Paul F. Eve, "An Essay Read before the Medical Society of Augusta, Jan. 10th, 1839," *SMSJ* 3 (Mar. 1839): 329.

56. Myddelton Michel, "On the Dependence of Menstruation upon the Development and Expulsion of Ova," *CMJR* (1848): 21–27. For another dissection of an enslaved woman, see William Blanding Diary, 24 July 1807, Blanding Papers, SCL.

57. Charles Witsell, "Case of Enormous Polypus of the Uterus Treated with the Muriated Tincture of Iron," *CMJR* 15 (1860): 326–28.

58. Creel, *"Peculiar People,"* 311–13. Cutting open the dead was not entirely unknown in some African societies. According to Creel, Mende practitioners performed a postmortem investigation in which the spleen of the deceased was removed in order to test for evidence of witchcraft. On Anglo-American Christian attitudes, see Robert L. Blakely and Judith M. Harrington, "Grave Consequences: The Opportunistic Procurement of Cadavers at the Medical College of Georgia," in Blakely and Harrington, *Bones in the Basement,* 165, 168.

59. Roediger, "And Die in Dixie," 167.

60. E. D. Fenner, "Dirt-Eating among Negroes," *Southern Medical Reports* 1 (1849): 194, quoted in Haller, "Negro and the Southern Physician," 242.

61. Love, *One Blood,* 44, 62–69.

62. Fry, *Night Riders in Black Folk History,* 170–211. Laura Steward interview, in Rawick, supp., ser. 1, 4:593. Cornelius Garner told of a near-escape from "a passel o' young Baltimore Doctors" whom he described as "Klu Klux"; see *Weevils,* 104. Although both Gladys-Marie Fry and Spencie Love document suspicion of white medical science in African American oral tradition, Fry tends to emphasize white social control and manipulation of African American supernaturalism, while Love emphasizes the underlying experiential truths of white medical abuse in African American legends.

63. Annie L. Burton, *Memories of Childhood's Slavery Days,* in Gates, *Six Women's Slave Narratives,* 5–6. See also Rawick, supp., ser. 1, 11:175.

64. Stewart Culin, "Concerning Negro Sorcery in the United States," *JAF* 3 (Oct.–Dec. 1890): 285.

65. *Norfolk Herald,* 18 Nov. 1831, in Greenberg, *Confessions of Nat Turner,* 19. For an analysis of Turner's dissection as a denial of Turner's capacity for honor, see Greenberg, *Honor and Slavery,* 98–107.

66. Greenberg, *Confessions of Nat Turner,* 19; Drewry, *Southampton Insurrection,* 102; F. Roy Johnson, *Nat Turner Story,* 210. Both Johnson and Drewry cite local sources for the claims about the disposition of Turner's body, but they do not cite any specific source in making these allegations.

67. Piersen, "White Cannibals, Black Martyrs," 147–59.

68. Equiano, *Life of Olaudah Equiano,* 22; John Thornton, *Africa and Africans in the Making of the Atlantic World,* 161; Miller, *Way of Death,* 266, 389.

69. William Piersen argues that the persistence of the "white cannibal" myths among Africans rested ultimately on their truth as a "mythopoeic analogy" of "chattel slavery as a kind of economic cannibalism" (Piersen, *Black Legacy,* 12).

70. See Chapter 3.

71. "Voudouism in Virginia," n.d., clipping in George William Bagby Scrapbook, 1866–76, George William Bagby Papers, VHS, 110.

72. 30 Apr. 1846, Plantation Journal, Walker Papers, SHC.

73. Deborah Gray White, *Ar'n't I A Woman,* 79; Fox-Genovese, *Within the Plantation Household,* 306–7, 315–16; Bush, *Slave Women in Caribbean Society,* 75–76.

74. Schwarz, *Twice Condemned,* 94–113; Phillips, *American Negro Slavery,* 458. South Carolina State Archive Records also contain numerous poisoning cases indexed under slave crime. See, for example, William Cain Petition, 1829, Reports and Petitions, South Carolina Department of Archives, Columbia.

75. *Weevils,* 318.

76. Rawick, 15:148.

77. "Petition in Regard to a Slave." See also Wyatt-Brown, *Southern Honor,* 423–24. Africans in the French Louisiana colonies also held reputations as knowledgeable poisoners. See Gwendolyn Midlo Hall, *Africans in Colonial Louisiana,* 162–65.

78. Leroy Beuford Petition, 1800, #173 and #174, Reports and Petitions, South Carolina Department of Archives, Columbia.

79. S. A. Townes to Geo. Franklin Townes, 10 Dec. 1835, folder 13, box 1, Townes Family Papers, SCL.

80. Recipe Book, William Gibbons Jr., Telfair Family Papers, GHS; 28 July 1826, Plantation Journal, Walker Papers, SHC.

81. The use of reptile parts is explained in the Marrinda Jane Singleton interview, in *Weevils,* 267. Brimstone was used in conjuring mixtures to remove a conjure spell, to break up a home, to drive a person insane, to prevent disease, and to predict a whipping. Bluestone (copper sulfate) was also a popular material used in conjuration to ensure safety and protection, to "make a fight" and produce harm, to detect a conjurer, to win a lover's affection, to mix with black haw roots as a contraceptive, or to cure venereal disease and scrofula. On the potential uses of bluestone and brimstone in conjuration, see Puckett, *Folk Beliefs of the Southern Negro,* 230, 235, 237, 240, 246, 269, 274, 280, 293, 297, 326, 331, 385, 384; Hurston, "Hoodoo in America," 367, 380, 388. It is likely, however, that these ingredients had already been assembled for a specific purpose and were not merely being stored for future use.

82. The root of the poke or pokeweed plant itself is poisonous, although it was commonly used in folk medicine for poultices. See Chapter 3.

83. Trial of Delphy, 10 June 1816, Louisa Co., Governor's Office, Wilson Cary Nicholas, box 232, Executive Papers, State Records, LV.

84. For a discussion of the "natural connection" between poisoning and insurrection, see Schwarz, *Twice Condemned,* 112.

85. Letters and petitions regarding the case of George, 2 July 1791, *Calendar of Virginia State Papers,* 5:334–38.

86. Confessions made before John Floyd and Henry Edmundson, 2 Apr. 1812, Montgomery Co., Governor's Office, James Barbour, box 185, Executive Papers, State Records, LV.

87. Corporation of Charleston, *An Account of the Late Intended Insurrection,* 23–24, 38. The authors of this contemporary report assumed Pritchard's native country was Angola. Douglas Egerton's recent study of Denmark Vesey presents strong evidence that Pritchard had been put onto a slaving vessel in an East African port near the island of Zanzibar. The planter who purchased him described Pritchard as an East African "priest" who boarded the ship with a bag of "conjuring implements." See Egerton, *He Shall Go Out Free,* 118.

88. *Macon v. State,* 4 Humphney 421, Apr. 1844, in Catterall, *Judicial Cases Concerning American Slavery,* 2:520–21, 423.

89. "An Act Directing the Trial of Slaves Committing Capital Crimes," 1748, chap. 38, in Hening, *Statutes at Large,* 104–5. See also Savitt, *Medicine and Slavery,* 175.

90. Fox-Genovese, *Within the Plantation Household,* 306. See also Frey and Wood, *Come Shouting to Zion,* 62 n. 135; Philip D. Morgan, *Slave Counterpoint,* 612–19.

91. "An Act to Prohibit the Employment of Slaves and Free Persons of Colour from Compounding or Dispensing of Medicines," 1835, *Acts of the General Assembly of the State of Georgia* (Milledgeville, 1836), and "Penal Code," 1860, *Acts of the General Assembly of the State of Georgia,* Nov./Dec. 1860, both in *Slav. Stat.*

92. Schwarz, *Twice Condemned,* 102, also discusses the efforts of slaveholders to use the medicine laws to benefit from the work of enslaved healers while keeping their activities under control.

93. "An Act Directing the Trial of Slaves Committing Capital Crimes," 1748, chap. 38, in Hening, *Statutes at Large,* 105.

94. "An Act to Prevent the Sale of Poisonous Drugs to Free Negroes and Slaves," 1856, chap. 51, *Acts of the General Assembly of Virginia,* session 1855–56 (Richmond, 1856), in *Slav. Stat.;* "Of Dealing with Slaves and Suffering Them to Go at Large," 1860, chap. 104, in *Code of Virginia,* 2d ed., 512.

95. Guild, *Black Laws of Virginia,* 1792, chap. 41; "An Act Reducing into One, the Several Acts Concerning Slaves, Free Negroes and Mulattoes," 1819, chap. 3, *Revised Code of the Laws of Virginia,* 427; "Offences by Negroes," 1849, chap. 200, *Code of Virginia,* 754; "Of Dealing with Slaves and Suffering Them to Go at Large," 1860, chap. 104, *Code of Virginia,* 2d ed., 512.

96. Genovese, *Roll, Jordan, Roll,* 32.

97. Schwarz, *Twice Condemned,* 113.

98. Trial of Roger, 4 Nov. 1754, King George Co., County Court Order Book, 1751–65 (microfilm reel 24), 373; Trial of Isaac and Quash, 29 May 1759, Cumberland Co., County Court Order Book, 1758–62 (microfilm reel 23), 56–57; Trial of Mill, 20 Aug. 1771, Loudoun Co., County Court Order Book, 1770–73 (microfilm reel 71), 211, all in State Records, LV. These cases, with many others involving poisoning and medicine, are also discussed in Schwarz, *Twice Condemned,* 99, 105.

99. "An Act Prescribing the Punishment of Slaves, Free Negroes and Mulattoes

for Poisoning or Attempting to Poison and for Selling Medicines," 1843, chap. 87, *Acts of the General Assembly of Virginia,* session 1842–43 (Richmond, 1843), in *Slav. Stat.* For a general discussion of the role of law in southern slavery and planter-class hegemony, see Genovese, *Roll, Jordan, Roll,* 25–49.

100. Watson, *Black Folk Medicine,* 1–15.

CHAPTER 7

1. Nathaniel Hooe to William Harrison, 16 Apr. 1834, Correspondence between Hooe and William A. Harrison, UVL.

2. The importance of "character" as a pervasive theme in slaveholders' assessments of enslaved African Americans as workers and as property is fully analyzed in Gross, "'Pandora's Box.'"

3. Owens, *This Species of Property,* 37.

4. Cartwright, "Diseases and Peculiarities of the Negro Race," 331–34.

5. Stowe, "Obstetrics and the Work of Doctoring," 562.

6. On the representation and social construction of disease, see Fee and Fox, *AIDS;* Gilman, *Disease and Representation;* Rosenberg, *Explaining Epidemics,* 310–14.

7. Articles featuring advice on plantation management appeared frequently, for example, in *De Bow's Review of the Southern and Western States* (particularly from the early 1850s on) and in the *Southern Cultivator* (beginning in the mid-1840s). See also Breeden, *Advice among Masters;* McKee, "Ideals and Realities," 199–204.

8. Nathaniel Hooe to William Harrison, 14 Mar. 1834, Correspondence between Hooe and William A. Harrison, UVL.

9. Louis Manigault to Charles Manigault, 8 Jan. 1854, Manigault Papers, DUL.

10. Holmes, "Typhoid Fever," 60. For a similar argument that slaves, like children, required regulation in their food, clothing, exercise, and sleep, see Cartwright, "Disease and Peculiarities of the Negro Race," 67.

11. J. T. Cooper to R. Habersham & Son, 30 June 1848, Manigault Family Papers, SCHS.

12. McKee, "Ideals and Realities," 203–7; Singleton, "Archaeology of Slave Life," 165–67; Singleton, "Archaeology of Slavery in North America," 124.

13. James R. Sparkman to Benjamin Allston, 10 Mar. 1858, quoted in Easterby, *South Carolina Rice Plantation,* 348–49. The concept of "medical police" emerged in Germany during the late seventeenth and early eighteenth centuries. It referred to oversight of a nation's health and welfare so as to promote the wealth and power of the state. See Rosen, *From Medical Police to Social Medicine,* 120–41, 142–58.

14. Simons, *Planter's Guide and Family Book of Medicine,* 210.

15. Rosengarten, *Tombee,* 495.

16. 4 Apr. 1851, Massie, Slave Record Book, 20, LV; see also 34.

17. Harris, "Cases in Obstetric Practice," 773. See also William M. Post, "Report of a Case of Placenta Proevia," *CMJR* 10 (1855): 463-66.

18. L. G. Cabell to Bowker Preston, 8 Oct. 1834, Preston Papers, UVL.

19. Cartwright, "Remarks on Dysentery among Negroes," 162.

20. Louis Manigault to Charles Manigault, 22 Nov. 1852, Manigault Papers, DUL.

21. J. T. Cooper to R. Habersham & Son, 30 June 1848, Manigault Family Papers, SCHS.

22. Louis Manigault to Charles Manigault, 24 Dec. 1854, Manigault Papers, DUL.

23. Gavin Diary, 19 Mar. 1861, SHC.

24. Roswell King Jr. to Pierce Butler, 7 Oct. 1821, Butler Papers, HSP.

25. L. G. Cabell to Bowker Preston, 8 Oct. 1834, Preston Papers, UVL.

26. J. C. Nott, "Description of the Double Inclined Plane," *SMSJ* 3 (May 1839): 462-70. Nott complained that the man insisted on removing his dressing when confined in an apparatus designed to heal the broken leg.

27. *SMSJ* 3 (1847): 205; *SMSJ* 4 (Jan. 1848): 27; L. A. Dugas, "Extirpation of a Cervical Tumor," *SMSJ* 9 (Jan. 1853): 42-45. For a discussion of the derogatory tone with which white physicians discussed their African American patients in medical journals, see Savitt, *Medicine and Slavery,* 302-5.

28. William A. Patteson, "On the Operation of Hysterotomy," *VMJ* 6 (1856): 1-6. A pessary was a rubber or glass device worn in the vagina to support the uterus. See Brodie, *Contraception and Abortion in Nineteenth-Century America,* 218, 221-23.

29. Pendleton, "On the Comparative Fecundity of the Caucasian and African Races," 351, 356; John H. Morgan, "Essay on the Causes of the Production of Abortion among Our Negro Population," 117. Historians' discussions of abortifacient use among enslaved women rest heavily on these two antebellum medical journal articles. On abortion among enslaved women, see Deborah Gray White, *Ar'n't I a Woman?,* 84-86; Gutman, *Black Family in Slavery and Freedom,* 80-82; Ross, "African-American Women and Abortion"; Hine and Wittenstein, "Female Slave Resistance," 292-93.

30. Charles C. Jones, *Negro Myths from the Georgia Coast,* 27-31; for additional examples of the trickster feigning illness, see 94-96, 102-7. See also Christensen, *Afro-American Folk Lore,* 27-28, 43-44, 81.

31. Charles C. Jones, *Negro Myths from the Georgia Coast,* 49.

32. Christensen, *Afro-American Folk Lore,* 77-78.

33. Charles C. Jones, *Negro Myths from the Georgia Coast,* 19-20.

34. Pretended illness also proved useful in other dangerous situations, such as escape from slavery, when black men and women used popular fears of contagious diseases to decrease their contact with suspicious white strangers. See Pennington, *Fugitive Blacksmith,* 223-24; William Craft and Ellen Craft, *Running a Thousand Miles for Freedom, or The Escape of William and Ellen Craft from Slavery,* in Bontemps, *Great Slave Narratives,* 295.

35. See, for example, Natalie Delage Sumter's anger toward a driver who worked field laborers in the "Heat of the day" (Sumter Diary, 1 July 1840, SCL). On field labor and pregnancies, see Campbell, "Work, Pregnancy, and Infant Mortality"; Savitt, *Medicine and Slavery*, 83–110.

36. Friend Diary, 24 Sept. 1849, Friend Family Papers, VHS.

37. Rosengarten, *Tombee*, 488.

38. Ibid., 530, 488.

39. Ibid., 497.

40. Deborah Gray White, *Ar'n't I a Woman?*, 79–82. See also Hine and Wittenstein, "Female Slave Resistance," 289–300; Angela Davis, "Reflections on the Black Woman's Role," 95; Stampp, *Peculiar Institution*, 104. For a comparison with slave women feigning sickness and pregnancy in the Caribbean, see Bush, *Slave Women in Caribbean Society*, 61–62. Bush suggests that the smaller emphasis on the "natural increase" of slave populations among Caribbean slaveholders meant that enslaved women there had less success with feigned pregnancy as a mode of resisting work.

41. Rawick, 15:57.

42. Kemble, *Journal of a Residence*, 277.

43. Mellon, *Bullwhip Days*, 97. See also Rosengarten, *Tombee*, 497, 666; James L. Smith, *Autobiography*, 21–24.

44. Bibb, *Narrative of the Life and Adventures of Henry Bibb*, 122.

45. Botkin, *Lay My Burden Down*, 83. See also Eliza Smith interview, letter to *American Missionary*, n.s. 7 (Sept. 1863): 209–10, reprinted in Blassingame, *Slave Testimony*, 364.

46. 11 Feb. 1859, Massie, Slave Record Book, 3, LV.

47. Nathaniel Hooe to William Harrison, 16 Apr. 1834, Correspondence between Hooe and William A. Harrison, UVL.

48. Kemble, *Journal of a Residence*, 277.

49. Rawick, 15:57.

50. Levine argues that moralistic tales within African American folklore provided realistic warnings of the dangers of pride and forgetting one's place in a white supremacist context; see Levine, *Black Culture and Black Consciousness*, 97.

51. Dance, *Shuckin' and Jivin'*, 186–87.

52. Moton, "Folklore and Ethnology," 75.

53. Parsons, *Folk-Lore of the Sea Islands*, 62. Another version of this story, in which the enslaved man upon discovery ran away and was never seen again, is collected in "The Cripple Slave," box A676, folder: South Carolina, Negro Lore, Stories, WPA Folklore Project, LC.

54. Merrill, "Essay on Some of the Distinctive Peculiarities of the Negro Race," 30.

55. Brevard Diary, 19 Oct., 10 Nov. 1860, 26 Jan. 1861, SCL.

56. Nathaniel Hooe to William Harrison, 8 June 1835, Correspondence between Hooe and William A. Harrison, UVL.

57. Harriott Pinckney to W. Winningham, 4 Feb. 1855, Pinckney Papers, SCL.

58. Socrates Maupin to Addison Maupin, 31 May 1849, Maupin Papers, UVL (emphasis added).

59. Alex. Yuille to John Peter Mettauer, 9 Aug. 1839, Mettauer Papers, VHS. See also Roswell King to Pierce Butler, 5 June 1814, Butler Papers, HSP.

60. Susan Hubard to Robert Hubard, 8 Mar. 1843, Hubard-Randolph Family Papers, UVL.

61. Ewell, *Planter's and Mariner's Medical Companion,* 154; See also Cooper, *Treatise of Domestic Medicine,* 1–23. For a brief and selective history of the development of hypochondria as a disease in the United States and Britain, see Baur, *Hypochondria,* 21–30. According to Baur some eighteenth-century British physicians believed that hypochondria was spreading out of the leisured classes and beginning to affect the working class as well.

62. An exception appears in the advertisement by Dr. T. Stillman quoted in Chapter 6. One of the conditions recruited among "sick negroes" was "confirmed hypochondriasm."

63. Gavin Diary, 2 Feb. 1859, SHC.

64. Rosengarten, *Tombee,* 10 June 1850, 500.

65. Charles Cotesworth Pinckney, 1929 address to the Agricultural Society of South Carolina, quoted in Creel, *"Peculiar People,"* 170.

66. A. R. Bagshaw to Charles Manigault, 14 Aug. 1844, Manigault Papers, DUL.

67. 9 June 1861, Greenwood Plantation Journal, LC (emphasis in original).

68. Deborah Gray White, *Ar'n't I A Woman?,* 82–83, discusses the historian's dilemma in sorting out feigned illness from enslaved women's impaired health.

69. Kemble, *Journal of a Residence,* 136.

70. 24 Mar. 1838, Butler Island, Plantation Hospital Book, Louisiana State Museum, New Orleans.

71. Rosengarten, *Tombee,* 558.

72. Ibid., 521.

73. Ibid., 598.

74. Louis Manigault to Charles Manigault, 25, 27 Feb. 1854, Manigault Papers, DUL; Haller Nutt, 8 Nov. 1843, Araby Plantation Journal, Nutt Papers, DUL; F. Nasworthy to George Noble Jones, 1 Nov. 1854, Jones Papers, DUL.

75. Roswell King Jr. to Thomas Butler, 24 Jan. 1830, Butler Papers, HSP.

76. Louis Manigault to Charles Manigault, 17, 19, 23 Apr. 1853, Manigault Papers, DUL.

77. Nathaniel H. Hooe to William Harrison, 16 Apr. 1834, Correspondence between Hooe and William A. Harrison, UVL.

78. Rosengarten, *Tombee,* 497; see 501, 627.

79. Rawick, 14:312–13.

80. S. A. Townes to George F. Townes, 22 June 1834, and J. A. Townes to Rachael Townes, 26 Apr. 1834, Townes Family Papers, SCL.

81. See, for example, Dr. I. I. I[nney] to Richard E. Byrd, 10 Apr. 1852, Meade-Funsten Papers, UVL.

82. W. H. Taylor, "Case of Catalepsy," *VMJ* 7 (1856): 51 (emphasis added).

83. McLoud, "Hints on the Medical Treatment of Negroes," 3, Theses, WHL.

84. Ibid., 4.

85. Ibid., 13–14.

86. "Address of Samuel A. Cartwright," 732–33.

87. McLoud, "Hints on the Medical Treatment of Negroes," 6, 9, Theses, WHL. For a West Indian comparison, see also [David Collins], *Practical Rules,* 227, 229.

88. The patient-centered style of observation popular in the early nineteenth century had changed by the late nineteenth century to a system of normative measurements based on the notion of a universalized "healthy" subject. See Warner, *Therapeutic Perspective,* 263–64; Stowe, "Seeing Themselves at Work."

89. McLoud, "Hints on the Medical Treatment of Negroes," 4–5, Theses, WHL.

90. Ibid., 10–11. McLoud believed an unpleasant remedy would be especially effective in cases where, he charged, slaves complained of illness in order to receive the common remedy of whiskey or camphorated spirits.

91. Thomas W. Hollaway to Joel Berly, 12 May 1859, Berly Family Papers, SCL. The woman had been seeking to avoid the "cloddy bottoms," where the labor was more difficult.

92. McLoud, "Hints on the Medical Treatment of Negroes," 9–12, Theses, WHL.

93. Holmes, "Typhoid Fever," 62.

94. "Address of Samuel A. Cartwright," 732–33.

CONCLUSION

1. Lorde, *Burst of Light,* 120, 116.

2. Angela Davis, *Women, Culture, and Politics,* 54.

3. The issue of medical authority has for several decades been an important focus of feminist historical scholarship. From the medicalization of childbirth to the relationships between Victorian women and their doctors, feminist historians have charted the junctures between social power and the changing practice and theory of medicine. For the most part, historians have focused on the two important areas of medical authority that nineteenth-century middle-class Americans recognized: the domestic authority of white laywomen and the professional authority of white male doctors. The distinctive notion of sacred authority in African American doctoring suggests the importance of religion as a foundation for alternative concepts of healing authority arising in working-class and subordinate groups. Important works on gender, authority, and medicine in the antebellum United States include Leavitt, *Brought to Bed;* Smith-Rosenberg, *Disorderly Conduct,* 197–244; Morantz-Sanchez, *Sympathy and Science.*

4. Mary Ross interview, 1941, box 2, folder 6, items 371, 373, WPA Folklore Collections, UVL.

5. Egypt, Masuoka, and Johnson, *Unwritten History of Slavery*, 180.

6. *Weevils*, 131.

7. Rawick, 14:61.

8. Logan, *Motherwit*, 89–90.

9. Faulkner, *Days When the Animals Talked*, 34.

10. Julian J. Chisolm, "President's Address upon Retiring from the Chair," 10 Dec. 1867, typescript, Chisolm Papers, WHL, 2.

11. *Index and Appeal*, 24 Apr. 1875, newspaper clipping in Speeches Delivered by George William Bagby, "The Old Virginia Negro," George William Bagby Papers, VHS.

12. Blanton, *Medicine in Virginia in the Eighteenth Century*, 171.

13. Julian J. Chisolm, "President's Address upon Retiring from the Chair," 10 Dec. 1867, typescript, Chisolm Papers, WHL, 4.

14. George William Bagby, "The Old Virginia Negro," George William Bagby Papers, VHS.

15. S. W. Douglas, "Difficulties and Superstitions Encountered in Practice among Negroes," manuscript, Waring files, WHL; also published in *Southern Medical Journal* 19 (1926): 736–38.

16. Raboteau, *Fire in the Bones*, 190–91. For a related argument about a secular "relationist paradigm" held by twentieth-century African American public health leaders, see David McBride, *From TB to AIDS: Epidemics among Urban Blacks since 1900* (Albany: State University of New York Press, 1991), 126, 139–40, 145.

Bibliography

UNPUBLISHED SOURCES

Duke University Library, Special Collections Department, Durham,
      North Carolina
   Archibald Boyd Papers
   Iveson Brookes Papers
   George Noble Jones Papers
   Louis Manigault Papers
   Haller Nutt Papers
      Journal of Araby Plantation
   Rockingham Plantation Journal
Georgia Historical Society, Savannah
   Georgia Infirmary Minute Books
   Jones Family Papers
   Savannah Historical Research Association Papers
   Telfair Family Papers
Historical Society of Pennsylvania, Philadelphia
   Butler Papers
Library of Congress, Washington, D.C.
   Manuscripts Division
      John Chesnutt Letterbook
      Duncan Clinch Papers
      Edward Frost Papers
      Greenwood Plantation Journal, 1858–64
      Joseph Merideth Toner Papers
         Noah Castle, "An Inaugural Dissertation on Cholera Infantum," thesis,
            Washington University of Baltimore, 1845, Dissertations
      U.S. Works Projects Administration (WPA) Folklore Project
         Traditional Folklore, Virginia, North Carolina, South Carolina, Georgia
   Archive of Folk Culture
      Recordings of Slave Narratives and Related Material
         John Henry Falk interview with Mrs. Laura Smalley, 1941, tape 3A,
            reference no. AFS 5096, A&B — 5498B2

Library of Virginia, Archives Research Service, Richmond
   William Massie, Slave Record Book, 1836–65, Nelson County, Personal Papers
      Collection, #20610
   Roslin Plantation Records, 1809–32
      William McKean, Letter Book, 1809–18, #23873
   State Records
      County Court Order Books
      Executive Papers, Letters Received (RG3)
      General Assembly (RG78)
Louisiana State Museum, Archives, New Orleans
   Butler Island, Plantation Hospital Book
South Carolina Department of Archives, Columbia
   Medical Committee Reports, S.C. General Assembly
   Reports and Petitions, selected documents
South Carolina Historical Society, Charleston
   T. P. Allen, Aetna Life Insurance Company Policy
   John Bennett Papers
   Cheves-Middleton Papers, Henry A. Middleton Jr.
      Weehaw Plantation Journal, 1855–61
   Louis D. De Saussure Papers
   Ford-Ravenel Papers
      Business and Plantation Correspondence
      Edmund Ravenel Plantation Papers
   Manigault Family Papers
   Henry Ravenel Medical Daybook
   Smith Family Papers
      Smithfield Plantation Book, 1851–61
   Wragg Family Papers
South Caroliniana Library, University of South Carolina, Columbia
   C. V. Barnes Account Book, vol. 1, and Prescription Book, vol. 2
   Berly Family Papers
   William Blanding Papers
   Bookman Family Remedy Book
   W. B. Boyd Account Book, 1858
   Keziah Goodwyn Hopkins Brevard Diary
   Cheves Family Papers
   N. C. Craig Papers
   Alexander McLeod Notebook, 1845–64 (photocopy)
   Robert Nesbitt Account Book
   Harriott Pinckney Papers
   E. J. Pugh Account Book
   Natalie Delage Sumter Diary (typescript)

John Peyre Thomas Medical Account Book, 1842–47

Townes Family Papers

John D. Warren Papers

Southern Historical Collection, University of North Carolina, Chapel Hill

Arnold and Screven Family Papers, #3419

Mary Jeffries Bethell Diary, #1737 (typescript)

Todd Robinson Caldwell Papers, #128

Confederate Papers, #172

Federal Writers' Project, Microfiche Collection

David Gavin Diary, vol. 1, #1103 (typescript)

Interview with Janie Cameron Riley and Moselle Cameron, 6 June 1975, transcript of interview B-63, Southern Oral History Program, #4007

Lenoir Family Papers, #426

Remedy Book

Elizabeth S. Martin Papers, #1023

Riddick Family Papers, #633

John Steele Papers #327

Mary Henderson Diary

John Walker Papers, #2300

Plantation Journal, 1824–1832 (typescript)

Earl Gregg Swem Library, William and Mary Special Collections, College of William and Mary, Williamsburg, Virginia

Jerdone Family Papers

University of Virginia Library, Albert H. Small Special Collections Library, Charlottesville

Letters of William Taylor Barry, #2569

Papers of Henry James Brown, #9930

Correspondence between Hooe and William A. Harrison, #10548

Hubard-Randolph Family Papers, #4717a–b

Farm Notebook of Fountain Humphreys, #1623

Papers of Socrates Maupin, #2769 a–b

Meade-Funsten Papers, #3039

Papers of Bowker Preston, #247

Letters of L. C. Randolph, #5885

WPA Folklore Collections, Virginia Writers' Project, #1547

Virginia Historical Society, Richmond

Elizabeth (Lumpkin) Motley Bagby Papers

Commonplace Book, 1824–32 (photocopy)

George William Bagby Papers

Thomas Chrystie Papers

Cocke Family Papers

Mary Banister Cookbook, 1834–36

Philip St. George Cocke Papers
  Plantation Account Books
Cushwa Family Papers
Douthat Family Papers
  Prescriptions
Friend Family Papers
  Charles Friend Diary
Grinnan Family Papers
Holladay Family Papers
Massie Family Papers
  Thomas Eugene Massie Commonplace Book, 1854
John Peter Mettauer Papers
Robert Morris Diary, 1845-48 (photocopy)
Philip Turner Southall Account Book
Wickham Family Papers
Waring Historical Library, Medical University of South Carolina, Charleston
Julian J. Chisolm Papers
William L. McCaa, "Observations on the Manner of Living and Diseases of the
  Slaves on the Wateree River," thesis, University of Pennsylvania, 1822
Theses, Medical College of the State of South Carolina
  M. L. McLoud, "Hints on the Medical Treatment of Negroes," 1850
  H. W. Moore, "A Thesis on Plantation Hygiene," February 1856 (typescript)
Joseph I. Waring Research Files
  James H. Hammond, "Plantation Manual of James H. Hammond of Beach
  Island, South Carolina," ca. 1834 (typescript)

PUBLISHED PRIMARY SOURCES

"Address of Samuel A. Cartwright." *New Orleans Medical and Surgical Journal*
  2 (May 1846): 424-733.
Albert, Octavia V. Rogers. *The House of Bondage, or Charlotte Brooks and Other
  Slaves.* New York: Hunt & Eaton, 1890. Reprint, Schomburg Library of
  Nineteenth-Century Black Women Writers, New York: Oxford University Press,
  1988.
Bass, Ruth. "Mojo." In Dundes, *Mother Wit from the Laughing Barrel,* 380-87.
  First published in *Scribner's Magazine* 87 (1930): 83-90.
Berkeley, Edmund, and Dorothy Smith Berkeley, ed. *The Reverend John Clayton:
  A Parson with a Scientific Mind.* Charlottesville: University Press of Virginia for
  the Virginia Historical Society, 1965.
Berlin, Jean V., ed. *A Confederate Nurse: The Diary of Ada W. Bacot, 1860-1863.*

Women's Diaries and Letters of the Nineteenth-Century South Series. Columbia: University of South Carolina Press, 1994.

Bibb, Henry. *Narrative of the Life and Adventures of Henry Bibb, An American Slave, Written by Himself.* New York, 1849. Reprinted in Osofsky, *Puttin' on Ole Massa,* 51–171. Page citations are to the reprint edition.

Blassingame, John W., ed. *Slave Testimony: Two Centuries of Letters, Speeches, Interviews, and Autobiographies.* Baton Rouge: Louisiana State University Press, 1977.

Bontemps, Arna, ed. *Great Slave Narratives.* Boston: Beacon, 1969.

Botanico-Medical Recorder, or Impartial Advocate of Botanic Medicine. Vols. 6–8. Columbus, Ohio, 1838–40.

Botkin, B. A. *Lay My Burden Down: A Folk History of Slavery.* Chicago: University of Chicago Press, 1945. Reprint, Athens: Delta, by arrangement with University of Georgia Press, 1994.

Breeden, James O., ed. *Advice among Masters: The Ideal in Slave Management in the Old South.* Westport, Conn.: Greenwood Press, 1980.

Brickell, John. *The Natural History of North-Carolina.* 1737. Reprint, New York: Johnson Reprint, 1969.

Brown, John. *Slave Life in Georgia: A Narrative of the Life, Sufferings, and Escape of John Brown, a Fugitive Slave.* London: W. M. Watts, 1855. Reprint, edited by F. N. Boney, Savannah: Beehive Press, 1972.

Brown, William Wells. *The Narrative of William W. Brown.* Boston: Anti-Slavery Office, 1847. Reprinted in *Five Slave Narratives.*

Bruce, Henry Clay. *The New Man: Twenty-Nine Years a Slave, Twenty-Nine Years a Free Man.* York, Pa.: P. Anstadt & Sons, 1895. Reprint, Miami: Mnemosyne Pub. Co., 1969.

Buchan, William. *Domestic Medicine; or, A Treatise on the Prevention and Cure of Diseases by Regimen and Simple Medicines.* 17th ed. Halifax, N.C.: Abraham Hadge, 1801.

Calendar of Virginia State Papers and Other Manuscripts. Vol. 5, *2 July 1790– 10 Aug. 1792.* Richmond: Rush U. Derr, 1885.

Cartwright, Samuel A. "Diseases and Peculiarities of the Negro Race." *De Bow's Review* 11 (1851): 65–69, 331–34, 504–8.

———. "The Diseases of Negroes: Pulmonary Congestions, Pneumonia, &c., No. II." *De Bow's Review* 11 (1851): 209–13.

———. "Dr. Cartwright on the Caucasians and the Africans." *De Bow's Review* 25 (1858): 45–56.

———. "Remarks on Dysentery among Negroes." *New Orleans Medical and Surgical Journal* 11 (September 1854): 145–63.

———. "Serpent Worship." *De Bow's Review* 31 (1861): 97–99.

Catterall, Helen Tunncliff, ed. *Judicial Cases Concerning American Slavery and the Negro*. Vols. 2, 3. Washington, D.C.: Carnegie Institution of Washington, 1929, 1932. Reprint, New York: Octagon Books, 1968.

Charleston Medical Journal and Review. Vols. 3–4, 6–10, 13–15. Charleston: 1848–49, 1851–55, 1858–60.

Chesnutt, Charles W. "Superstitions and Folklore of the South." In Dundes, *Mother Wit from the Laughing Barrel*, 369–76. First published in *Modern Culture* 13 (1901): 231–35.

Christensen, A. M. H. *Afro-American Folk Lore: Told Round Cabin Fires on the Sea Islands of South Carolina*. 1892. Reprint, New York: Negro Universities Press, 1969.

"Code of Medical Ethics, adopted at the late Meeting of the National Medical Convention." *Southern Medical and Surgical Journal* 3 (September 1847): 538.

The Code of Virginia. Richmond: William F. Ritchie, 1849.

The Code of Virginia. 2d ed. Richmond: Ritchie, Dunnavant & Co., 1860.

[Collins, David]. *Practical Rules for the Management and Medical Treatment of Negro Slaves in the Sugar Colonies by a Professional Planter*. London: J. Barfield, 1811. Reprint, Freeport, N.Y.: Books for Libraries Press, 1971.

Cooper, Thomas. *A Treatise of Domestic Medicine, Intended for Families*. Reading, Pa.: George Getz, 1824.

The Corporation of Charleston. *An Account of the Late Intended Insurrection Among a Portion of the Blacks of this City*. Charleston: A. E. Miller, 1822. Printed in the *Sixteenth Annual Report of the American Society for Colonizing the Free People of Colour of the United States*. Washington, D.C., 1833.

Coxe, John Redman. *The Philadelphia Medical Dictionary*. 2d ed. Philadelphia: Fry for Dobson, 1817.

Dancer, Thomas. *The Medical Assistant, or Jamaica Practice of Physic: Designed Chiefly for the Use of Families and Plantations*. 2d ed. St. Jago de la Vega: John Lunan, 1809.

De Bow's Review. Vols. 1–32. New Orleans, January 1846–August 1862.

Douglass, Frederick. *Narrative of the Life of Frederick Douglass, an American Slave: Written by Himself*. Boston: Anti-Slavery Office, 1845. Reprint, Chicago: Signet, 1968.

Drago, Edmund L., ed. *Broke by the War*. Columbia: University of South Carolina Press, 1991.

Dundes, Alan, ed. *Mother Wit from the Laughing Barrel: Readings in the Interpretation of Afro-American Folklore*. New York: Garland, 1981.

Easterby, J. H., ed. *The South Carolina Rice Plantation as Revealed in the Papers of Robert F. Allston*. Chicago: University of Chicago Press, 1945.

Egypt, Ophelia Settle, J. Masuoka, and Charles S. Johnson, eds. *Unwritten History of Slavery: Autobiographical Account of Negro Ex-Slaves*. Nashville, Tenn.: Social Science Institute, Fisk University, 1945. Reprint, Westport, Conn.: Greenwood Press, 1972.

Equiano, Olaudah. *The Life of Olaudah Equiano.* Edited by Paul Edwards. White Plains, N.Y.: Longman, 1988.

Ewell, James. *The Planter's and Mariner's Medical Companion.* Baltimore: P. Mauro, 1813.

Faulkner, William J. *The Days When the Animals Talked: Black American Folktales and How They Came to Be.* Chicago: Follett Pub. Co., 1977.

Five Slave Narratives: A Compendium. New York: Arno Press and the New York Times, 1968.

Folger, Alfred M. *The Family Physician, Being a Domestic Medical Work.* Spartanburg, S.C.: Z. D. Cottrell, G. H. Joyce, 1845.

Gates, Henry Louis, Jr., ed. *Six Women's Slave Narratives.* Schomburg Library of Nineteenth-Century Black Women Writers. New York: Oxford University Press, 1988.

Georgia Blister and Critic. Vols. 1–2. Atlanta, 1854–55.

Georgia Writers' Project, Savannah Unit, ed. *Drums and Shadows: Survival Studies among the Georgia Coastal Negroes.* Athens: University of Georgia Press, 1940.

Guild, June Purcell. *Black Laws of Virginia: A Summary of the Legislative Acts of Virginia Concerning Negroes from Earliest Times to the Present.* Richmond: Whittet & Shepperson, 1936.

Gunn, John C. *Gunn's Domestic Medicine: A Facsimile of the First Edition.* 1830. Reprint, Knoxville: University of Tennessee Press, 1986.

Hall, Julien A. "Negro Conjuring and Tricking," *Journal of American Folklore* 10 (July–September 1897): 241–43.

Harris, S. N. "Cases in Obstetric Practice." *Charleston Medical Journal and Review* 7 (1852): 773–74.

———. "Report on the Treatment of Some Cases of Cholera Occurring on Savannah River." *Charleston Medical Journal and Review* 4 (1849): 581–85.

Harriss, Juriah. "What Constitutes Unsoundness in the Negro?" *Savannah Journal of Medicine* 1 (September 1858): 145–52; (January 1859): 289–95; 2 (May 1859): 10–16.

Hening, William Waller, ed. *The Statutes at Large: Being a Collection of All the Laws of Virginia.* Vol. 6. 1819. Reprint, Charlottesville: University of Virginia Press, 1969.

Herron, Leonora, and Alice M. Bacon. "Conjuring and Conjure Doctors." In Dundes, *Mother Wit from the Laughing Barrel,* 359–68.

Holmes, W. Fletcher. "Typhoid Fever, as observed in Newberry District, S.C." *Charleston Medical Journal and Review* 7 (1852): 58–67.

Jacobs, Harriet A. *Incidents in the Life of a Slave Girl: Written by Herself.* 1861. Reprint, edited by Jean Fagan Yellin, Cambridge, Mass.: Harvard University Press, 1987.

Johnson, Clifton H., ed. *God Struck Me Dead: Religious Conversion Experiences and Autobiographies of Ex-Slaves.* Philadelphia: United Church Press, 1969.

Johnson, F. Roy. *The Fabled Doctor Jim Jordan: A Story of Conjure.* Murfreesboro, N.C.: Johnson Pub. Co., 1963.

Jones, Charles C. *Negro Myths from the Georgia Coast: Told in the Vernacular.* Boston: Houghton Mifflin, 1888.

Journal of American Folklore. Vols. 1–32. Boston, 1888–1919.

Journal of the Commons House of Assembly, March 28, 1749–March 19, 1750. Edited by James H. Easterby. Columbia: South Carolina Archives Dept., 1962.

Journal of the Commons House of Assembly, November 12, 1754–September 23, 1755. Edited by Terry W. Lipscomb. Columbia: University of South Carolina Press, 1986.

Keckley, Elizabeth. *Behind the Scenes, or Thirty Years a Slave, and Four Years in the White House.* New York: G. W. Carleton 1868. Reprint, New York: Oxford University Press, 1988.

Kemble, Frances Anne. *Journal of a Residence on a Georgian Plantation in 1838–1839.* 1863. Reprint, edited by John A. Scott, Athens: University of Georgia Press, 1984.

Kemper, Charles E. "Documents Relating to the Boundaries of the Northern Neck." *Virginia Magazine of History and Biography* 28 (October 1920): 306–7.

Lewis, Henry Clay. *Odd Leaves from the Life of a Louisiana Swamp Doctor.* 1850. Reprint, Baton Rouge: Louisiana State University Press, 1997.

Lyell, Charles. *A Second Visit to the United States of North America.* Vol 1. New York: Harper & Bros., 1849.

McCaw, James B. "On the Present Condition of the Medical Profession in Virginia." *Virginia Medical and Surgical Journal* 3 (October 1853): 42–47.

McCoy, Ambrose. "Voodooism in the South." *Louisville Medical News,* December 1884, 380–81.

McKain, W. J. "Strangulation of the Jejunum, Produced by an Encysted Tumour of the Mesentery." *Charleston Medical Journal and Review* 3 (1848): 276–79.

Medical Society of the State of North Carolina, Transactions. Raleigh, 1849–60.

Mellon, James, ed. *Bullwhip Days: The Slaves Remember.* New York: Weidenfeld & Nicolson, 1988.

Merrill, A. P. "An Essay on Some of the Distinctive Peculiarities of the Negro Race." *Southern Medical and Surgical Journal* 12 (January 1856): 21–36; (February 1856): 80–90; (March 1856): 147–56.

Morgan, John H. "An Essay on the Causes of the Production of Abortion among Our Negro Population." *Nashville Journal of Medicine and Surgery* 19 (1860): 117–23.

Moton, R. R. "Folklore and Ethnology: Sickness in Slavery Days." *Southern Workman* 28 (1899): 74–75.

New Orleans Medical and Surgical Journal. Vols. 1–17. New Orleans, 1844–60.

Northup, Solomon. *Twelve Years a Slave: Narrative of Solomon Northup.* New York, 1853. Reprinted in Osofsky, *Puttin' On Ole Massa,* 225–406. Page citations are to the reprint edition.

O'Neall, John Belton. *The Negro Law of S.C. Collected and Digested by John Belton O'Neall.* Columbia, S.C.: John H. Bowman, 1848.

Osofsky, Gilbert, ed. *Puttin' On Ole Massa: The Slave Narratives of Henry Bibb, William Wells Brown, and Solomon Northup.* New York: Harper & Row, 1969.

Parsons, Elsie Worthington Clews, ed. *Folk-Lore of the Sea Islands, South Carolina.* New York: American Folk-Lore Society, 1923.

Pendleton, E. M. "On the Comparative Fecundity of the Caucasian and African Races." *Charleston Medical Journal and Review* 6 (1851): 351–56.

Pennington, James W. C. *The Fugitive Blacksmith.* London: Charles Gilpin, 1849. Reprinted in Bontemps, *Great Slave Narratives,* 193–267.

Perdue, Charles L., Jr., Thomas E. Barden, and Robert K. Phillips. *Weevils in the Wheat: Interviews with Virginia Ex-Slaves.* Charlottesville: University Press of Virginia, 1976.

Peters, Erskine. *Lyrics of the Afro-American Spiritual: A Documentary Collection.* Westport, Conn.: Greenwood Press, 1993.

"Petition in Regard to a Slave, 1773." *Virginia Historical Magazine* 18 (1910): 394–96.

Pettigrew, Thomas Joseph. *On Superstitions Connected with the History and Practice of Medicine and Surgery.* London: John Churchill, 1844.

Porcher, Francis Peyre. *Resources of the Southern Fields and Forests, Medical, Economical and Agricultural.* Charleston: Walker, Evans & Cogswell, 1869.

Rawick, George P., ed. *The American Slave: A Composite Autobiography.* Vol. 1, *From Sundown to Sunup: The Making of the Black Community,* by George P. Rawick. Westport, Conn.: Greenwood Press, 1972.

———. *The American Slave: A Composite Autobiography.* Vols. 2, 3, *South Carolina Narratives.* Westport, Conn.: Greenwood Press, 1972.

———. *The American Slave: A Composite Autobiography.* Vols. 12, 13, *Georgia Narratives.* Westport, Conn.: Greenwood Press, 1972.

———. *The American Slave: A Composite Autobiography.* Vols. 14, 15, *North Carolina Narratives.* Westport, Conn.: Greenwood Press, 1972.

———. *The American Slave: A Composite Autobiography.* Supplement, ser. 1, vols. 3, 4, *Georgia Narratives.* Westport, Conn.: Greenwood Press, 1977.

———. *The American Slave: A Composite Autobiography.* Supplement, ser. 1, vol. 11, *North Carolina and South Carolina Narratives.* Westport, Conn.: Greenwood Press, 1977.

The Revised Code of the Laws of Virginia. Vol. 1. Richmond: Thomas Ritchie, 1819.

Roper, Moses. *A Narrative of the Adventures and Escape of Moses Roper, from American Slavery*. Philadelphia: Merrihew & Gunn, 1838. Reprint, Philadelphia: Rhistoric Publications, 1969.

Rosengarten, Theodore, ed. *Tombee: Portrait of a Cotton Planter, with the Plantation Journal of Thomas B. Chaplin, 1822–1890*. New York: Quill, William Morrow & Co., 1986.

Savannah Journal of Medicine. Vols 1–2. Savannah, 1858–59.

Shryock, Richard H., ed. *Letters of Richard D. Arnold, M.D., 1808–1876*. Durham, N.C.: Seeman Press, 1929. Reprinted in *Historical Papers, Published by the Trinity College Historical Society*, ser. 16 (Durham, N.C.: Duke University Press, 1936).

Simons, J. Hume. *The Planter's Guide and Family Book of Medicine*. Charleston: M'Carter & Allen, 1848.

Sims, J. Marion. "On the Treatment of Vesico-Vaginal Fistula." *American Journal of the Medical Sciences*, n.s., no. 45 (January 1852): 59–82.

———. *The Story of My Life*. Edited by H. Marion Sims. New York: Appleton, 1885.

———. "Two Cases of Vesico-Vaginal Fistula, Cured." *New-York Medical Gazette and Journal of Health* 5 (January 1854): 1–7.

Slave Narratives: A Folk History of Slavery in the United States. Vol. 12, *Georgia Narratives*. 1941. Reprint, St. Clair Shores, Mich.: Scholarly Press, 1976.

Smith, James L. *Autobiography of James L. Smith*. Norwick, Conn: The Bulletin, 1881. Electronic ed., Chapel Hill: University of North Carolina, 2000.

Southern Journal of Medicine and Pharmacy. Vols. 1–2. Charleston, 1846–47.

Southern Medical and Surgical Journal. Vols. 1–16. Augusta, Ga., 1845–60.

Southern Medical Reformer. Vol. 1. Petersburg, Va., 1848.

Southern Medical Reformer and Review. Vols. 6, 10. Macon, Ga., 1857, 1860.

Southern Medical Reports. Vols. 1–2. New Orleans, 1849–50.

Southern Planter. Vols. 1–20. Richmond, 1841–60.

State Slavery Statutes, 1789–1860. Virginia, North Carolina, South Carolina, Georgia. Frederick, Md.: University Press of America Microfiche Series, 1989.

Steiner, Roland. "Braziel Robinson Possessed of Two Spirits." *Journal of American Folklore* 13 (July–September 1900): 226–28. Reprinted in Dundes, *Mother Wit from the Laughing Barrel*, 377–79.

———. "Observations on the Practice of Conjuring in Georgia." *Journal of American Folklore* 14 (July–September 1901): 173–80.

Stethoscope and Virginia Medical Gazette: A Monthly Journal of Medicine and the Collateral Sciences. Vol. 1. Richmond, 1851.

Stroyer, Jacob. *My Life in the South*. Salem, Mass.: Newcomb & Gauss, 1898.

Thomsonian Recorder, or Impartial Advocate of Botanic Medicine and the Principles Which Govern the Thomsonian Practice. Vols. 1–2. Columbus, Ohio, 1833–34.

Thornton, Phineas. *The Southern Gardener and Receipt Book.* Newark, N.J.: A. L. Dennis, 1845.

Tidyman, P[hilip]. "A Sketch of the most remarkable Diseases of the Negroes of the Southern States, with an account of the method of treating them, accompanied by physiological observations." *Philadelphia Journal of the Medical and Physical Sciences,* n.s. 3, 12 (1826): 306-38.

"Virginia Council Journals, 1726-1753." *Virginia Magazine of History and Biography* 34 (April 1926): 103-4.

Virginia Medical and Surgical Journal. Vols. 1-5. Richmond, 1853-55.

Virginia Medical Journal. Vols. 6-13. Richmond, 1856-59.

Wells, Ida B. *A Red Record* (1895). In *Southern Horrors and Other Writings,* edited by Jacqueline Jones Royster, 73-157. Boston: Bedford/St. Martins Press, 1997.

Yetman, Norman R., ed. *Life under the "Peculiar Institution": Selections from the Slave Narrative Collection.* New York: Holt, Rinehart and Winston, 1970.

SECONDARY SOURCES

Abel, Emily K. *Hearts of Wisdom: American Women Caring for Kin, 1850-1940.* Cambridge, Mass.: Harvard University Press, 2000.

Abrahams, Roger D., ed. *Afro-American Folktales: Stories from Black Traditions in the New World.* New York: Pantheon, 1985.

Anderson, Martha G., and Christine Mullen Kreamer. *Wild Spirits, Strong Medicine: African Arts and the Wilderness.* New York: Center for African Art; Seattle: University of Washington Press, 1989.

Arens, W., and Ivan Karp, eds. *Creativity of Power: Cosmology and Action in African Societies.* Washington, D.C.: Smithsonian Institution Press, 1989.

Asante, Molefi Kete. *The Afrocentric Idea.* Philadelphia: Temple University Press, 1987.

Axelsen, Diana E. "Women as Victims of Medical Experimentation: J. Marion Sims' Surgery on Slave Women, 1845-1850." *SAGE* 2 (1985): 10-13.

Bankole, Katherine. *Slavery and Medicine: Enslavement and Medical Practices in Antebellum Louisiana.* New York: Garland, 1998.

Baur, Susan. *Hypochondria: Woeful Imaginations.* Berkeley: University of California Press, 1988.

Bay, Mia. *The White Image in the Black Mind: African-American Ideas about White People, 1830-1925.* New York: Oxford University Press, 1999.

Beauvoir-Dominique, Rachel. "Underground Realms of Being: Vodoun Magic." In Cosentino, *Sacred Arts of Haitian Vodou,* 153-77.

Beckles, Hilary. "Black Female Slaves and White Households in Barbados." In Gaspar and Hine, *More Than Chattel,* 111-25.

Bederman, Gail. *Manliness and Civilization: A Cultural History of Gender and*

Race in the United States, 1880–1917. Chicago: University of Chicago Press, 1995.

Behrendt, Stephen D. "The British Slave Trade, 1785–1807: Volume, Profitability, and Mortality." Ph.D. diss., University of Wisconsin, Madison, 1993.

Bell-Scott, Patricia, Beverly Guy-Sheftall, Jacqueline Jones Royster, Janet Sims-Wood, Miriam DeCosta-Willis, and Lucie Fultz, eds. *Double Stitch: Black Women Write about Mothers and Daughters.* Boston: Beacon, 1991.

Berlin, Ira. *Many Thousands Gone: The First Two Centuries of Slavery in North America.* Cambridge, Mass.: Harvard University Press, 1998.

Berlin, Ira, and Philip D. Morgan. "Introduction: The Slaves' Economy: Independent Production by Slaves in the Americas." *Abolition and Slavery* 12 (May 1991): 1–27.

Blakely, Robert L., and Judith M. Harrington. *Bones in the Basement: Post-Mortem Racism in Nineteenth-Century Medical Training.* Washington, D.C.: Smithsonian Institution Press, 1997.

Blanton, Wyndham B. *Medicine in Virginia in the Eighteenth Century.* Richmond: Garrett & Massie, 1931. Reprint, New York: AMS Press, 1980.

———. *Medicine in Virginia in the Nineteenth Century.* Richmond: Garrett & Massie, 1933.

Blassingame, John W. *The Slave Community: Plantation Life in the Antebellum South.* Rev. and enl. ed. New York: Oxford University Press, 1979.

———. "Status and Social Structure in the Slave Community: Evidence from New Sources." In *Perspectives and Irony in American Slavery,* edited by Harry P. Owens, 137–51. Jackson: University Press of Mississippi, 1976.

Bleser, Carol, ed. *Secret and Sacred: The Diaries of James Henry Hammond, a Southern Slaveholder.* New York: Oxford University Press, 1988.

Boles, John B. *Black Southerners, 1619–1869.* Lexington: University Press of Kentucky, 1983.

Boney, F. N. "Slaves as Guinea Pigs: Georgia and Alabama Episodes." *Alabama Review* 37 (January 1984): 45–51.

Brandon, George. *Santeria from Africa to the New World: The Dead Sell Memories.* Bloomington: Indiana University Press, 1993.

———. "The Uses of Plants in Healing in an Afro-Cuban Religion, Santeria." *Journal of Black Studies* 22 (September 1991): 55–76.

Braude, Ann. *Radical Spirits: Spiritualism and Women's Rights in Nineteenth-Century America.* Boston: Beacon, 1989.

Breeden, James O. "Body Snatchers and Anatomy Professors: Medical Education in Nineteenth-Century Virginia." *Virginia Magazine of History and Biography* 83 (July 1975): 321–45.

———. "Thomsonianism in Virginia." *Virginia Magazine of History and Biography* 82 (April 1974): 150–80.

Breen, T. H., and Stephen Innes. *"Myne Owne Ground": Race and Freedom on Virginia's Eastern Shore, 1640–1676.* New York: Oxford University Press, 1980.

Brodie, Janet Farrell. *Contraception and Abortion in Nineteenth-Century America.* Ithaca, N.Y.: Cornell University Press, 1994.

Brown, David H. "Conjure/Doctors: An Exploration of a Black Discourse in America, Antebellum to 1940." *Folklore Forum* 23 (1990): 3–46.

Brown, Elsa Barkley. "Negotiating and Transforming the Public Sphere: African American Political Life in the Transition from Slavery to Freedom." *Public Culture* 7 (fall 1994): 107–46.

——. "'What Has Happened Here': The Politics of Difference in Women's History and Feminist Politics." *Feminist Studies* 18 (summer 1992): 295–312.

Brown, Kathleen M. *Good Wives, Nasty Wenches, and Anxious Patriarchs: Gender, Race, and Power in Colonial Virginia.* Chapel Hill: University of North Carolina Press, 1996.

Burnside, Madeleine. *Spirits of the Passage: The Transatlantic Slave Trade in the Seventeenth Century.* New York: Simon & Schuster, 1997.

Bush, Barbara. "Hard Labor: Women, Childbirth, and Resistance in British Caribbean Slave Societies." In Gaspar and Hine, *More Than Chattel,* 193–217.

——. *Slave Women in Caribbean Society, 1650–1838.* Bloomington: Indiana University Press, 1990.

Butler, Jon. *Awash in a Sea of Faith: Christianizing the American People.* Cambridge, Mass.: Harvard University Press, 1990.

——. "The Dark Ages of American Occultism, 1760–1848." In *The Occult in America: New Historical Perspectives,* edited by Howard Kerr and Charles L. Crow, 58–78. Urbana: University of Illinois Press, 1983.

Bynum, Victoria E. *Unruly Women: The Politics of Social and Sexual Control in the Old South.* Chapel Hill: University of North Carolina Press, 1992.

Byrd, W. Michael, and Linda A. Clayton. *An American Health Dilemma: A Medical History of African Americans and the Problem of Race.* New York: Routledge, 2000.

Cadwallader, D. E., and F. J. Wilson. "Folklore Medicine among Georgia's Piedmont Negroes after the Civil War." *Georgia Historical Quarterly* 49 (1965): 217–27.

Campbell, John. "As 'A Kind of Freeman'?: Slaves' Market-Related Activities in the South Carolina Upcountry, 1800–1860." *Slavery and Abolition* 12 (May 1991): 131–69.

——. "Work, Pregnancy, and Infant Mortality among Southern Slaves." *Journal of Interdisciplinary History* 14 (spring 1984): 793–812.

Carby, Hazel. "Ideologies of Black Folk: The Historical Novel of Slavery." In McDowell and Rampersad, *Slavery and the Literary Imagination,* 125–43.

——. *Reconstructing Womanhood: The Emergence of the Afro-American Woman Novelist.* New York: Oxford University Press, 1987.

Carrigan, Jo Ann. "Early Nineteenth Century Folk Remedies." *Louisiana Folklore Miscellany* 1 (January 1960): 43–64.

Cayleff, Susan E. *Wash and Be Healed: The Water-Cure Movement and Women's Health.* Philadelphia: Temple University Press, 1987.

Chappell, Buford S. "'Doctor Caesar' and His Cure for Poisons and Rattle-snake Bites." *Journal of the South Carolina Medical Association* 71 (June 1975): 183–87.

Chireau, Yvonne. "Conjure and Christianity in the Nineteenth Century: Religious Elements in African American Magic." *Religion and American Culture* 7 (summer 1997): 225–46.

———. "The Uses of the Supernatural: Toward a History of Black Women's Magical Practices." In *A Mighty Baptism: Race, Gender, and the Creation of American Protestantism,* edited by Susan Juster and Lisa MacFarlane, 171–88. Ithaca, N.Y.: Cornell University Press, 1996.

Clinton, Catherine. *The Plantation Mistress: Woman's World in the Old South.* New York: Pantheon, 1982.

Cody, Cheryll Ann. "Cycles of Work and of Childbearing: Seasonality in Women's Lives on Low Country Plantations." In Gaspar and Hine, *More Than Chattel,* 61–77.

———. "A Note on Changing Patterns of Slave Fertility in the South Carolina Rice District, 1735–1865." *Southern Studies* 16 (1977): 457–63.

Collins, Patricia Hill. *Black Feminist Thought: Knowledge, Consciousness, and the Politics of Empowerment.* New York: Routledge, 1991.

———. "The Meaning of Motherhood in Black Culture and Black Mother-Daughter Relationships." In Bell-Scott et al., *Double Stitch,* 42–60.

Conser, Walter H., Jr. *God and the Natural World: Religion and Science in Antebellum America.* Columbia: University of South Carolina Press, 1993.

Cosentino, Donald J., ed. *Sacred Arts of Haitian Vodou.* Los Angeles: UCLA Fowler Museum of Cultural History, 1995.

Cosslett, Tess, ed. *Science and Religion in the Nineteenth Century.* New York: Cambridge University Press, 1984.

Creel, Margaret Washington. "Gullah Attitudes towards Life and Death." In Holloway, *Africanisms in American Culture,* 69–97.

———. *"A Peculiar People": Slave Religion and Community-Culture among the Gullahs.* New York: New York University Press, 1988.

Crellin, John K., and Jane Philpott. *Herbal Medicine Past and Present.* Vol. 1, *Trying to Give Ease.* Durham, N.C.: Duke University Press, 1990.

Curtin, Philip D. *The Image of Africa: British Ideas and Action, 1780–1850.* Madison: University of Wisconsin Press, 1964.

———. *The Rise and Fall of the Plantation Complex: Essays in Atlantic History.* New York: Cambridge University Press, 1990.

Dance, Daryl Cumber. *Shuckin' and Jivin': Folklore from Contemporary Black Americans.* Bloomington: Indiana University Press, 1978.

Davidoff, Leonore. "Class and Gender in Victorian England: The Diaries of Arthur J. Munby and Hannah Cullwick." *Feminist Studies* 5 (spring 1979): 87–141.

Davis, Angela. "Reflections on the Black Woman's Role in the Community of Slaves." *Massachusetts Review* 13 (winter–spring 1972): 81–103.

———. *Women, Culture, and Politics.* New York: Vintage, 1989.

Deas-Moore, Vennie. "Home Remedies, Herb Doctors, and Granny Midwives." *World and I,* January 1987, 474–85.

Diamond, Timothy. *Making Gray Gold: Narratives of Nursing Home Care.* Chicago: University of Chicago Press, 1992.

Drewry, William Sidney. *The Southampton Insurrection.* Washington, D.C., Neale, 1900. Reprint, Murfreesboro, N.C.: Johnson Pub. Co., 1968.

Du Bois, William E. B. *The Souls of Black Folk.* In *Three Negro Classics.* New York: Avon, 1965.

Duden, Barbara. *The Woman beneath the Skin: A Doctor's Patients in Eighteenth-Century Germany.* Cambridge, Mass: Harvard University Press, 1991.

Duffy, John. *The Healers: The Rise of the Medical Establishment.* New York: McGraw-Hill, 1976.

———. "Medical Practice in the Ante Bellum South." *Journal of Southern History* 25 (February 1959): 53–72.

Dusinberre, William. *Them Dark Days: Slavery in the American Rice Swamps.* New York: Oxford University Press, 1996.

Edwards, Laura F. *Gendered Strife and Confusion: The Political Culture of Reconstruction.* Urbana: University of Illinois Press, 1997.

Egerton, Douglas R. *He Shall Go Out Free: The Lives of Denmark Vesey.* Madison, Wisc.: Madison House Publishers, 1999.

Elkins, Stanley M. *Slavery: A Problem in American Institutional and Intellectual Life.* Chicago: University of Chicago Press, 1959.

Fanon, Frantz. *A Dying Colonialism.* Translated by Haakon Chevalier. New York: Grove Press, 1965.

Faust, Drew. "Culture, Conflict, and Community: The Meaning of Power on an Ante-Bellum Plantation," *Journal of Social History* 14 (fall 1980): 83–97.

Fee, Elizabeth, and Daniel Fox, eds. *AIDS: The Burdens of History.* Berkeley: University of California Press, 1988.

Feierman, Steven. "Struggles for Control: The Social Roots of Health and Healing in Modern Africa." *African Studies Review* 28 (June/September 1985): 73–147.

Feierman, Steven, and John M. Janzen, eds. *The Social Basis of Health and Healing in Africa.* Berkeley: University of California Press, 1992.

Ferguson, Leland. "'The Cross Is a Magic Sign': Marks on Eighteenth-Century Bowls from South Carolina." In Singleton, *"I, Too, Am America,"* 116–31.

———. *Uncommon Ground: Archaeology and Early African America, 1650–1800.* Washington, D.C.: Smithsonian Institution Press, 1992.

Fields, Barbara Jeanne. *Slavery and Freedom on the Middle Ground: Maryland during the Nineteenth Century.* New Haven: Yale University Press, 1985.

———. "Slavery, Race, and Ideology in the United States of America." *New Left Review,* May/June 1990, 95–118.

Fields, Mamie Garvin. *Lemon Swamp and Other Places: A Carolina Memoir.* New York: Free Press, 1983.

Fisher, Walter. "Physicians and Slavery in the Antebellum Southern Medical Journal." *Journal of the History of Medicine and Allied Sciences* 23 (1968): 36–49.

Fogel, Robert William. *Without Consent or Contract: The Rise and Fall of American Slavery.* New York: Norton, 1989.

Foster, Steven, and James A. Duke. *A Field Guide to Medicinal Plants: Eastern and Central North America.* Boston: Houghton Mifflin, 1990.

Fox-Genovese, Elizabeth. *Within the Plantation Household: Black and White Women of the Old South.* Chapel Hill: University of North Carolina Press, 1988.

Frazier, E. Franklin. *The Negro Church in America.* New York: Schocken Books, 1964.

Fredrickson, George. *The Black Image in the White Mind: The Debate on Afro-American Character and Destiny, 1817–1914.* New York: Harper & Row, 1972.

Frey, Sylvia R., and Betty Wood. *Come Shouting to Zion: African American Protestantism in the American South and British Caribbean to 1830.* Chapel Hill: University of North Carolina Press, 1998.

Friedman, Jean E. *The Enclosed Garden: Women and Community in the Evangelical South, 1830–1900.* Chapel Hill: University of North Carolina Press, 1985.

Fry, Gladys-Marie. *Night Riders in Black Folk History.* Knoxville: University of Tennessee Press, 1975.

Gaspar, David Barry, and Darlene Clark Hine, eds. *More Than Chattel: Black Women and Slavery in the Americas.* Bloomington: Indiana University Press, 1996.

Geggus, David P. "Slave and Free Colored Women in Saint Domingue." In Gaspar and Hine, *More Than Chattel,* 259–78.

Genovese, Eugene D. "The Medical and Insurance Costs of Slaveholding in the Cotton Belt." *Journal of Negro History* 45 (July 1960): 141–55.

———. *Roll, Jordan, Roll: The World the Slaves Made.* New York: Vintage, 1976.

Gevitz, Norman, ed. *Other Healers: Unorthodox Medicine in America.* Baltimore: Johns Hopkins University Press, 1988.

Gilman, Sander L. "Black Bodies, White Bodies: Toward an Iconography of Female Sexuality in Late Nineteenth-Century Art, Medicine, and Literature." In *Race, Writing, and Difference,* edited by Henry L. Gates, 223–61. Chicago: University of Chicago Press, 1986.

———. *Disease and Representation: Images of Illness from Madness to AIDS.* Ithaca, N.Y.: Cornell University Press, 1988.

Gomez, Michael A. *Exchanging Our Country Marks: The Transformation of African Identities in the Colonial and Antebellum South.* Chapel Hill: University of North Carolina Press, 1998.

Good, Byron J. *Medicine, Rationality, and Experience: An Anthropological Perspective.* New York: Cambridge University Press, 1994.

Good, Byron J., and Mary-Jo Del Vecchio Good. "The Semantics of Medical Discourse." In *Sciences and Cultures,* vol. 5, *Sociology of the Sciences,* edited by Everett Mendelsohn and Yehuda Elkana, 177–212. Boston: D. Reidel, 1981.

Goodson, Martia Graham. "Medical-Botanical Contributions of African Slave Women to American Medicine." *Western Journal of Black Studies* 11 (1987): 198–203.

Gorn, Eliott. "Folk Beliefs of the Slave Community." In Numbers and Savitt, *Science and Medicine in the Old South,* 295–326.

Gould, Stephen Jay. *The Mismeasure of Man.* Rev. and exp. ed. New York: Norton, 1996.

Greenberg, Kenneth S. *Honor and Slavery.* Princeton: Princeton University Press, 1996.

———, ed. *The Confessions of Nat Turner and Related Documents.* Boston: Bedford Books, 1996.

Grimé, William Ed. *Ethno-Botany of the Black Americans.* Algonac, Mich.: Reference Publications, 1979.

Gross, Ariela. *Double Character: Slavery and Mastery in the Antebellum Southern Courtroom.* Princeton: Princeton University Press, 2000.

———. "'Pandora's Box': Slave Character on Trial in the Antebellum Deep South." *Yale Journal of Law and the Humanities* 7 (spring 1995): 101–45.

Gutman, Herbert G., *The Black Family in Slavery and Freedom, 1750–1925.* New York: Vintage, 1976.

Hall, Gwendolyn Midlo. *Africans in Colonial Louisiana: The Development of Afro-Creole Culture in the Eighteenth Century.* Baton Rouge: Louisiana State University Press, 1992.

Haller, John S. "The Negro and the Southern Physician: A Study of Medical and Racial Attitudes, 1800–1860." *Medical History* 16 (1972): 239–54.

Hand, Wayland D. "The Folk Healer: Calling and Endowment." *Journal of the History of Medicine and Allied Sciences* 26 (July 1971): 263–75.

Hein, Wolfgang-Hagen, ed. *Botanical Drugs of the Americas in the Old and New Worlds: Invitational Symposium at the Washington-Congress, 1983.* Stuttgart:

Wissenschaftliche Verlagsgesellschaft, International Society for the History of Pharmacy, 1983.

Herskovits, Melville. *The Myth of the Negro Past*. Boston: Beacon, 1958.

Hill, Carole E., and Holly Mathews. "Traditional Health Beliefs and Practices among Southern Rural Blacks: A Complement to Biomedicine." In *Perspectives on the American South: An Annual Review of Society, Politics, and Culture*, edited by Merle Black and John Shelton Reed, 307–22. New York: Gordon & Breach, 1981.

Hine, Darlene Clark, and Kate Wittenstein. "Female Slave Resistance: The Economics of Sex." In Steady, *Black Woman Cross-Culturally*, 289–99.

Holloway, Joseph E., ed. *Africanisms in American Culture*. Bloomington: Indiana University Press, 1990.

Hudson, Larry E., Jr., ed. *Working toward Freedom: Slave Society and Domestic Economy in the American South*. Rochester, N.Y.: University of Rochester Press, 1994.

Hufford, David J. "Folk Healers." In *Handbook of American Folklore*, edited by Richard M. Dorson, 306–13. Bloomington: Indiana University Press, 1983.

Humez, Jean McMahon, ed. *Gifts of Power: The Writings of Rebecca Jackson, Black Visionary, Shaker Eldress*. Amherst: University of Massachusetts Press, 1981.

Hunt, Nancy Rose. *A Colonial Lexicon: Of Birth Ritual, Medicalization, and Mobility in Congo*. Durham, N.C.: Duke University Press, 1999.

Hunter, Tera W. *To 'Joy My Freedom: Southern Black Women's Lives and Labors after the Civil War*. Cambridge, Mass.: Harvard University Press, 1997.

Hurston, Zora Neale. "Hoodoo in America." *Journal of American Folklore* 44 (October–December 1931): 317–417.

———. *Mules and Men*. Philadelphia: Lippincott, 1935. Reprint, Bloomington: Indiana University Press, 1978.

———. *The Sanctified Church: The Folklore Writings of Zora Neale Hurston*. Berkeley, Calif.: Turtle Island, 1981.

———. *Tell My Horse: Voodoo and Life in Haiti and Jamaica*. Philadelphia: Lippincott, 1938. Reprint, New York: Harper & Row, 1990.

Isaac, Rhys. *The Transformation of Virginia, 1740–1790*. Chapel Hill: University of North Carolina Press, 1982.

Jackson, Bruce. "The Other Kind of Doctor: Conjure and Magic in Black American Folk Medicine." In *American Folk Medicine: A Symposium*, edited by Wayland D. Hand, 259–72. Berkeley: University of California Press, 1976.

Janzen, John M. *The Quest for Therapy in Lower Zaire*. Berkeley: University of California Press, 1978.

Johnson, Charles S. *Shadow of the Plantation*. Chicago: University of Chicago Press, 1934.

Johnson, F. Roy. *The Nat Turner Story.* Murfreesboro, N.C.: Johnson Pub. Co., 1970.

Johnson, Guy B. *Folk Culture on St. Helena Island, South Carolina.* Chapel Hill: University of North Carolina Press, 1930. Reprint, Hatboro, Pa.: Folklore Associates, 1968.

Johnson, Michael P. "Smothered Slave Infants: Were Slave Mothers at Fault?" *Journal of Southern History* 47 (November 1981): 493-520.

———. "Work, Culture, and the Slave Community: Slave Occupations in the Cotton Belt in 1860." *Labor History* 27 (summer 1986): 325-55.

Johnson, Walter. *Soul by Soul: Life inside the Antebellum Slave Market.* Cambridge, Mass.: Harvard University Press, 1999.

Jones, Jacqueline. *Labor of Love, Labor of Sorrow: Black Women, Work, and the Family, from Slavery to the Present.* New York: Vintage, 1985.

———. "Race, Sex, and Self-Evident Truths: The Status of Slave Women during the Era of the American Revolution." In *Half Sisters of History: Southern Women and the American Past,* edited by Catherine Clinton, 18-35. Durham, N.C.: Duke University Press, 1994.

Jones, James H. *Bad Blood: The Tuskegee Syphilis Experiment.* New York: Free Press, 1981.

Jones, Norrece T., Jr. *Born a Child of Freedom, Yet a Slave: Mechanisms of Control and Strategies of Resistance in Antebellum South Carolina.* Hanover, N.H.: University Press of New England, Wesleyan University Press, 1990.

Jordan, Winthrop. *White over Black: American Attitudes toward the Negro, 1550-1812.* New York: Norton, 1968.

Joyner, Charles. *Down by the Riverside: A South Carolina Slave Community.* Chicago: University of Illinois Press, 1984.

Karras, Alan L. "The Atlantic World as a Unit of Study." In *Atlantic American Societies: From Columbus through Abolition, 1492-1888,* edited by Alan L. Karras and J. R. McNeill, 1-15. New York: Routledge, 1992.

Kaufman, Martin. *Homeopathy in America: The Rise and Fall of a Medical Heresy.* Baltimore: Johns Hopkins University Press, 1971.

Kelley, Jennifer Olsen, and J. Lawrence Angel. "Life Stresses of Slavery." *American Journal of Physical Anthropology* 74 (1987): 199-211.

Kelley, Robin D. G. "Notes on Deconstructing 'The Folk.'" *American Historical Review* 97 (December 1992): 1400-1408.

———. "'We Are Not What We Seem': Rethinking Black Working-Class Opposition in the Jim Crow South." *Journal of American History* 80 (June 1993): 75-112.

Kerber, Linda J. "Separate Spheres, Female Worlds, Women's Place: The Rhetoric of Women's History." *Journal of American History* 75 (June 1988): 9-39.

Kett, Joseph. *The Formation of the American Medical Profession: The Role of Institutions, 1780-1860.* New Haven: Yale University Press, 1968.

Kincaid, Jamaica. "In History." *Callaloo* 20 (1997): 1–7.

King, Wilma. *Stolen Childhood: Slave Youth in Nineteenth-Century America.* Bloomington: Indiana University Press, 1995.

Kiple, Kenneth F., ed. *The African Exchange: Toward a Biological History.* Durham, N.C.: Duke University Press, 1987.

Kiple, Kenneth F., and Virginia Himmelsteib King. *Another Dimension of the Black Diaspora: Diet, Disease, and Racism.* New York: Cambridge University Press, 1981.

Kiple, Kenneth F., and Virginia H. Kiple. "Slave Child Mortality: Some Nutritional Answers to a Perennial Puzzle." *Journal of Social History* 10 (spring 1977): 284–309.

Kirkland, James, Holly F. Mathews, C. W. Sullivan III, and Karen Baldwin, eds. *Herbal and Magical Medicine: Traditional Healing Today.* Durham, N.C.: Duke University Press, 1992.

Kleinman, Arthur. "The Meaning Context of Illness and Care: Reflections on a Central Theme in the Anthropology of Medicine." In *Sciences and Cultures,* vol. 5, *Sociology of the Sciences,* edited by Everett Mendelsohn and Yehuda Elkana, 161–76. Boston: D. Reidel, 1981.

———. "What Is Specific to Western Medicine?" In *Companion Encyclopedia of the History of Medicine,* edited by W. F. Bynum and Roy Porter, 1:15–23. London: Routledge, 1993.

Lacy, Virginia Jayne, and David Edwin Harrell Jr. "Plantation Home Remedies: Medicinal Recipes from the Diaries of John Pope." *Tennessee Historical Quarterly* 22 (1963): 259–65.

LaGuerre, Michel. *Afro-Caribbean Medicine.* South Hadley, Mass.: Bergin & Garvey, 1987.

Leavitt, Judith Walzer. *Brought to Bed: Childbearing in America, 1750–1950.* New York: Oxford University Press, 1986.

Lebsock, Suzanne. *The Free Women of Petersburg: Status and Culture in a Southern Town, 1784–1860.* New York: Norton, 1984.

Levine, Lawrence W. *Black Culture and Black Consciousness: Afro-American Folk Thought from Slavery to Freedom.* New York: Oxford University Press, 1977.

Lichtenstein, Alex. " 'That Disposition to Theft, With Which They Have Been Branded': Moral Economy, Slave Management, and the Law." *Journal of Social History* 21 (spring 1989): 413–40.

Logan, Onnie Lee. *Motherwit: An Alabama Midwife's Story.* New York: Plume, 1989.

Lorde, Audre. *A Burst of Light: Essays by Audre Lorde.* Ithaca, N.Y.: Firebrand, 1988.

Love, Spencie. *One Blood: The Death and Resurrection of Charles R. Drew.* Chapel Hill: University of North Carolina Press, 1996.

McCandless, Peter. *Moonlight, Magnolias, and Madness: Insanity in South*

Carolina from the Colonial Period to the Progressive Era. Chapel Hill:
University of North Carolina Press, 1996.

McClure, Susan A. "Parallel Usage of Medicinal Plants by Africans and Their
Caribbean Descendants." *Economic Botany* 36 (1982): 291–301.

McCurry, Stephanie. *Masters of Small Worlds: Yeoman Households, Gender
Relations, and the Political Culture of the Antebellum South Carolina Low
Country.* New York: Oxford University Press, 1995.

McDaniel, George W. *Hearth and Home: Preserving a People's Culture.*
Philadelphia: Temple University Press, 1982.

McDowell, Deborah E., and Arnold Rampersad, eds. *Slavery and the Literary
Imagination: Selected Papers from the English Institute, 1987.* Baltimore: Johns
Hopkins University Press, 1989.

MacGaffey, Wyatt. "Complexity, Astonishment, and Power: The Visual Vocabulary
of Kongo Minkisi." *Journal of Southern African Studies* 14 (1988): 188–203.

———. "The Eyes of Understanding: Kongo Minkisi." In *Astonishment and
Power,* 20–103. Washington, D.C.: Smithsonian Institution Press, for the
National Museum of African Art, 1993.

McGregor, Deborah Kuhn. *From Midwives to Medicine: The Birth of American
Gynecology.* New Brunswick, N.J.: Rutgers University Press, 1998.

McKee, Larry. "The Earth Is Their Witness." *The Sciences* (March/April 1995):
36–41.

———. "The Ideals and Realities behind the Design and Use of Nineteenth-
Century Virginia Slave Cabins." In *The Art and Mystery of Historical
Archaeology: Essays in Honor of James Deetz,* edited by Anne Elizabeth Yentsch
and Mary C. Beaudry, 195–214. Boca Raton: CRC Press, 1992.

McMillen, Sally G. *Motherhood in the Old South: Pregnancy, Childbirth, and
Infant Rearing.* Baton Rouge: Louisiana State University Press, 1990.

———. "'No Uncommon Disease': Neonatal Tetanus, Slave Infants, and the
Southern Medical Profession." *Journal of the History of Medicine and Allied
Sciences* 46 (1991): 291–314.

Marks, Bayly E. "Skilled Blacks in Antebellum St. Mary's County, Maryland."
Journal of Southern History 53 (November 1987): 537–65.

Marshall, Mary Louise. "Plantation Medicine." *Bulletin of the Medical Library
Association* 26 (January 1938): 115–28.

Mbiti, John S. *African Religions and Philosophy.* New York: Praeger, 1969.

Miller, Joseph C. *Way of Death: Merchant Capitalism and the Angolan Slave Trade,
1730–1830.* Madison: University of Wisconsin Press, 1988.

Mintz, Sidney, and Michel-Rolph Trouillot. "The Social History of Haitian
Vodou." In Cosentino, *Sacred Arts of Haitian Vodou,* 123–47.

Mitchell, Faith. *Hoodoo Medicine: Sea Island Herbal Remedies.* Illustrated by
Naomi Steinfeld. Berkeley, Calif.: Reed, Cannon and Johnson, 1978.

Mitchell, Martha Carolyn. "Health and the Medical Profession in the Lower South, 1845–1860." *Journal of Southern History* 10 (November 1944): 424–46.

Morais, Herbert M. *The History of the Afro-American in Medicine.* International Library of Afro-American Life and History. Cornwells Heights, Pa.: Publisher's Agency, 1976.

Morantz-Sanchez, Regina Markell. *Sympathy and Science: Women Physicians in American Medicine.* New York: Oxford, 1985.

Morgan, Edmund Sears. *American Slavery, American Freedom: The Ordeal of Colonial Virginia.* New York: Norton, [1975].

Morgan, Philip D. *Slave Counterpoint: Black Culture in the Eighteenth-Century Chesapeake and Lowcountry.* Chapel Hill: University of North Carolina Press, 1998.

———. "Work and Culture: The Task System and the World of Lowcountry Blacks, 1700 to 1880." *William and Mary Quarterly* 39 (October 1982): 563–99.

Morrison, Toni. *Playing in the Dark: Whiteness and the Literary Imagination.* New York: Vintage, 1992.

Morton, Julia F. *Folk Remedies of the Low Country.* Miami: E. A. Seeman, 1974.

Morton, Patricia. *Disfigured Images: The Historical Assault on Afro-American Women.* New York: Praeger, 1991.

Moss, Kay K. *Southern Folk Medicine, 1750–1820.* Columbia: University of South Carolina Press, 1999.

Murphy, Lamar Riley. *Enter the Physician: The Transformation of Domestic Medicine, 1760–1860.* History of American Science and Technology Series. Tuscaloosa: University of Alabama Press, 1991.

Newton, James E., and Ronald L. Lewis. *The Other Slaves: Mechanics, Artisans, and Craftsmen.* Boston: G. K. Hall, 1978.

Numbers, Ronald L. *Prophetess of Health: Ellen G. White and the Origins of Seventh-Day Adventist Health Reform.* Rev. and enl. ed. Knoxville: University of Tennessee Press, 1992.

Numbers, Ronald L., and Darrel W. Amundsen, eds. *Caring and Curing: Health and Medicine in the Western Religious Traditions.* New York: Macmillan, 1986.

Numbers, Ronald L., and Todd L. Savitt, eds. *Science and Medicine in the Old South.* Baton Rouge: Louisiana State University Press, 1989.

Owens, Leslie H. *This Species of Property: Slave Life and Culture in the Old South.* New York: Oxford University Press, 1976.

Painter, Nell Irvin. "Soul Murder and Slavery: Toward a Fully Loaded Cost Accounting." In *U.S. History as Women's History: New Feminist Essays,* edited by Linda K. Kerber, Alice Kessler-Harris, and Kathryn Kish Sklar, 125–46. Chapel Hill: University of North Carolina Press, 1995.

Patterson, Bishop J. O, Rev. German R. Ross, and Mrs. Julia Mason Atkins, eds. *History and Formative Years of the Church of God in Christ, with Excerpts from*

the *Life and Works of Its Founder.* Memphis: Church of God in Christ
Publishing House, 1969.

Payne-Jackson, Arvilla, and John Lee. *Folk Wisdom and Mother Wit: John Lee, an
African American Herbal Healer.* Westport, Conn.: Greenwood Press, 1993.

Peek, Philip M. *African Divination Systems: Ways of Knowing.* Bloomington:
Indiana University Press, 1991.

Pernick, Martin S. *A Calculus of Suffering: Pain, Professionalism, and Anesthesia
in Nineteenth-Century America.* New York: Columbia University Press, 1985.

————. "The Patient's Role in Medical Decisionmaking: A Social History of
Informed Consent in Medical Therapy." In *Making Health Care Decisions: The
Ethical and Legal Implications of Informed Consent in the Patient-Practitioner
Relationship,* vol. 3, *Appendices: Studies on the Foundations of Informed
Consent,* by President's Commission for the Study of Ethical Problems in
Medicine and Biomedical and Behavioral Research, 1–35. Washington, D.C.:
GPO, 1982.

Phillips, Ulrich Bonnell. *American Negro Slavery: A Survey of the Supply,
Employment, and Control of Negro Labor as Determined by the Plantation
Regime.* New York: Appleton, 1918.

Piersen, William D. *Black Legacy: America's Hidden Heritage.* Amherst: University
of Massachusetts Press, 1993.

————. *Black Yankees: The Development of an Afro-American Subculture in
Eighteenth-Century New England.* Amherst: University of Massachusetts Press,
1988.

————. "White Cannibals, Black Martyrs: Fear, Depression, and Religious Faith
as Causes of Suicide among New Slaves." *Journal of Negro History* 62 (April
1977): 147–59.

Pollard, Leslie J. *Complaint to the Lord: Historical Perspectives on the African
American Elderly.* London: Associated University Presses, 1996.

Postell, William D. *The Health of Slaves on Southern Plantations.* Baton Rouge:
Louisiana State University Press, 1951.

Puckett, Newbell Niles. *Folk Beliefs of the Southern Negro.* Montclair, N.J.:
Patterson Smith, 1968.

Raboteau, Albert J. "The Afro-American Traditions." In Numbers and Amundsen,
Caring and Curing, 539–62.

————. *A Fire in the Bones: Reflections on African-American Religious History.*
Boston: Beacon, 1995.

————. *Slave Religion: The "Invisible Institution" in the Antebellum South.* New
York: Oxford University Press, 1978.

Reverby, Susan M. *Ordered to Care: The Dilemma of American Nursing, 1850–
1945.* Cambridge: Cambridge University Press, 1987.

Risse, Guenter B. "Transcending Cultural Barriers: The European Reception of

Medicinal Plants from the Americas." In Hein, *Botanical Drugs of the Americas in the Old and New Worlds,* 31–42.

Risse, Guenter B., Ronald L. Numbers, and Judith Walzer Leavitt, eds. *Medicine without Doctors: Home Health Care in American History.* New York: Science History Publications, 1977.

Roberts, Dorothy. *Killing the Black Body: Race, Reproduction, and the Meaning of Liberty.* New York: Pantheon, 1997.

Robertson, Claire. "Africa into the Americas? Slavery and Women, the Family, and the Gender Division of Labor." In Gaspar and Hine, *More Than Chattel,* 3–29.

Robinson, Beverly J. "Africanisms and the Study of Folklore." In Holloway, *Africanisms in American Culture,* 211–24.

———. "Faith Is the Key and Prayer Unlocks the Door: Prayer in African American Life." *Journal of American Folklore* 110 (fall 1997): 408–14.

Roediger, David R. "And Die in Dixie: Funerals, Death, and Heaven in the Slave Community, 1700–1865." *Massachusetts Review* 22 (spring 1981): 163–83.

Rosen, George. *From Medical Police to Social Medicine: Essays on the History of Health Care.* New York: Science History Publications, 1974.

Rosenberg, Charles. *The Care of Strangers: The Rise of America's Hospital System.* New York: Basic Books, 1987.

———. *The Cholera Years: The United States in 1832, 1849, and 1866.* Chicago: University of Chicago Press, 1962.

———. *Explaining Epidemics and Other Studies in the History of Medicine.* Cambridge: Cambridge University Press, 1992.

———. "The Therapeutic Revolution: Medicine, Meaning, and Social Change in Nineteenth-Century America." *Perspectives in Biology and Medicine* 21 (summer 1977): 485–506.

Ross, Loretta J. "African-American Women and Abortion: A Neglected History." *Journal of Health Care for the Poor and Underserved* 3 (fall 1992): 274–84.

Rothstein, William G. *American Physicians in the Nineteenth Century: From Sects to Science.* Baltimore: Johns Hopkins University Press, 1992.

Ryan, Mary P. *Cradle of the Middle Class: The Family in Oneida County, New York, 1790–1865.* Cambridge: Cambridge University Press, 1981.

Savitt, Todd L. *Fevers, Agues, and Cures: Medical Life in Old Virginia.* Richmond: Virginia Historical Society, 1990.

———. *Medicine and Slavery: The Diseases and Health Care of Blacks in Antebellum Virginia.* Chicago: University of Illinois Press, 1978.

———. "Medicine in the Old South: The Special Problem of Slavery." Paper presented to the Second Barnard-Millington Symposium on Science and Medicine in the South, Jackson, Miss., 17–19 March 1983.

———. "Politics in Medicine: The Georgia Freedmen's Bureau and the Organization of Health Care." *Civil War History* 28 (1982): 45–64.

———. "Slave Life Insurance in Virginia and North Carolina." *Journal of Southern History* 43 (November 1977): 583–600.

———. "The Use of Blacks for Medical Experimentation and Demonstration in the Old South." *Journal of Southern History* 48 (August 1982): 331–48.

Savitt, Todd L., and James Harvey Young, eds. *Disease and Distinctiveness in the American South.* Knoxville: University of Tennessee Press, 1988.

Schlotterbeck, John T. "The Internal Economy of Slavery in Rural Piedmont Virginia," *Slavery and Abolition* 12 (May 1991): 170–81.

Scholten, Catherine M. "'On the Importance of the Obstetrick Art': Changing Customs of Childbirth in America, 1760–1825." *William and Mary Quarterly* 34 (July 1977): 426–45.

Schwartz, Marie Jenkins. "'At Noon, Oh How I Ran': Breastfeeding and Weaning on Plantation and Farm in Antebellum Virginia and Alabama." In *Discovering the Women in Slavery: Emancipating Perspectives on the American Past,* edited by Patricia Morton, 241–59. Athens: University of Georgia Press, 1996.

Schwarz, Phillip. *Twice Condemned: Slaves and the Criminal Laws of Virginia, 1705–1865.* Baton Rouge: Louisiana State University Press, 1988.

Scott, Anne Firor. *The Southern Lady: From Pedestal to Politics, 1830–1930.* Chicago: University of Chicago Press, 1970.

Scott, James C. *Domination and the Arts of Resistance: Hidden Transcripts.* New Haven: Yale University Press, 1990.

Shammas, Carole. "Black Women's Work and the Evolution of Plantation Society in Virginia." *Labor History* 26 (winter 1985): 5–28.

Shaw, Stephanie J. "Mothering under Slavery in the Antebellum South." In *Mothering: Ideology, Experience, and Agency,* edited by Evelyn Nakano Glenn, Grace Chang, and Linda Rennie Forcey, 237–58. New York: Routledge, 1994.

Sheridan, Richard B. *Doctors and Slaves: A Medical and Demographic History of Slavery in the British West Indies, 1680–1834.* New York: Cambridge University Press, 1985.

Shick, Tom W. "Healing and Race in the South Carolina Low Country." In *Africans in Bondage: Studies in Slavery and the Slave Trade,* edited by Paul E. Lovejoy, 107–24. Madison: African Studies Program, University of Wisconsin, University of Wisconsin Press, 1986.

Shryock, Richard H. "Medical Practice in the Old South." *South Atlantic Quarterly* 29 (1930): 160–78.

Shultz, Suzanne M. *Body Snatching: The Robbing of Graves for the Education of Physicians in Early Nineteenth-Century America.* Jefferson, N.C.: McFarland, 1992.

Sikes, Lewright. "Medical Care for Slaves: A Preview of the Welfare State." *Georgia Historical Quarterly* 52 (1968): 405–13.

Silverman, Kenneth. *The Life and Times of Cotton Mather.* New York: Columbia University Press, 1985.

Simpson, George Eaton. *Black Religions in the New World.* New York: Columbia University Press, 1978.

Singleton, Theresa, "The Archaeology of Slave Life." In *Before Freedom Came: African-American Life in the Antebellum South,* edited by Edward D. C. Campbell Jr., with Kym S. Rice, 155–75. Richmond: Museum of the Confederacy; Charlottesville: University Press of Virginia, 1991.

———. "The Archaeology of Slavery in North America." *Annual Review of Anthropology* 24 (1995): 119–40.

———, ed. *The Archaeology of Slavery and Plantation Life.* New York: Academic Press, 1985.

———. *"I, Too, Am America": Archaeological Studies of African-American Life.* Charlottesville: University Press of Virginia, 1999.

Smith, Dorothy E. *The Everyday World as Problematic: A Feminist Sociology.* Boston: Northeastern University Press, 1987.

Smith, Julia Floyd. *Slavery and Rice Culture in Low Country Georgia, 1750–1860.* Knoxville: University of Tennessee Press, 1985.

Smith, Margaret Charles, and Linda Janet Holmes. *Listen to Me Good: The Life Story of an Alabama Midwife.* Columbus: Ohio State University Press, 1996.

Smith, Theophus H. *Conjuring Culture: Biblical Formations of Black America.* New York: Oxford University Press, 1994.

Smith-Rosenberg, Carroll. *Disorderly Conduct: Visions of Gender in Victorian America.* New York: Oxford University Press, 1985.

Snow, Loudell F. "Sorcerers, Saints, and Charlatans: Black Folk Healers in Urban America." *Culture, Medicine, and Psychiatry* 2 (1978): 69–106.

———. *Walkin' over Medicine.* Boulder, Colo.: Westview Press, 1993.

Sobel, Mechal. *Trabelin' On: The Slave Journey to an Afro-Baptist Faith.* Westport, Conn.: Greenwood Press, 1979. Reprint, Princeton: Princeton University Press, 1988.

Sobo, Elisa Janine. *One Blood: The Jamaican Body.* Albany: State University of New York Press, 1993.

Stampp, Kenneth M. *The Peculiar Institution: Slavery in the Ante-Bellum South.* New York: Knopf, 1956.

Starr, Paul. *The Social Transformation of American Medicine.* New York: Basic Books, 1982.

Steady, Filomina Chioma, ed. *The Black Woman Cross-Culturally.* Cambridge, Mass.: Schenkman, 1981.

Steckel, Richard. "Birth Weights and Infant Mortality among American Slaves." *Explorations in Economic History* 23 (April 1986): 173–98.

———. "A Dreadful Childhood: The Excess Mortality of American Slaves." *Social Science History* 10 (winter 1986): 427–65.

Stephens, Lester D. *Science, Race, and Religion in the American South: John*

Bachman and the Charleston Circle of Naturalists, 1815–1895. Chapel Hill: University of North Carolina Press, 1999.

Stevenson, Brenda E. *Life in Black and White: Family and Community in the Slave South.* New York: Oxford University Press, 1996.

Stewart, Mart A. *"What Nature Suffers to Groe": Life, Labor, and Landscape on the Georgia Coast, 1680–1920.* Athens: University of Georgia Press, 1996.

Stowe, Steven M. "Obstetrics and the Work of Doctoring in the Mid-Nineteenth-Century American South." *Bulletin of the History of Medicine* 64 (1990): 540–66.

———. "Seeing Themselves at Work: Physicians and the Case Narrative in the Mid-Nineteenth-Century American South." *American Historical Review* 101 (February 1996): 41–79.

Stuckey, Sterling. *Slave Culture: Nationalist Theory and the Foundations of Black America.* New York: Oxford University Press, 1987.

———. "Through the Prism of Folklore: The Black Ethos in Slavery." *Massachusetts Review* 9 (summer 1968): 417–37.

Sullivan, Lawrence E., ed. *Healing and Restoring: Health and Medicine in the World's Religious Traditions.* New York: Macmillan, 1989.

Swados, Felice. "Negro Health on the Ante Bellum Plantations." *Bulletin of the History of Medicine* 10 (1941): 460–72.

Tadman, Michael. *Speculators and Slaves: Masters, Traders, and Slaves in the Old South.* Madison: University of Wisconsin Press, 1989.

Terry, Jennifer, and Jacqueline Urla, eds. *Deviant Bodies: Critical Perspectives on Difference in Science and Popular Culture.* Bloomington: Indiana University Press, 1995.

Thompson, Robert Farris. *Flash of the Spirit: African and Afro-American Art and Philosophy.* New York: Random House, 1982.

———. "From the Isle beneath the Sea: Haiti's Africanizing Vodou Art." In Cosentino, *Sacred Arts of Haitian Vodou,* 91–119.

———. "Icons of the Mind: Yoruba Herbalism Arts in Atlantic Perspective." *African Arts* 8 (1975): 52–59, 89–90.

———. "Kongo Influences on African American Artistic Culture." In Holloway, *Africanisms in American Culture,* 148–84.

Thornton, John. *Africa and Africans in the Making of the Atlantic World, 1400–1680.* Cambridge: Cambridge University Press, 1992.

Troester, Rosalie Riegle. "Turbulence and Tenderness: Mothers, Daughters, and 'Othermothers' in Paule Marshall's *Brown Girl, Brownstones.*" In Bell-Scott et al., *Double Stitch,* 163–72.

Ulrich, Laurel Thatcher. *A Midwife's Tale: The Life of Martha Ballard, Based on Her Diary, 1785–1812.* New York: Vintage, 1990.

Valverde, José-Louise. "The Aztec Herbal of 1552." In Hein, *Botanical Drugs of the Americas in the Old and New Worlds,* 15–27.

Van Deburg, William L. *Slavery and Race in American Popular Culture*. Madison: University of Wisconsin Press, 1984.

Vlach, John Michael. *Back of the Big House: The Architecture of Plantation Slavery*. Chapel Hill: University of North Carolina Press, 1993.

Voeks, Robert A. *Sacred Leaves of Candomblé: African Magic, Medicine, and Religion in Brazil*. Austin: University of Texas Press, 1997.

Wahl, Jenny Bourne. *The Bondsman's Burden: An Economic Analysis of the Common Law of Southern Slavery*. New York: Cambridge University Press, 1998.

Walker, Margaret. *Jubilee*. New York: Bantam Books, 1966.

Wall, Bennett H. "Medical Care of Ebenezer Pettigrew's Slaves." *Mississippi Valley Historical Review* 37 (1950): 451–70.

Waring, Joseph I. *A History of Medicine in South Carolina, 1825–1900*. Vol. 2. Charleston: South Carolina Medical Association, 1967.

Warner, John Harley. *Against the Spirit of the System: The French Impulse in Nineteenth-Century American Medicine*. Princeton: Princeton University Press, 1998.

———."Idea of Southern Medical Distinctiveness: Medical Knowledge and Practice in the Old South." In Numbers and Savitt, *Science and Medicine in the Old South*, 179–205.

———. "A Southern Medical Reform: The Meaning of the Antebellum Argument for Southern Medical Education." In Numbers and Savitt, *Science and Medicine in the Old South*, 206–25.

———. *The Therapeutic Perspective: Medical Practice, Knowledge, and Identity in America, 1820–1885*. Cambridge, Mass.: Harvard University Press, 1986.

Watson, Wilbur H., ed. *Black Folk Medicine: The Therapeutic Significance of Faith and Trust*. New Brunswick, N.J.: Transaction Books, 1988.

Webber, Thomas L. *Deep Like the Rivers: Education in the Slave Quarter Community, 1831–1865*. New York: Norton, 1978.

Weiner, Marli F. *Mistresses and Slaves: Plantation Women in South Carolina, 1830–80*. Urbana: University of Illinois Press, 1998.

Wenger, Etienne. *Communities of Practice: Learning, Meaning, and Identity*. New York: Cambridge University Press, 1998.

Wertz, Richard W., and Dorothy C. Wertz. *Lying-In: A History of Childbirth in America*. New York: Free Press, 1977.

Westmacott, Richard. *African-American Gardens and Yards in the Rural South*. Knoxville: University of Tennessee Press, 1992.

White, Deborah Gray. *Ar'n't I a Woman?: Female Slaves in the Plantation South*. New York: Norton, 1985.

White, Richard Donn. "'We Didn Know No Clinic': An Ethnomedicinal Study of Plant Use in Central Mississippi." Ph.D. diss., Miami University, 1994.

White, Shane, and Graham White. *Stylin': African American Expressive Culture from Its Beginnings to the Zoot Suit.* Ithaca, N.Y.: Cornell University Press, 1998.

Whitten, David O. "The Medical Care of Slaves on South Carolina Rice Plantations." M.A. thesis, University of South Carolina, 1963.

Wilkie, Laurie A. "Secret and Sacred: Contextualizing the Artifacts of African-American Magic and Religion." *Historical Archaeology* 31 (1997): 81–106.

———. "Transforming African American Ethnomedical Traditions: A Case Study from West Feliciana." *Louisiana History* 37 (fall 1996): 457–71.

Williams, Patricia J. *The Alchemy of Race and Rights: Diary of a Law Professor.* Cambridge, Mass.: Harvard University Press, 1991.

Williams, Raymond. *Keywords: A Vocabulary of Culture and Society.* Rev. ed. New York: Oxford University Press, 1983.

Wood, Betty. *Women's Work, Men's Work: The Informal Slave Economies of Lowcountry Georgia.* Athens: University of Georgia Press, 1995.

Wood, Peter. *Black Majority: Negroes in Colonial South Carolina from 1670 through the Stono Rebellion.* New York: Norton, 1974.

———. "People's Medicine in the Early South." *Southern Exposure* 6 (1978): 50–53.

Woodson, Carter G. *The Negro in Our History.* Washington, D.C.: Associated Publishers, 1922.

Wright, Gavin. *The Political Economy of the Cotton South: Households, Markets, and Wealth in the Nineteenth Century.* New York: Norton, 1978.

Wyatt-Brown, Bertram. *Southern Honor: Ethics and Behavior in the Old South.* New York: Oxford University Press, 1982.

Yetman, Norman R. "The Background of the Slave Narrative Collection." *American Quarterly* 19 (fall 1967): 534–53.

Young, Jeffrey Robert. *Domesticating Slavery: The Master Class in Georgia and South Carolina, 1670–1837.* Chapel Hill: University of North Carolina Press, 1999.

———. "Ideology and Death on a Savannah River Rice Plantation, 1833–1867: Paternalism amidst 'a Good Supply of Disease and Pain.'" *Journal of Southern History* 59 (November 1993): 673–706.

Index

elders, 26; curtailing black healers, 160, 165–67

Lawson, Dave, 116

Lewis (slave healer), 61, 82, 217 (n. 2)

Lewis, Henry Clay, 153–54

Life insurance: for slaves, 23–24

Light root, 72

Little, Archibald Alexander, 24

Littlejohn, Chana, 179, 182

Long, Crawford, 152

Lorde, Audre, 193

Louisiana, 9, 126; New Orleans, 32, 62

Lowcountry (Ga., S.C.), 7, 9, 76, 81, 99, 120, 195

Lucy (slave), 151

Lyell, Charles, 135, 136

Lymus (slave of William Harrison), 183

McCaa, William, 49

McCaw, James, 47

MacDonald, Sarah, 126

McDowell, Emma, 100

McElveen, A. J., 32

MacGaffey, Wyatt, 102, 103, 104

McKain, W. F., 138

McKean, William, 84–85, 87, 88

McKee, Larry, 173

McLoud, M. L., 188, 189, 190

McLurg, James, 26

Malvina (slave healer), 131

Manigault, Charles, 25, 124

Manigault, Louis, 114, 124, 126, 172, 174–75, 186

Manigault family, 131, 133, 136, 185

Manson, Roberta, 129

Markie (slave), 180

Marmar (slave of William Harrison), 169–70

Maryland, 72, 97

Massie, Thomas, 28

Massie, Thomas Eugene, 149

Massie, William, 27, 136, 174

Maupin, Socrates, 183

Meaning-centered framework, 11, 206 (n. 39)

Measles, 124

Medical College of South Carolina, 10

Medical journals, southern, 10, 45, 47, 146, 175–76

Medical schools, southern, 8, 10, 20, 152–54, 241 (n. 49)

Medical science: racial theories in, 1–2, 22, 29, 151, 152, 153, 171, 189; and theory of specificity, 144, 204 (n. 17); obstetrics and gynecology, 151; and dissection of black bodies, 152, 153–56, 157; and autopsy, 154–56, 242 (n. 58)

Medical Society of South Carolina, 197

Medicinal plants. *See names of individual plants*

Mental illness, 27, 94, 96

Merrill, A. P., 49

Mesmerism, 44, 213 (nn. 49, 50)

Meteor shower of 1833, 48–49

Mettauer, John Peter, 27

Michel, Myddleton, 156

Middleton, Henry A., Jr., 135

Midwives, 2, 45, 51, 53, 55, 58, 76, 112, 231 (n. 2); in conflict with white doctors, 45, 51, 140; payment to, 100, 111–12; status of, in slave community, 129, 130; mobility of enslaved, 130, 236 (n. 94). *See also* Slave women: as plantation health workers

Mike (slave of David Gavin), 116

Miller, L. G., 72

Mills Plantation (Ga.), 89–90

Miner, Felix, 23

Minkisi, 11, 40–41, 79, 95, 102–4

Mississippi, 22, 81, 104

Mitchell, Faith, 74

Mitchell, Isabella, 163

Mobley, Bob, 130
Moll (slave of Thomas Chaplin), 25
Moore, Fannie, 128
Moore, H. W., 139
Morgan, John, 176–77
Morgan, Philip D., 42, 212 (n. 31)
Morrison, Toni, 50, 212 (n. 35)
Mullein, 63
Murphy, John, 114–15
Mustard seed, 68

Nancy (slave of Manigaults), 186
Native Americans, 2, 53, 63–64, 98, 218
    (n. 16), 219 (n. 22)
Neal, James, 28
Ned (conjure doctor), 91, 104
Nelson, Eliza, 72, 73
Newby, Harriet, 122–23
Nichols, Lila, 161–62
Night doctors, 157, 242 (n. 62)
North Carolina, 8, 22, 46, 69, 81, 129,
    223 (n. 5); Edenton, 51; Durham,
    102
Northup, Solomon, 33, 57, 115
Nott, Josiah C., 176

Obeah, 41, 81
Okra, 63
Old Divinity, 81
Opium, 151
Opossum ear plant, 62
Orature, African American, 177, 181,
    210 (n. 70)
Osanyin, 77
Overseers, 89, 114–15, 124, 181

Papan (slave healer), 64, 218 (n. 20)
Parker, Ann, 102
Parsons, Elsie Clews, 182
Paternalism, 25, 141, 197
Patience (slave of William Jerdone),
    36–38, 39–40, 59

Patton, James, 142, 143
Peach tree, 57, 74, 79
Peggy (slave of Thomas Chaplin),
    185–86
Pendleton, E. M., 176, 177
Pennington, James W. C., 15, 30, 148
Pennyroyal, 63, 65
Perry, Matilda Henrietta, 106
Peter (slave patient), 188
Peter (slave of Thomas Chaplin), 96
Pharmocosm, 38–40, 59, 90, 94, 107,
    199; healing and harming processes
    of, 39–41, 59, 95, 107, 212 (n. 31)
Phillips, Ulrich B., 16
Pinckney, Charles, 17, 21
Pinckney, Charles Cotesworth, 184–85
Pinckney, Harriott, 183
Pine, 61, 67, 74
Plantain, 63, 68
Planter's and Mariner's Medical Com-
    panion, 47, 68, 184
Planter's Guide and Family Book of
    Medicine, 173
Pneumonia, 74, 175
Polypody, 64
Poisoning, 60–61, 113, 159–60, 165–66,
    223 (n. 2); domestic slaves accused
    of, 142, 160–62, 163; conjure doctors
    accused of, 142, 162–64
Pokeweed, 74, 163, 221 (n. 63)
Polygenesis, 1
Pompey (slave), 142
Postmortem examination. *See* Autopsy;
    Dissection: of black bodies
Pregnancy. *See* Childbearing, slave
    women's
Preston, Bowker, 175
Pricy (slave of Thomas Holloway), 190
Proctor, Jenny, 30, 33, 148
Property principle, 16, 18, 29–34, 33,
    141, 191, 198
Proslavery arguments, 1, 4, 15, 26, 49;

CPSIA information can be obtained
at www.ICGtesting.com
Printed in the USA
LVHW111916130821
695223LV00021B/2276